Chemokine Receptors and AIDS

INFECTIOUS DISEASE AND THERAPY

Series Editor

Burke A. Cunha

Winthrop-University Hospital, Mineola, and
State University of New York School of Medicine
Stony Brook, New York

1. Parasitic Infections in the Compromised Host, *edited by Peter D. Walzer and Robert M. Genta*
2. Nucleic Acid and Monoclonal Antibody Probes: Applications in Diagnostic Methodology, *edited by Bala Swaminathan and Gyan Prakash*
3. Opportunistic Infections in Patients with the Acquired Immunodeficiency Syndrome, *edited by Gifford Leoung and John Mills*
4. Acyclovir Therapy for Herpesvirus Infections, *edited by David A. Baker*
5. The New Generation of Quinolones, *edited by Clifford Siporin, Carl L. Heifetz, and John M. Domagala*
6. Methicillin-Resistant *Staphylococcus aureus*: Clinical Management and Laboratory Aspects, *edited by Mary T. Cafferkey*
7. Hepatitis B Vaccines in Clinical Practice, *edited by Ronald W. Ellis*
8. The New Macrolides, Azalides, and Streptogramins: Pharmacology and Clinical Applications, *edited by Harold C. Neu, Lowell S. Young, and Stephen H. Zinner*
9. Antimicrobial Therapy in the Elderly Patient, *edited by Thomas T. Yoshikawa and Dean C. Norman*
10. Viral Infections of the Gastrointestinal Tract: Second Edition, Revised and Expanded, *edited by Albert Z. Kapikian*
11. Development and Clinical Uses of Haemophilus b Conjugate Vaccines, *edited by Ronald W. Ellis and Dan M. Granoff*
12. *Pseudomonas aeruginosa* Infections and Treatment, *edited by Aldona L. Baltch and Raymond P. Smith*
13. Herpesvirus Infections, *edited by Ronald Glaser and James F. Jones*
14. Chronic Fatigue Syndrome, *edited by Stephen E. Straus*
15. Immunotherapy of Infections, *edited by K. Noel Masihi*
16. Diagnosis and Management of Bone Infections, *edited by Luis E. Jauregui*
17. Drug Transport in Antimicrobial and Anticancer Chemotherapy, *edited by Nafsika H. Georgopapadakou*
18. New Macrolides, Azalides, and Streptogramins in Clinical Practice, *edited by Harold C. Neu, Lowell S. Young, Stephen H. Zinner, and Jacques F. Acar*
19. Novel Therapeutic Strategies in the Treatment of Sepsis, *edited by David C. Morrison and John L. Ryan*
20. Catheter-Related Infections, *edited by Harald Seifert, Bernd Jansen, and Barry M. Farr*
21. Expanding Indications for the New Macrolides, Azalides, and Streptogramins, *edited by Stephen H. Zinner, Lowell S. Young, Jacques F. Acar, and Harold C. Neu*
22. Infectious Diseases in Critical Care Medicine, *edited by Burke A. Cunha*
23. New Considerations for Macrolides, Azalides, Streptogramins, and Ketolides, *edited by Stephen H. Zinner, Lowell S. Young, Jacques F. Acar, and Carmen Ortiz-Neu*
24. Tickborne Infectious Diseases: Diagnosis and Management, *edited by Burke A. Cunha*
25. Protease Inhibitors in AIDS Therapy, *edited by Richard C. Ogden and Charles W. Flexner*
26. Laboratory Diagnosis of Bacterial Infections, *edited by Nevio Cimolai*
27. Chemokine Receptors and AIDS, *edited by Thomas R. O'Brien*

Chemokine Receptors and AIDS

edited by
Thomas R. O'Brien
National Cancer Institute
Rockville, Maryland

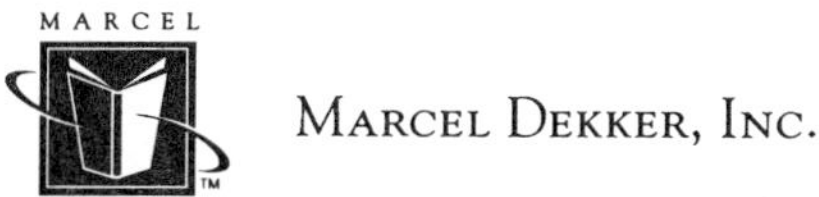

Marcel Dekker, Inc. New York • Basel

ISBN: 0-8247-0636-6

This book is printed on acid-free paper.

Headquarters
Marcel Dekker, Inc.
270 Madison Avenue, New York, NY 10016
tel: 212-696-9000; fax: 212-685-4540

Eastern Hemisphere Distribution
Marcel Dekker AG
Hutgasse 4, Postfach 812, CH-4001 Basel, Switzerland
tel: 41-61-261-8482; fax: 41-61-261-8896

World Wide Web
http://www.dekker.com

The publisher offers discounts on this book when ordered in bulk quantities. For more information, write to Special Sales/Professional Marketing at the headquarters address above.

Current printing (last digit):
10 9 8 7 6 5 4 3 2 1

PRINTED IN THE UNITED STATES OF AMERICA

Preface

The past few years have seen dramatic advances in our understanding of how human immunodeficiency virus type 1 (HIV-1) enters cells. Chemokines (chemoattractant cytokines) and chemokine receptors form a complex system that is essential to inflammation. Some chemokine receptors also act as HIV-1 coreceptors, which allow the virus to enter lymphocytes, macrophages, and other target cells in consort with the CD4 protein. As a result, certain chemokines can block HIV entry by attaching to their receptors. Although at least a dozen chemokine receptors (or closely related proteins) can serve as HIV-1 coreceptors, two receptors appear to be most important *in vivo*. CC-chemokine receptor 5 (CCR5), a receptor for the β–chemokines RANTES, MIP-1α, and MIP-1β, is the major coreceptor for HIV-1 strains that predominate during early infection. CXCR4, the receptor for the SDF-1 chemokine, is the major coreceptor for the more pathogenic, syncytium-inducing strains that often emerge in late infection.

Human genetic differences in the chemokine/chemokine receptor system can affect susceptibility to HIV-1 infection and the clinical course of those who have become infected. A mutant version of the *CCR5* gene has a 32 base-pair deletion (*CCR5-Δ32*) which renders it incapable of binding its ligand chemokines or HIV-1. The *CCR5-Δ32* allele is frequent in Caucasians of northern European descent, but is infrequent or absent in Asians and Africans. The identification of *CCR5-Δ32* led to investigations in epidemiologic cohorts to determine if susceptibility to HIV-1 infection or clinical prognosis after infection varied by *CCR5* genotype. *CCR5-Δ32* homozygotes (people with two copies of *CCR5-Δ32*) strongly resist HIV-1 infection, but this protection is not absolute and HIV-1 infection has now been documented in a handful of *CCR5-Δ32* homozygotes. *CCR5-Δ32* heterozygotes (people with one copy of *CCR5-Δ32*) are not protected against acquisition of HIV-1, but once infected they have a slower progression to

AIDS. Therefore, while a functional CCR5 is not an absolute requirement for HIV-1 infection, this coreceptor plays a key role in susceptibility to infection and the clinical course of those who become infected. The importance of CCR5 in clinical prognosis is further underscored by studies suggesting that genetic polymorphisms in the *CCR5* promoter region, presumably linked to CCR5 cellular expression, also predict the course of HIV-1 infection.

Polymorphisms in other genes have also been linked to HIV-1 prognosis. The *CCR2*-64I allele has a frequency of 10–15% in Caucasians and African Americans. Although *CCR2*-64I genotype is not associated with reduced susceptibility to HIV-1 infection, heterozygosity for *CCR2*-64I is associated with slower progression to AIDS. CCR2 is a minor HIV-1 coreceptor and the mechanism underlying the *CCR2*-64I effect is yet unknown. Polymorphisms in genes outside the chemokine-chemokine receptor system have also been linked to HIV-1 infection. For example, human leukocyte antigen (HLA) haplotype has been associated with the clinical prognosis of HIV-1-infected patients.

Insights into the roles played by chemokines, chemokine receptors, and human genetic variability promise to yield new therapeutic options for HIV-1 infected patients. The goal of HIV-1 therapy is to minimize HIV-1 replication and, thereby, halt or reverse the loss of CD4+ lymphocytes. Current combination therapies, which chiefly target two HIV-1 enzymes (reverse transcriptase and protease), can reduce HIV-1 RNA to undetectable levels. These regimens have led to dramatic improvements in patient survival, but additional therapies are needed because HIV-1 strains that are resistant to these drugs frequently develop. As chemokine receptors are integral to HIV-1 replication, novel therapies that target CCR5 and CXCR4 are particularly attractive. A number of such strategies are currently under investigation, including gene therapy to prevent chemokine expression, the downregulation of CCR5 expression on CD4+ lymphocytes, and the blockade of chemokine receptors. If one or more such therapies prove successful, it would likely provide a major addition to the treatment of HIV-1 infection.

The discoveries about the relationship between chemokine receptors, human genetics, and AIDS carry enormous implications, and I hope that this book will prove useful to a variety of readers. For the virologist, epidemiologist, or clinician specializing in AIDS, this volume seeks to provide a comprehensive, yet comprehensible, review of recent seminal work in their field. Basic scientists and epidemiologists whose primary interest lies in the study of other infectious agents may also find the paradigm presented here useful, as it is likely that the insights gained by applying genetic epidemiology to the study of infectious diseases have just begun.

Thomas R. O'Brien

Contents

Contributors

Laurent Abel, M.D., Ph.D. Director of Research, Human Genetics of Infectious Diseases, INSERM U550, Necker Medical School, Paris, France

David H. Adams, M.D., F.R.C.P., F. Med. Sci. Professor, MRC Centre for Immune Regulation, Queen Elizabeth Hospital and University of Birmingham, Birmingham, England

Susan Buchbinder, M.D. Director, HIV Research Section, San Francisco Department of Health, San Francisco, California

J. Scott Cairns, Ph.D. Senior Scientist, Division of AIDS, National Institute of Allergy and Infectious Diseases, Bethesda, Maryland

Mary Carrington, Ph.D. Senior Scientist, Intramural Research Support Program, SAIC-Frederick, National Cancer Institute, Frederick, Maryland

Michael Dean, Ph.D. Chief, Human Genetics Section, Laboratory of Genomic Diversity, National Cancer Institute, Frederick, Maryland

M. Patricia D'Souza, Ph.D. Scientist, Vaccine Clinical Research Branch, Division of AIDS, National Institute of Allergy and Infectious Diseases, Bethesda, Maryland

Eric A. Engels, M.D., M.P.H. Investigator, Viral Epidemiology Branch, Division of Cancer Epidemiology and Genetics, National Cancer Institute, Rockville, Maryland

Bodduluri Haribabu, Ph.D. Associate Research Professor, Department of Medicine, Duke University Medical Center, Durham, North Carolina

Maureen P. Martin, M.D. Scientist, Intramural Research Support Program, SAIC-Frederick, National Cancer Institute, Frederick, Maryland

Nelson L. Michael, M.D., Ph.D. Chief, Department of Molecular Diagnostics and Pathogenesis, Division of Retrovirology, Walter Reed Army Institute of Research, Rockville, Maryland

Thomas R. O'Brien, M.D., M.P.H. Senior Investigator, Viral Epidemiology Branch, Division of Cancer Epidemiology and Genetics, National Cancer Institute, Rockville, Maryland

Giuseppe Pantaleo, M.D. Professor, Department of Internal Medicine, Centre Hospitalier Universitaire Vaudois, University of Lausanne, Lausanne, Switzerland

Ricardo M. Richardson, Ph.D. Associate Research Professor, Department of Medicine, Duke University Medical Center, Durham, North Carolina

Douglas D. Richman, M.D. Professor, Departments of Pathology and Medicine, San Diego VA Healthcare System and University of California, San Diego and La Jolla, California

G. Paolo Rizzardi, M.D. Department of Internal Medicine, Centre Hospitalier Universitaire Vaudois, University of Lausanne, Lausanne, Switzerland

Haynes W. Sheppard, Ph.D. Research Scientist, Viral and Rickettsial Disease Laboratory, California Department of Health Services, Berkeley, California

Philip L. Shields, M.B.Ch. B., B.S.C., Ph.D., M.R.C.P. Clinical Research Fellow, Liver Research Laboratories, Department of Medicine, Queen Elizabeth Hospital and University of Birmingham, Birmingham, England

Ralph Snyderman, M.D. Chancellor of Health Affairs, Departments of Medicine and Immunology, Duke University Medical Center, Durham, North Carolina

1

Chemokines and Chemokine Receptor Interactions and Functions

Philip L. Shields and David H. Adams

Queen Elizabeth Hospital and University of Birmingham, Birmingham, England

INTRODUCTION

The immune system needs to provide a constant vigil over tissues throughout the body in order to mount a rapid and effective response to foreign invasion by pathogens. Leukocytes, and in particular lymphocytes, play a crucial role in this process by providing immunosurveillance of tissues and by co-ordinating a rapid inflammatory response when foreign antigen is detected. When T cells are activated by dendritic cells presenting their specific antigen in the lymph node, they undergo a process of proliferation and differentiation to become effector (memory) T cells. These effector cells acquire new migratory tendencies as a consequence of expression of specific cell surface receptors. The pattern of this expression depends on the nature and site of the activating signal and will determine how readily and to which tissues cells are recruited. The recruitment of circulating cells from the blood stream into tissues requires, firstly, that the leukocyte recognizes endothelium in the target tissue, secondly, that it binds to the endothelium, and, thirdly, that it migrates through the endothelium into tissue. This process is regulated by a co-ordinated sequence of molecular interactions in which one set of molecules, classically selectins, induces the flowing cell to roll or bump on the vessel wall allowing it to pick up signals from the endothelium that activate leukocyte adhesion molecules called integrins. Integrins promote arrest and firm adhesion to the vessel wall. The most important integrin-activating signals come from the chemokine family of cytokines that activate specific G-protein-linked receptors on the leukocyte. Once the cell has come to a halt it can then migrate through the endothelium into tissue in response to local chemotactic signals, also provided by chemokines.

The chemokine family comprises a rapidly expanding number of structurally related proteins that signal through G-protein-linked transmembrane spanning receptors on leukocytes. Chemokines lead to a dramatic morphological change in leukocytes within only a few seconds, characterised by actin polymerisation, cytoskeletal reorganization, and the induction of migration. Chemokines are, however, more than just simple chemotactic factors. The large number of chemokines and chemokine receptors provides a sophisticated network for regulating leukocyte migration, which allows specific cells to be recruited to particular tissue compartments in response to local signals. Chemokines are involved in all aspects of leukocyte development, from the release of stem cells from the bone marrow to thymic differentiation of T lymphocytes, as well as lymphoid tissue homeostasis and inflammatory responses. In addition, there is also evidence that they may have a role in influencing other cell types (e.g., promoting angiogenesis and tumor growth).

CHEMOKINES

Chemokines are small (8-10kd) proteins containing four conserved cysteines, linked by disulphide bonds. They are subdivided into families depending on the relative position of cysteine residues within the mature protein. CXC or alpha chemokines are distinguished by the presence of an amino acid between the first two cysteines whereas the cysteines are adjacent in CC or beta chemokines (Figure 1). Alpha chemokines can be further divided according to whether they contain a glutamic acid-leucine-arginine (ELR) sequence preceding the CXC portion. Structural distinctions are important as they determine the ability of chemokines to attract specific leukocyte subsets. The alpha chemokines containing the ELR sequence act predominantly on neutrophils, the prototype example of which is interleukin (IL)-8, whereas alpha chemokines without the ELR sequence (e.g., interferon inducible protein (IP)-10 and monokine induced by gamma interferon (MIG)) act on T cells. Beta-chemokines, for example monocyte chemotactic protein (MCP)-1, macrophage inflammatory protein. (MIP)-1α, MIP-1β, and eotaxin, act on lymphocytes, monocytes, eosinophils, and mast cells. Two chemokines that do not conform to this classification (and may be members of separate families) are lymphotactin, which lacks the first and the third cysteines in this 4-cysteine motif, and fractalkine in which the first two cysteines are separated by 3 amino acids (CXXXC). CXC chemokine genes are located on chromosome 4, whereas CC chemokine genes are clustered on chromosome 17. Genes for fractalkine and lymphotactin are positioned on chromosome 12 and 1 respectively. Table 1 summarizes the classification of chemokines and their receptors and the cell types for which they are chemotactic.

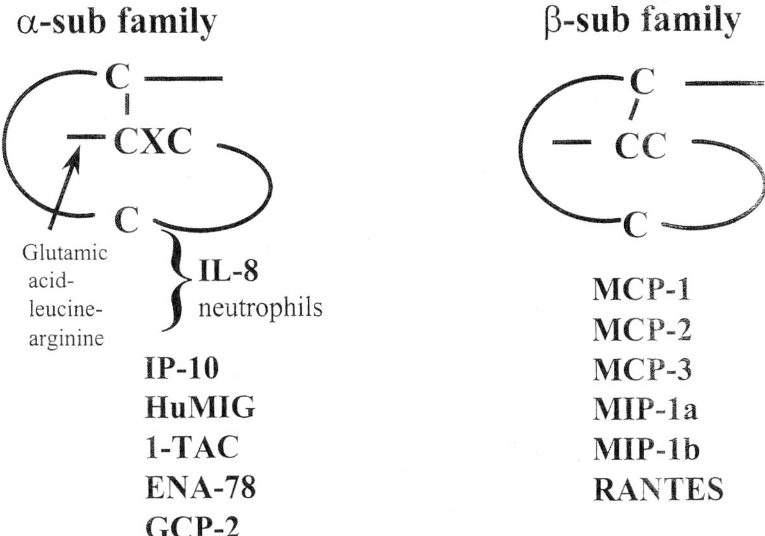

Figure 1 Chemokines may be divided into alpha and beta chemokine families depending on the relative position of cysteine residues within the mature protein. Alpha or CXC chemokines have an amino acid between the first two cysteines whereas in beta or CC chemokines, the cysteines are adjacent. Alpha chemokines may be further divided according to the presence of a glutamic acid-leucine-arginine (ELR) motif preceding the CXC portion. ELR containing chemokines are chemotactic for neutrophils and include IL-8.

CHEMOKINE PRODUCTION

Chemokines are produced by a wide variety of cell types, including immune cells and endothelial cells, and may be rapidly induced following stimulation by a variety of agents. These include bacterial lipopolysaccharide (LPS), viruses and proinflammatory cytokines such as Il-1α, IL-1β, interferon (IFN)-γ and tumor necrosis factor (TNF)-α (1).

The cellular source of chemokines is variable; MCP-1 and IL-8 are almost universally expressed, whereas platelet factor 4 (PF4), platelet basic protein (PBP) and connective tissue activating protein (CTAP)-111 are produced only by platelets (2). Activated T cells have been reported to express a range of chemokines at both the mRNA and protein levels. Chemokine secretion by T cells is to some extent subset dependent with increased levels produced by memory cytotoxic T (CD45RO+ CD8+) cells (3). Non-hematopoietic cells also secrete chemokines; endothelial cells are a potent source of many chemokines and there is increasing evidence for chemokine secretion by epithelial cells. The chemokines secreted in response to particular stimuli show differences between cell types. For instance, epithelial cells secrete large amounts of the CXC chemokines epithelial neutrophil

Table 1 The currently known chemokine receptors, the cell types on which they are expressed and their chemokine ligands.

Receptor	Cell Types	Ligands
CC Chemokines		
CCR1	Activated T cells, Monocytes, Eosinophils, Dendritic cells	MIP-1α, RANTES, MCP-3
CCR2	Monocytes, Macrophages, Activated T Cells	MCP1-5
CCR3	Eosinophils, Basophils, Activated T Cells (TH2)	Eotaxin, MCP-3, MCP-4, RANTES
CCR4	Activated T cells, Basophils, Platelets	TARC, MIP-1α, RANTES, MDC
CCR5	Activated T cells, Monocytes, Macrophages, Dendritic Cells	MIP-1α, MIP-1β, RANTES
CCR6	Dendritic Cells, T Cells	MIP-3αa
CCR7	B Cells, T Cells	SLC, MIP-3β
CCR8	Monocytes, Macrophages	I309
CCR9	Dendritic Cells, T Cells	TECK
CCR10	T Cells	CTACK
CXC Chemokines		
CXCR1	Neutrophils	IL-8, CGP-2
CXCR2	Neutrophils	IL-8, NAP-2, GROα, ENA-78
CXCR3	Activated T Cells (TH1)	IP-10, MIG, I-TAC
CXCR4	Naïve T Cells, B Cells, Macrophages	SDF-1α/β
CXCR5	B Cells	BCA-1
CXCR6	NK Cells, T Cells	CXCL16
Other		
XCR1	T Cells	Lymphotactin
CX3CR1	T Cells (CD8+), NK Cells	Fractalkine
Duffy Antigen	Red Blood Cells	CC and CXC Chemokines

activating protein (ENA)-78 and IL-8 in response to LPS and early response cytokines IL-1 and TNF, but epithelial cells fail to respond to IL-10 or IFN–γ. Because IL-8 and ENA-78 act predominantly on neutrophils this mechanism may be important in triggering early responses to bacterial penetration of the epithelial barrier (4). At sites of chronic inflammation, however, the endothelium will express IFN-γ dependent cytokines, such as IP-10, that promote lymphocyte and monocyte recruitment.

Infiltrating leukocytes, particularly monocytes and activated lymphocytes, are a major source of chemokines at sites of inflammation. The chemokines produced will determine the subsequent composition and duration of the inflammatory response. For example, CD8+ cytotoxic T-lymphocytes (CTLs) specific to myelin proteolipid protein peptide, a putative antigen in multiple sclerosis, secrete the chemokines MIP-1α, MIP-1β, IL-16, and IP-10 (5). These chemokines act predominantly on CD4+ T cells of the same T cell receptor (TCR) specificity (6). Thus, CD8+ cytotoxic T cells can promote and maintain inflammatory responses in multiple sclerosis by recruiting specific CD4 subsets. Certain viral epitopes have also been shown to promote the release of chemokines suggesting that this might be a more general function of CTLs (6-8).

The intracellular control mechanisms for chemokine release vary. Secretion of most chemokines requires transcription and protein synthesis resulting in a delay before their extracellular release. RANTES (regulated on activation, normal T expressed and secreted), however, is stored in preformed granules and rapidly released on activation. MIP-1α and RANTES co-localize within the cytolytic granules of HIV-1-specific CD8+ CTL (7) and following antigen-specific activation in-vitro, they are secreted together as a macromolecular complex containing sulfated proteoglycans, facilitating both lysis of HIV producing cells and the inhibition of free virus.

CHEMOKINE RETENTION AT SITES OF INFLAMMATION

If chemokines are to trigger adhesion and migration effectively at the endothelial surface, they must be retained at the vessel wall to allow interaction with circulating leukocytes. This immobilization is mediated by proteoglycans in the endothelial glycocalyx via interactions with glycosaminoglycan binding motifs (9). Chemokines show differential binding to proteoglycans. Because proteoglycans vary from site to site and with activation, this differential binding provides a mechanism by which tissues can selectively express a particular proadhesive factor enabling them to recruit specific leucocyte subsets. The system is highly sophisticated in the endothelium where chemokines secreted by sub-endothelial cells can be transported through the endothelial cells before being presented on proteoglycans in the glycocalyx (10). Proteoglycan binding is also important for retention and presentation in the extracellular matrix.

CHEMOKINE RECEPTOR CLASSIFICATION

Chemokines act via specific cell surface, seven transmembrane spanning G-protein-linked receptors (Figure 2). Five CXC chemokine receptors (CXCR1 to CXCR5), ten CC chemokine receptors (CCR1 to CCR10), and one CXXXC receptor have been identified so far in humans (Table 1). Most chemokine receptors are shared by more than one chemokine, such as CXCR3 which binds IP-10, MIG or IFN-inducible T cell alpha chemoattractant (I-TAC). A few have a restricted number of ligands such as CCR6 which binds MIP-3α and CXCR1, which binds IL-8 and granulocyte chemoattractant protein-2 (GCP-2). Some chemokines can also interact with more than one receptor (e.g., MIP-1α) suggesting a degree of redundancy and flexibility in the chemokine/chemokine receptor system. Engagement of chemokine receptors is associated with a calcium flux and G-protein dependent activation of phospholipases. The details of the downstream signals differ between cell types, so, for instance, IL-8 causes phospholipase D activation in lymphocytes, but not in neutrophils. There is also evidence that the consequences of receptor engagement is determined by the intracellular signals., Thus cytoskeletal rearrangement is a consequence of phospholipase C and Rho activation, whereas activation of protein tyrosine kinases is involved in cell activation and proliferation (11).

Chemokines also bind two types of non-signalling receptors that do not induce intracellular calcium fluxes. The Duffy antigen receptor for chemokines (DARC) on red blood cells is highly promiscuous and may act as a sump for mopping up excess CXC and CC chemokines in the circulation. Heparan sulphate proteoglycans are negatively charged molecules that will bind basic chemokine proteins, fixing them to extracellular matrix and to the surface of vascular endothelium. This mechanism allows a chemokine concentration gradient to be established away from a site of chemokine release, such as an inflammatory reaction (12).

CHEMOKINE – CHEMOKINE RECEPTOR INTERACTIONS

Role of Chemokines During the Multi-Step Process of Lymphocyte Migration through Endothelium

A multi-step process involving cell surface molecules on both leukocytes and vascular endothelium regulates leukocyte recruitment to tissue. As illustrated in Figure 3, chemokines play a crucial role in this process by triggering integrin- mediated adhesion and activating transendothelial migration into tissue (13). The first encounter between the flowing leukocyte and the vessel wall slows the cell by a process of transient tethering which induces the cell to roll or bump on the endothelium. This slowing is classically mediated by adhesion molecules, called selectins, which bind to carbohydrate containing receptors, although other molecules, such as vascular cell adhesion molecule (VCAM)-1 and mucosal addressin cell adhesion molecule (MAdCAM)-1, may be involved under certain conditions

Figure 2 Chemokine receptors are seven transmembrane spanning G-protein-linked cell surface receptors. These receptors may be shared or specific for their chemokine ligands.

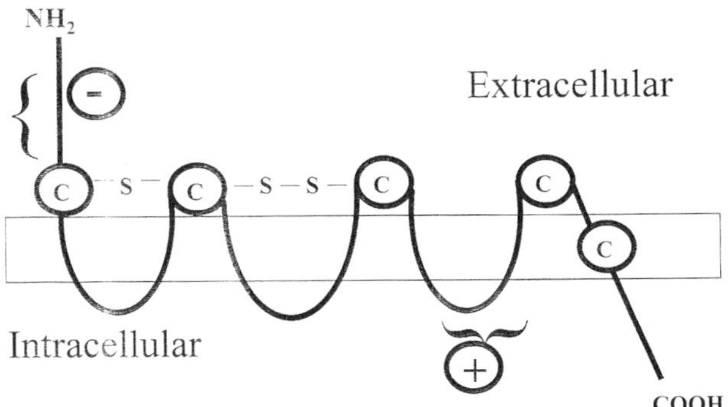

(14, 15). Although the cell may disengage after slowing, in the presence of an appropriate signal from a chemokine on the endothelium it comes to a halt, flattens and becomes strongly adherent to the vessel wall. This firm adhesion is mediated by the binding of leukocyte integrins to members of the immunoglobulin superfamily, such as intercellular adhesion molecule (ICAM)-1 and VCAM-1 on the endothelium. Over a period of minutes the cell migrates between the endothelial cells and enters the tissue, a process termed diapedesis. As well as triggering integrin-mediated adhesion, chemokines also facilitate recruitment by inducing morphological changes in the cell, characterised by the formation of cellular projections (uropods). Uropods are crucial for motility and cell adhesion receptors are redistributed to the tips of the uropods at the point of contact between the leukocyte and endothelium (16-18).

The attachment of leukocytes to the endothelium depends upon a very rapid increase in the affinity of leukocyte integrins for their endothelial ligands. Chemokines achieve this effect by rapidly inducing a conformational change in the integrin, which increases its affinity and avidity for counter-receptors (i.e., ICAM-1 and VCAM-1) and results in the conversion of rolling to arrest. (19, 20). This action was first demonstrated for IL-8. IL-8 triggers binding of the integrin lymphocyte function associated antigen (LFA-1) on neutrophils to its counter receptor ICAM-1 on endothelial cells. Subsequently, similar observations were made with T cells when MIP-1α and MIP-1β were shown to promote binding to ICAM-1 and VCAM-1 (9, 21, 22). Other chemokines have been shown also to have this property and to induce adhesion of human T cells to endothelial cells (22, 23). More recently, stromal cell derived factor (SDF-)1, secondary lymphoid tissue chemokine (SLC or 6-C-kine), MIP-1α, and MIP-1β have been shown to trigger adhesion to ICAM-1 and to induce arrest of rolling cells under flow conditions which more exactly mimic the *in vivo* situation within a blood vessel (24). Fractalkine

Figure 3 The role of chemokines in leukocyte-endothelial interactions and the subsequent migration of leukocytes into tissue. Interactions between chemokines and chemokine receptors on leukocytes are crucial in facilitating the multistep process of T cell adhesion to vascular endothelium, leading to integrin molecule activation, enhancing their binding to adhesion molecules ICAM-1 and VCAM-1. Chemokines also induce morphological changes in leukocytes and the formation of uropods. Cell adhesion receptors are redistributed to the tips of these projections, to the point of contact between leukocyte and endothelium. Chemokines bound to tissue heparan sulphate proteoglycans set up a concentration gradient across which leukocytes migrate to sites of inflammation.

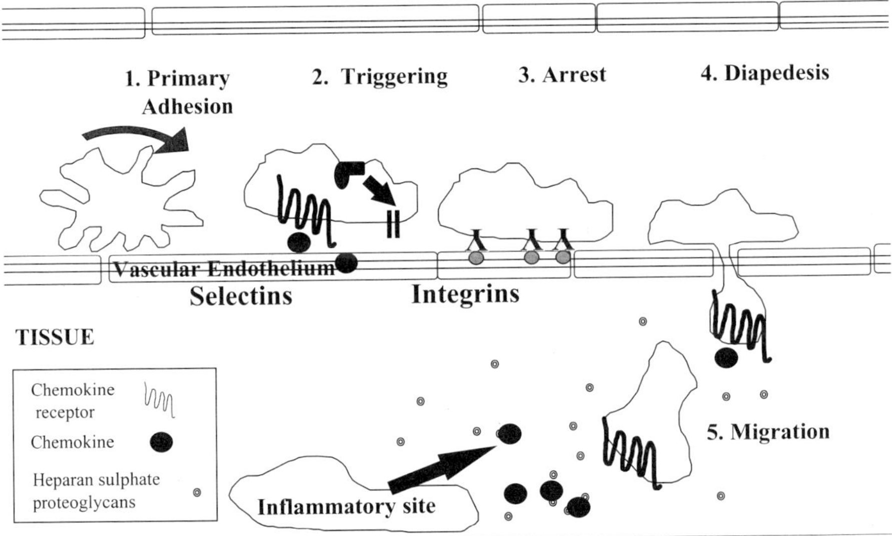

has also been shown to mediate the rapid capture, firm adhesion, and activation of circulating leukocytes under flow conditions. This adhesion was not inhibited by anti-integrin antibodies, suggesting an integrin independent, and therefore novel, pathway for leukocyte trafficking (25).

The Regulation of Chemokine Receptors on Leukocytes

Regulation with Maturation and Differentiation of Lymphocytes

Regulation of recruitment is not only controlled by the chemokines produced at sites of inflammation, but also by the levels of chemokine receptors expressed by leukocyte subsets. Thus some chemokines display preferential activity for particular leukocyte subsets. Lymphocytes can express most of the known chemokine receptors, but the levels of expression depend on the differentiation and activation status of the cell. During thymocyte maturation there are dramatic changes in the expression of several chemokine receptors including CCR4 and CCR7. These changes in chemokine receptor expression allow cells to be recruited and, as they mature, to migrate through the cortex, to the medulla, and into the circulation in response to different chemokines at each stage of maturation (26). Chemokines also play a role during B cell development within the bone marrow. The CXC chemokine SDF-1 is chemotactic for pre-B cells and may be involved in directing progenitor cells into appropriate maturation sites within the bone marrow (27, 28). In support of this function, mice lacking SDF-1 have poor lymphopoesis and reduced numbers of B cell precursors (29).

Chemokine / Chemokine Receptor Interactions in Lymphoid Organ Homeostasis

Secondary lymphoid tissues serve as a meeting place for antigen, antigen presenting cells, and antigen specific T cells so that an immune response may occur. Antigen bearing dendritic cells drain from peripheral sites of infection or inflammation to the T cell zones of lymph nodes where they present antigen to T cells in conjunction with MHC molecules. Naïve T cells enter lymphoid tissue from blood and spend several hours migrating through the T cell zone, making contact with multiple dendritic cells before re-entering the peripheral circulation. Resting B cells travel through lymphoid tissues by the same pathways as T cells, but home to B cell rich areas where they reside briefly before returning to the circulation. After antigen binding, B cells relocate to outer T cell zones promoting an encounter between antigen specific T and B cells. This highly orchestrated movement of T and B cells into and within secondary tissues depends on specific chemokine-chemokine receptor interactions (30, 31). Particular interest has focused on the CC chemokines thymus and activation regulated chemokine (TARC), EBV induced molecule-1 ligand chemokine (ELC, also known as MIP-3β), secondary lymphoid tissue chemokine (SLC, also known as 6-C-kine), liver and activation regulated chemokine (LARC), and dendritic cell chemokine (DC-CK1) that are all constitutively expressed within lymphoid tissues.

T Cell Recruitment and Positioning

SLC, and ELC, are both structurally related chemokines that bind CCR7 (32). SLC is strongly expressed by high endothelial venules in lymph nodes and by stromal cells in T cell areas of lymph nodes, spleen, and Peyer's patches. Thus, SLC appears to promote the homing of naïve T cells across high endothelial venules (HEVs) and into lymphoid T cell areas, as well as to stimulate the recruitment of dendritic cells to these areas (33). Mice with the paucity of lymph node T cells (*plt*) mutation, that spontaneously occurs in the DDD/l strain, are known to have a defect in T cell homing into lymph nodes and splenic white pulp (34, 35). The *plt* gene is on chromosome 4, syntenic to the region of human chromosome 9 that contains the linked SLC and ELC genes. Furthermore, SLC is largely absent and the expression of ELC greatly reduced in *plt* mice (36).

B Cell Recruitment and Positioning

Chemokines are also involved in recruiting and positioning B cells in lymphoid tissue. Mice lacking CXCR5 (BLR1), a chemokine receptor expressed by B lymphocytes, show defective formation of primary follicles and germinal centers in Peyer's patches and the spleen, as well as a loss of inguinal lymph nodes. CXCR5 deficient B cells enter T cell areas within lymphoid tissues, but fail to home to B cell areas (31). The chemokine ligand for CXCR5, BCA-1/BLC is highly expressed in lymphoid tissues and selectively recruits B lymphocytes (37, 38).

Dendritic Cell Recruitment

SLC and ELC are also involved in the homing of dendritic cells to lymphoid T cell zones (39). Maturing dendritic cells also up regulate CCR7 (the SLC and ELC receptor) and migrate to ELC in vitro (32, 40-44). Further support for the role of SLC and ELC in dendritic cell recruitment comes from the observations that dendritic cell numbers are greatly reduced in lymph nodes of *plt* mice (36). Immature dendritic cells have been shown to express a range of chemokine receptors, including CCR1, CCR5, CCR6, and CXCR1, which may participate in recruitment to inflamed tissues (40-43). Furthermore, differential expression of chemokine receptors may allow for their selective recruitment. For example, the MCP-3α receptor CCR6 is not expressed by monocyte derived dendritic cells, but is expressed at high levels by lung dendritic cells and by dendritic cells derived in vitro from CD34+ cord blood precursors (40, 42, 45).

Expression of inflammatory chemokine receptors promotes the recruitment of immature dendritic cells to sites of inflammation and also prevents them from leaving the area and migrating to draining nodes. This problem is overcome by changes in chemokine receptor expression that occur with activation and maturation of dendritic cells. Inflammatory chemokine receptors are downregulated during maturation, whereas CCR7 expression is increased promoting emigration out of peripheral tissue and subsequently into the lymph node (40-42, 46). From lymphatic vessels dendritic cells migrate into the T cell zone and become interdigitating cells. Interactions between SLC, ELC and their receptor CCR7, as well as between stromal cell factor and CXCR4, may play a role in this process (42).

Chemokines and Cell-Cell Interactions in Lymphoid Tissue

Once inside the lymphoid areas immune cells are required to interact and this process may also be controlled by chemokines. A novel CC chemokine named ABCD-1 is released from activated splenic B cells and dendritic cells. This chemokine is unusual in its specificity for attracting only activated T cells (47). ABCD-1 may, therefore, play an important role in the collaboration of dendritic cells and B-lymphocytes with T cells in immune responses.

Activation-Dependent Regulation of Chemokine Receptors on Leukocyte Subsets

The expression of chemokine receptors is carefully regulated on lymphocytes with activation. The activating signals and the environment in which the lymphocyte is activated both determine the patterns of chemokines expressed (11). There are fundamental differences between naïve T cells, which are yet to encounter their cognate antigen, and memory/effector cells. Naïve T cells express high levels of both L-selectin, an adhesion molecule that promotes binding to endothelium in lymph nodes, and CCR7. The ligands for CCR7 are two chemokines that are constitutively expressed in lymphoid tissue, SLC, which is found on high endothelial venules and ELC, which is made by interdigitating dendritic cells in the T cell areas of the lymph node (32). Thus, naïve T cells will be recruited to the T cell areas of lymphoid tissue where they can be efficiently activated by antigen presented by dendritic cells.

Regulation with Lymphocyte Activation

On activation the naïve T cell differentiates into an effector cell and receptors for inflammatory chemokines are upregulated, particularly CCR5, which binds RANTES, MIP-1α, and MIP-1β, and CXCR3, which binds the interferon dependent chemokines IP-10, I-Tac, and MIG. Thus, these effector cells can be rapidly recruited to sites of inflammation in tissue. The pattern of chemokine receptors expressed by effector cells is also determined by where the cell is activated. Chemokines not only attract effector cells to sites of inflammation, but they also determine which tissues those effector cells will preferentially migrate to. For example, effector T cells that are primed in the gut express low levels of CCR4, but high levels of CCR5 allowing them to respond to inflammatory chemokines in gut tissue. In contrast, effector cells that are primed in peripheral lymph nodes draining the skin express high levels of CCR4 which allows them to respond to TARC and macrophage derived chemokine (MDC) at sites of inflammation in the skin (48). Thus, the site of differentiation will determine which chemokine receptors are expressed and, thereby, the homing pattern of effector T cells. This process increases the efficiency of immune surveillance and ensures that effector cells are recruited to sites where they are most likely to encounter antigen.

After exposure to antigen, immunological memory is induced (i.e., the next time antigen is encountered there is a rapid response), suggesting the existence of memory T cells that are partially activated and able to orchestrate rapid secondary responses. These cells can be distinguished from naïve T cells by their expression of several cell surface molecules, including the CD45RO isoform, and by their enhanced ability to respond to antigen. Recent studies suggest that CD45RO+ cells can be divided into true memory cells and effector memory cells by their expression of certain chemokine receptors. CCR7 expressing true memory cells bear lymph node homing receptors, including L-selectin. True memory cells lack immediate effector function, but can efficiently stimulate dendritic cells and differentiate into CCR7 negative effector cells upon secondary stimulation. CCR7 negative memory cells express receptors for migration into inflamed tissues and display immediate effector function (49).

CCR5 (the receptor for MIP-1α, MIP-1β and RANTES)and CXCR3 (the receptor for IP-10, Mig and I-TAC) show increased expression on human peripheral blood memory CD45RO+ T cells (50). CCR5 and CXCR4 appear to denote an effector phenotype as these cells are predominantly CCR7 negative (49). Tissue infiltrating T cells in rheumatoid synovium which are predominantly of a memory phenotype have also been shown to express high levels of CXCR3 and CCR5 (51). CCR4 marks memory T cells, but its expression appears to be even more specific; skin homing memory T cells express high levels of this receptor, whereas gut homing memory T cells express low levels. CCR4 may, therefore, direct tissue specific T cell migration (48).

The role of the stromal cell derived factor (SDF)-1 receptor CXCR4 on mature lymphocytes is still poorly understood. SDF-1 is a potent chemotactic factor for freshly isolated peripheral blood lymphocytes (52) and, in flow-based assays that more closely mimic the *in vivo* situation within a blood vessel, it has been shown that both memory and naïve CD4+ cells respond to SDF-1α (24). Because SDF-1α is constitutively expressed in a wide variety of tissues, including liver, heart, lung, brain, muscle spleen and kidney (53), and because its expression is not altered by inflammatory stimuli, it may play a role in lymphocyte recirculation in normal tissues.

Regulation with TCR Triggering

There is evidence for a further layer of sophistication to chemokine receptor regulation with activation. Whereas activation and differentiation in secondary lymphoid tissue increases expression of chemokine receptors that promote recruitment to tissue, subsequent engagement of the TCR at sites of chronic inflammation downregulates many of these receptors including CCR1, CCR2, CCR5, and CCR7. This downregulation may serve to immobilise the lymphocyte at the site of antigen exposure in tissue (54).

Regulation of Chemokine Receptors on Functional Th1 / Th2 Cell Subsets

Unlike naïve T cells, antigen primed memory T cells are heterogeneous and include cells with different states of activation and polarisation. Functionally T cells can be subdivided into Th1 and Th2 cells based on their secretion of cytokines (55). Th1 cells produce pro-inflammatory cytokines (IL-2, IFN-γ and TNFβ) and activate both cellular responses and delayed type hypersensitivity. Th2 cells produce IL-4 and IL-10 and promote humoral and allergic responses (56). The cytokine milieu at the time of antigen priming, the co-stimulatory molecule expression, and the avidity of the T cell receptor/MHC peptide complex all influence whether cells differentiate down a Th1 or Th2 pathway. Th1 and Th2 cells produce cytokines mutually inhibitory for the differentiation and effector function of the reciprocal phenotype. It has recently been shown that several chemokine receptors are selectively expressed on Th1 cells which provides an explanation for their selective recruitment to tissues in certain inflammatory reactions (Figure 4).

In vitro, Th1 cells express CCR1, CCR5 and CXCR3, and migrate to their respective chemokines, which are: RANTES, MIP-1α, and MIP-1β for CCR1 and CCR5, and IP-10 and MIG for CXCR3 (57). Th1 cells are more than 10 times more responsive to IP-10 than Th2 cells, but Th1 cells fail to respond to the CCR3 ligand eotaxin. CXCR3 and CCR5 have been demonstrated on Th1 cells from rheumatoid synovial fluid and from the liver of patients with hepatitis C virus infection (58). The cytokines that influence T cell differentiation down a Th1 or Th2 pathway may also regulate the expression of both chemokines and chemokine receptors. *In vitro*, combinations of proinflammatory cytokines associated with a Th1 response (IFN-γ, TNF-α) may induce expression of the chemokines IP-10 and MIG. TNF-α also co-localises with these chemokines in the hepatocyte lobules and may account for their increased expression within the inflamed liver in chronic hepatitis C virus infection (58). IFN-α, which promotes Th1 polarisation

Figure 4 Chemokine receptors mark functional subsets of T lymphocytes. Unprimed, naïve Th0 cells are stimulated by dendritic cells (DC) within secondary lymphoid tissue. Dendritic cells present antigen in the groove of the MHC molecule to T cells and provide the relevant co-stimulatory signals. T cells then proliferate and differentiate down a Th1 or Th2 pathway depending on the local cytokine milieu. These T cells will then express specific combinations of chemokine receptors depending on their phenotype.

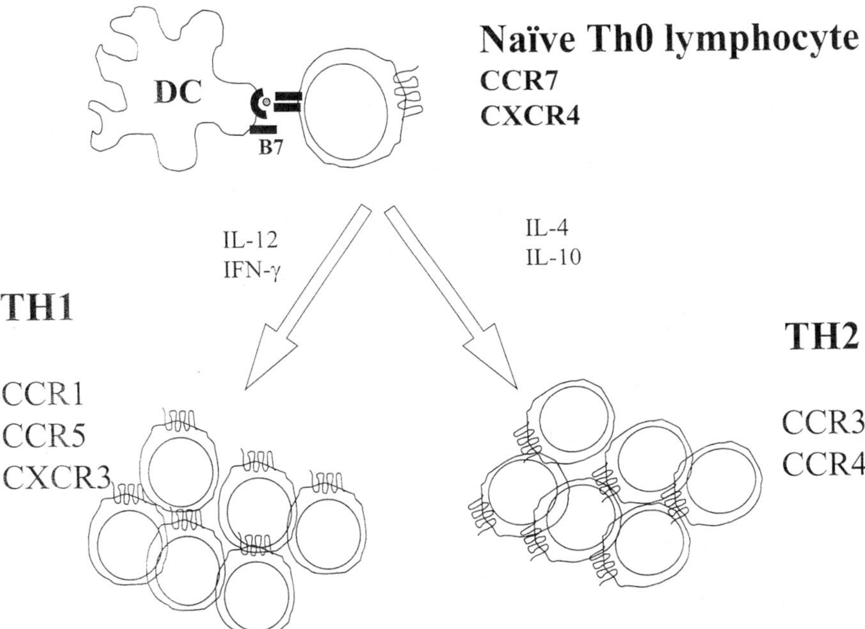

of human T cells (59) also inhibits expression of CCR3 and CCR4, chemokine receptors associated with a Th2 phenotype (60), whilst increasing expression of CXCR3, which is associated with Th1 cells. Furthermore, Th1 cells and monocytes/macrophages both express the receptors CCR1 and CCR5 which allows the recruitment and retention of macrophages and T cells to sites of chronic inflammation or delayed type hypersensitivity.

Th2 cells express a different array of chemokine receptors and have so far been shown to selectively express CCR3 (61), CCR4 (57, 62), and CCR8 (60). Antigen triggering (through TCR and CD28) leads to increased expression of CCR4 and CCR8, and reduced expression of CCR3 on Th2 cell lines, independent of IL-4. These cells also showed enhanced responses (intracellular calcium mobilisation) to chemokines I-309 (the ligand for CCR8) and TARC (for CCR4 andCCR8), and reduced responses to eotaxin (for CCR3). Thus, CCR4 and CCR8 may play an important role in the localization of activated Th2 cells at sites of antigenic challenge. Common expression of CCR3 by cell types including Th2 cells, eosinophils (63) and basophils (64) suggests that this chemokine receptor might act to bring together the different components of an allergic immune response (65).

In summary, there is now evidence for an elaborate network of chemokine/chemokine receptor interactions which provides a sophisticated mechanism that not only regulates leukocyte subset-specific recruitment to sites of inflammation, but also controls leukocyte recirculation during normal homeostasis.

Leukocyte Activation

In addition to regulating recruitment, some chemokines can also activate leukocytes. Thus, RANTES, MCP-1, and MIP-1α (66) have all been shown to co-stimulate activation of purified human T cells in response to TCR engagement. Furthermore, endogenously produced chemokines can provide co-stimulatory signals during human T cell activation suggesting that there is an autocrine and paracrine network promoting lymphocyte activation. RANTES induces a biphasic mobilization of Ca^+ in T cells. The first increase in cytosolic calcium is associated with chemotaxis (67). The second influx leads to activation of protein tyrosine kinases and a range of cellular responses, including IL-2 receptor expression, cytokine release, and T cell proliferation.

Activation of Non-Hemopoietic Cells: Chemokines and Angiogenesis

CXC chemokines are important regulators of angiogenesis (new blood vessel formation), which is fundamental to a variety of physiological and pathological processes, such as reproduction, embryonic development, tissue growth, and wound repair. An imbalance in neovascularization contributes to the pathogenesis of several diseases, including chronic inflammatory conditions and diabetic retinopathy. In addition, it is an essential factor in tumor growth and metastasis.

Several members of the CXC chemokine family can either promote or inhibit angiogenesis (68). Human platelet factor 4 (PF4) was the first chemokine reported to be angiostatic when it was shown to inhibit the growth of melanoma and colonic carcinomas (69). Subsequently, IL-8 was found to mediate angiogenesis in the absence of inflammation (70, 71) whereas other CXC chemokines (IP-10 and MIG) inhibited angiogenesis (70). Whether a CXC chemokine is angiogenic or angiostatic is determined by the presence or absence of a 3 amino acid glu-leu-arg (ELR) motif within the NH2 terminus of the molecule. The ELR motif was established as the critical structural/functional domain for determining angiogenic activity by site-directed mutagenesis (72). When the ELR motif in the angiogenic IL-8 protein was replaced with the corresponding sequence from the angiostatic chemokine IP-10 there was a switch from angiogenic to angiostatic activity. In complementary experiments a mutant form of MIG was constructed in which the insertion of the ELR motif resulted in a change from angiostatic to angiogenic activity. ELR-containing CXC chemokines that are angiogenic include Il-8, ENA-78, growth related oncogene (GRO)-α, GRO-β, GRO-γ, granulocyte chemotactic protein(GCP)-2, and platelet basic protein (PBP). The non-ELR angiostatic chemokines include PF-4, IP-10, MIG and SDF-1 (68, 73, 74).

In a model of human non-small cell lung cancer tumorigenesis in SCID mice, IL-8 promoted tumor growth (75). Neutralizing antibodies to IL-8 resulted in a 40% reduction in tumor size and a decline in tumor-associated vascular density. The reduction in tumour size in response to IL-8 neutralizing antibodies was paralleled by a decrease in spontaneous metastasis. The opposite findings have been seen with IP-10 (76-79), as IP-10 levels are inversely correlated with tumor growth. Reconstitution of intratumor IP-10 for a period of 8 weeks resulted in a significant inhibition of tumour growth, tumour-associated angiogenic activity, neovascularization, and spontaneous lung metastases, whereas, administration of an IP-10 neutralizing antibody for 10 weeks augmented tumour growth (78).

In addition to their angiogenic effects, there is evidence that chemokines can promote the growth of epithelial cells directly (80). Thus chemokines play several important roles in regulating tumour angiogenesis, growth, and metastatic potential. The CXC chemokines are likely to be important novel therapeutic targets for anti-cancer treatment.

INTERFERING WITH THE CHEMOKINE/CHEMOKINE RECEPTOR SYSTEM: KNOCKOUT AND ANIMAL MODELS

The study of animals that lack or over express chemokines or chemokine receptors has helped to delineate the relationships between chemokines and pathophysiological processes. MCP-1 knockout mice are unable to recruit monocytes in response to several inflammatory stimuli. In response to schistosoma mansoni, these animals have impaired delayed type hypersensitivity (DTH) responses and granuloma formation, as well as blunted secretion of IL-4, IL-5, and IFN-γ. Responses to *Mycobacterium tuberculosis* were not impaired in these mice suggesting that Th1 responses are intact (81). These studies are complemented by studies of animals in which CCR2, the main MCP-1 receptor, is knocked out. These mice also fail to recruit macrophages to inflammatory lesions and are unable to clear infection by intracellular bacteria such as *Listeria monocytogenes* (82).

Although MIP-1α has been shown to be a potent inhibitor of hemopoietic stem cell proliferation in vitro (83), MIP-1α knockout mice demonstrated no abnormalities in hematopoiesis or bone marrow function and seemed to develop normally (84). The putative role of MIP-1α in autoimmune disease is supported by the finding that these knockouts fail to develop coxsackie virus induced autoimmune myocarditis (85), which is mediated primarily by cytotoxic T lymphocytes. In contrast, control mice expressing MIP-1α developed severe myocarditis. Influenza virus infected MIP-1α knockout mice had reduced pneumonitis and delayed clearance of the virus compared to infected normal mice. These studies suggest that MIP-1α is likely to be required for the efficient recruitment of immunocompetent T cells to sites of inflammation *in vivo* and in the clearance of viral infections.

Mice lacking CCR1, a MIP-1α receptor which also interacts with RANTES, MIP-5, MCP-2, and MCP-3, have impaired trafficking and proliferation of myeloid progenitor cells. Mature neutrophils from these animals fail to migrate in response to MIP-1α. These mice also have accelerated mortality when challenged with *Aspergillus fumigatus*, a fungus controlled predominantly by neutrophils. In addition, CCR1 knockout mice have abnormal responses to Schistosoma mansoni, as manifested by increased IFN-γ and decreased IL-4 production (i.e. impaired Th2 responses) during this infection (86). Because several chemokines can bind to the same receptor and several receptors may bind a chemokine, it is important to compare results in animals deficient of the receptors as well as of the chemokines themselves.

One example in which a single receptor appears to mediate the function of a single chemokine is the CXCR4 receptor and SDF-1. Mice lacking either the SDF-1 gene or the gene encoding CXCR4 have impairment of both B cell lymphopoesis and bone marrow myelopoesis. These findings support functional studies suggesting that this chemokine is involved in lymphopoesis in the bone marrow. However, these animals have pointed out a crucial role of CXCR4 and SDF-1 in vascular development. SDF-1 is expressed in developing vascular endothelial cells and CXCR4 knockout mice die in utero with defective vascular development, haematopoesis and cardiogenesis. CXCR4 and SDF-1 are responsible for the formation of a mature vascular system by regulating vascular branching and remodelling in endothelial cells (29, 87).

Studies in eotaxin deficient mice have confirmed this chemokine's role in the generation of peripheral blood eosinophilia and antigen induced allergic responses. Eotaxin enhances the strength of the early eosinophil recruitment after antigen challenge in models of asthma and stromal keratitis, and plays a role in regulating the number of eosinophils in the peripheral circulation (88).The role of the IL-8 receptor in regulating myeloid progenitor cells has been suggested using IL-8R knockouts (89). These mice develop lymphadenopathy due to an increase in B cells, as well as splenomegally due to an increase in metamyelocytes, band, and mature neutrophils (90). In addition, impaired neutrophil recruitment to sites of inflammation in these animals confirms the functional studies and suggests that the IL-8 receptor may be useful as a therapeutic target in inflammatory disease (90).

CHEMOKINES AND THEIR RECEPTORS IN DISEASE

Chemokines play a crucial role in regulating the accumulation and the activation of leukocytes in tissues and, thereby, dictate the nature of the infiltrate in acute and chronic inflammation. Because there are so many chemokines, many of which are widely expressed, until recently it has been difficult to draw functional conclusions from studies of chemokine expression in disease. However, the development of monoclonal antibodies that recognise chemokine receptors has greatly enhanced our understanding of the role of chemokines. By studying chemokine and chemokine receptor expression together one can more accurately delineate the functionally important chemokines in any given situation.

Early studies showed high levels of some chemokines in particular situations. For example, in acute bacterial pneumonia there is a huge influx of neutrophils into the lung associated with high levels of the neutrophil chemoattractant IL-8 in bronchoalveolar fluid (91). In rheumatoid arthritis high levels of MIP-1α and MIP-1ß were found in synovial fluid associated with a mononuclear cell infiltrate (92). In chronic hepatitis C virus infection, characterised by T cell infiltration of the liver, there is increased expression of the chemokines IP-10 and Mig. T cells infiltrating the liver express high levels of CXCR3 and CCR5 compared with autologous circulating T cells, suggesting that the ligands of these two receptors play a role in the selective recruitment of T cells to the inflamed liver. Moreover, the anatomical distribution of the chemokines and receptor-bearing infiltrating cells suggests that different chemokine receptor/chemokine interactions may determine the extent and severity of the infiltration (58). Similar observations have been made in multiple sclerosis where CCR5 and CXCR3 appear to be particularly important (93). The role played by chemokines and chemokine receptors in the pathogenesis of a range of disease states will now be described in more detail.

Atherosclerosis

Chemokines play a significant role in atherogenesis (reviewed in references 94 and 95). Immune cells infiltrate vascular lesions from the earliest stages and the intimal fatty streak is characterized by the presence of T lymphocytes and macrophages, which differentiate into foam cells after ingesting lipoprotein particles. Given the polyclonal nature of the T cell infiltrate, the presence of T cells in atheromatous plaques is due to active recruitment of these cells rather than clonal antigen mediated expansion in situ (96, 97). Several chemokines, including MCP-1, MCP-4, RANTES, PARC, and ELC, are expressed within atherosclerotic plaques and have been implicated in the recruitment of mononuclear cells (98, 99). Animal models provide direct evidence of a role for chemokines in the pathogenesis of atherosclerosis because over expression of MCP-1 accelerates atheroma development (100, 101), whereas mice lacking the MCP-1 receptor CCR2 show reduced atheroma formation (102). In human studies, CCR2 expression is increased on monocytes in hypercholesterolemic patients compared with normocholesterolemic controls suggesting a mechanism for monocyte recruitment to the vessel wall during atherogenesis (103).

Reperfusion Injury

Re-establishing blood flow to ischaemic tissues provokes an inflammatory response, known as reperfusion injury, which exacerbates ischaemic damage. Reperfusion injury is involved in the pathogenesis of multiple organ failure after hypovolemia, myocardial infarction, stroke, and graft dysfunction after organ transplantation. Chemokines play an important role during this process and several chemokines, including IL-8 and MCP-1, can be induced during re-oxygenation of hypoxic endothelial cells *in vitro* (104). In animal models reperfusion injury is associated with local IL-8 production, neutrophil infiltration, and tissue destruction. The administration of neutralizing monoclonal antibody against IL-8 prevents neutrophil infiltration and tissue injury (105). IL-8 is released into the plasma of patients following acute myocardial infarction and subsequently binds to red blood cells, resulting in only a transient rise of plasma IL-8 and a more prolonged increase of erythrocyte bound IL-8 (106).

Asthma and Other Allergic Disorders

Asthma, allergic rhinitis, and atopic dermatitis are characterised by the selective accumulation and activation of T cells, eosinophils, and mast cells. The role of chemokines in allergic disease was first suggested after it was found that RANTES and MCP-3 were able to activate eosinophils and basophils, thereby causing chemotaxis and the release of histamine and leukotrienes (107). Several chemokines are increased in the bronchoalveolar lavage fluid of asthmatics (108) including eotaxin, which is responsible for the selective recruitment of eosinophils and basophils (109, 110). In addition, T cells with Th2 properties are also found at sites of allergic inflammation and these Th2 cells express high levels of the eotaxin receptor CCR3 (111). Thus, pathophysiologically relevant leukocytes sharing the CCR3 receptor are capable of being recruited together to the site of allergic inflammation by the same chemokines. T cells in non-allergic infiltrates and in tissues lacking eosinophils, such as rheumatoid arthritis synovium or the liver in chronic viral hepatitis, do not express CCR3 (111).

Other Auto-Immune and Inflammatory Conditions

Chemokines are clearly of paramount importance in the recruitment of immune cells to inflammatory lesions in several diseases. Psoriasis, a chronic inflammatory disorder characterised by neutrophil, macrophage, and T-cell infiltration of the skin, is associated with increased expression of several chemokines (including MIG and IP-10) within dermal papillae (112–117). Ulcerative colitis and Crohn's disease are chronic inflammatory conditions affecting the gastrointestinal tract. Ulcerative colitis involves the large bowel only, whereas Crohn's disease can involve any part of the gastrointestinal tract from mouth to anus. Macrophages and lymphocytes infiltrate the bowel and there may also be neutrophil infiltration during acute exacerbations. Several chemokines are up regulated within inflamed lesions in the bowel wall in these conditions (reviewed in reference 118), including IL-8, MCP-1, MIP-1α, MIP-1β, IP-10, RANTES, and ENA-78.

Multiple sclerosis (MS) is a T cell dependent chronic inflammatory disease that affects the central nervous system. Chemokines (IP-10, Mig and RANTES) have been found at increased levels in the CSF of patients during MS attacks (119) and several chemokines (IP-10, MIP-1α and MCP-1) are expressed within demyelinating lesions themselves (93;120).Their chemokine receptors, CXCR3 and the IP-10/Mig receptor, are expressed on T cells in virtually every perivascular inflammatory infiltrate in active MS lesions. CCR5, a RANTES receptor, is present on T cells, macrophages, and microglia in actively demyelinating MS brain lesions. Compared with circulating T cells, T cells in the cerebral spinal fluid are enriched for cells expressing CXCR3 or CCR5 (119). T cells that express CXCR3 are also increased in the peripheral blood of patients with relapsing–remitting MS and both CXCR3 and CCR5 expressing T cells are increased in progressive MS compared with controls (93). Expression of these specific chemokines and receptors allow for the selective recruitment of Th1 cells to MS lesions.

Infectious Diseases

All infectious diseases that induce an inflammatory response are associated with increased chemokine expression. Here we will focus on diseases with more specific associations with chemokines and where chemokines have a direct role in pathogenesis.

HIV

The role of chemokines in HIV is reviewed elsewhere in this book so we will only mention briefly their role in HIV infection. The discovery that certain chemokines (MIP-1α, MIP-1β and RANTES) produced by CD8 cells could suppress the infection of T cells with an M-(monocyte/macrophage) tropic HIV-1 strain (121) and accelerated the search for a receptor for these chemokines. The receptor CCR5 was subsequently shown to be a coreceptor with CD4 for the M-tropic strain (122). In a similar way the chemokine SDF-1 blocked infection with T-tropic HIV strains that infect CD4+ T cells (123), and CXCR4 was also identified as the co-receptor for these strains (124). The importance of these discoveries was emphasized when it was found that individuals who were resistant to HIV-1 infection despite multiple exposures were often homozygous for a mutation in the *CCR5* gene in which a 32bp deletion (*CCR5-Δ32*) produces a truncated protein that cannot be expressed on the cell surface. This mutant conferred resistance to HIV-1 and at the same time was not obviously deleterious to the individual, presumably because the important physiological functions mediated by CCR5 could be compensated for by CCR1 which binds many of the same chemokines. The *CCR5-Δ32* allele is relatively common in individuals of Northern European descent (125). A second rarer mutation has also been described in which the mutant *CCR5* contains a premature stop codon at position 303 resulting in a truncated protein which also confers resistance to HIV-1 (126). Later during the course of infection T-tropic variants of HIV-1 can emerge capable of using CCR3, CCR2 and CCR5 as well as CXCR4 (127). The fusion of the fields of chemokine biology and HIV has and will continue to result in rapid advances in both areas. Furthermore, the chemokines and their receptors will provide potential targets and allow for a number of therapeutic interventions against HIV. Further relationships between chemokines, their receptors and HIV infection are described in greater detail throughout subsequent chapters.

Plasmodium Malaria

The promiscuous erythrocyte chemokine receptor, DARC is a receptor for Plasmodium vivax, the organism responsible for plasmodium malaria. This receptor also binds several CC and CXC chemokines and is thought to act as a sump for excess soluble chemokines within the circulation (128).

Virally Induced Chemokines and Chemokine Receptors

Many pathogenic viruses express cytokines or cytokine receptors which either help the organism enter mammalian cells or which subvert the immune response. Chemokine receptors are expressed by several viruses and many of these can bind known chemokines. The US28 gene product of human cytomegalovirus, is a chemokine receptor which binds several chemokines and a gene product from herpesvirus saimiri binds human IL-8 (129). Furthermore the Kaposi's sarcoma associated herpesvirus (human herpesvirus 8) encodes a chemokine receptor that stimulates cell proliferation and angiogenesis providing a mechanism for virus proliferation in the host (130, 131).

CONCLUSIONS

The dominant role of chemokines is to regulate the migration and recruitment of specific leukocyte subsets to particular tissues. They play a critical role in the generation of cellular inflammation as part of the protective responses to invading pathogens and the pathological processes associated with infection and immune-mediated diseases. In addition there is now compelling evidence that they are crucial for lymphoid organ homeostasis and the development of the cellular immune system. The ability to define specific functional leukocyte subsets based on their expression of particular patterns of chemokine receptors has greatly enhanced our understanding of how immune responses are regulated. Chemokines are more than simple chemotactic factors, because they are also implicated in leukocyte activation, angiogenesis, and anti-microbial functions. In addition the discovery that chemokine receptors are critical co-factors for the entry of the HIV virus into mammalian cells has opened up a new field of chemokine research and given impetus to attempts to establish therapeutic agents that modulate chemokine release or inhibit the activation of chemokine receptors.

ADDENDUM

The speed of developments in the chemokine field has been such that this chapter inevitably omits new and important details. In addition to the references listed below, the interested reader is directed to Nature Immunology 2001;2:92-136, which includes a series of outstanding reviews covering all aspects of chemokine biology.

REFERENCES

1. Strieter, R.M., T.J. Standiford, G.B. Huffnagle, L.M. Colletti, N.W. Lukacs, and S.L. Kunkel. 1996. The good, the bad, and the ugly - the role of chemokines in models of human-disease - commentary. *Journal of Immunology 156*:3583.
2. Baggiolini, M., D. Dewald, and B. Moser. 1994. Interleukin-8 and related chemotactic cytokines: CXC and CC chemokines. *Adv.Immunol. 55*:97.
3. Conlon, K., A. Lloyd, U. Chattopadhyay, N. Lukacs, S. Kunkel, T. Schall, D. Taub, C. Morimoto, J. Osborne, J. Oppenheim, H. Young, D. Kelvin, and J. Ortaldo. 1995. Cd8(+) and cd45ra(+) human peripheral-blood lymphocytes are potent sources of macrophage inflammatory protein 1-alpha, interleukin-8 and rantes. *European Journal of Immunology 25*:751.
4. Lukacs, N.W., S.L. Kunkel, R. Allen, H.L. Evanoff, C.L. Shaklee, J.S. Sherman, M.D. Burdick, and R.M. Strieter. 1995. Stimulus and cell-specific expression of c-x-c and c-c chemokines by pulmonary stromal cell-populations. *American Journal Of Physiology-Lung Cellular And Molecular Physiology 12*:L 856.
5. Biddison, W.E., D.D. Taub, W.W. Cruikshank, D.M. Center, E.W. Connor, and K. Honma. 1997. Chemokine and matrix metalloproteinase secretion by myelin proteolipid protein-specific CD8+ T cells: potential roles in inflammation. *J.Immunol. 158*:3046.
6. Biddison, W.E., W.W. Cruikshank, D.M. Center, C.M. Pelfrey, D.D. Taub, and R.V. Turner. 1998. CD8+ myelin peptide-specific T cells can chemoattract CD4+ myelin peptide-specific T cells: importance of IFN-inducible protein 10. *J.Immunol. 160*:444.

7. Wagner, L., O.O. Yang, E.A. Garcia-Zepeda, Y. Ge, S.A. Kalams, B.D. Walker, M.S. Pasternack, and A.D. Luster. 1998. Beta-chemokines are released from HIV-1-specific cytolytic T-cell granules complexed to proteoglycans. *Nature 391*:908.
8. Price, D.A., A.K. Sewell, T. Dong, R. Tan, P.J. Goulder, S.L. Rowland-Jones, and R.E. Phillips. 1998. Antigen-specific release of beta-chemokines by anti-HIV-1 cytotoxic T lymphocytes. *Curr.Biol. 8*:355.
9. Tanaka, Y., D.H. Adams, S. Hubscher, H. Hirano, U. Siebenlist, and S. Shaw. 1993. T-cell adhesion induced by proteoglycan-immobilized cytokine MIP-1β. *Nature 361*:79.
10. Middleton, J., S. Neil, J. Wintle, I. Clark-Lewis, H. Moore, C. Lam, M. Auer, E. Hub, and A. Rot. 1997. Transcytosis and surface presentation of IL-8 by venular endothelial cells. *Cell 385:* 385-395.
11. Ward, S.G., K. Bacon, and J. Westwick. 1998. Chemokines and T lymphocytes: more than an attraction. *Immunity. 9*:1.
12. Tanaka, Y., K. Kimata, D.H. Adams, and S. Eto. 1998. Modulation of cytokine function by proteoglycans: sophisticated models for the regulation of cellular responses to cytokines. *Proceedings of the Association of American Physicians 110*:118.
13. Adams, D.H. and S. Shaw. 1994. Leucocyte endothelial interactions and regulation of leucocyte migration. *Lancet 343*:831.
14. Picker, L.J. 1994. Control of lymphocyte homing. *Curr.Opin.Immunol. 6*:394.
15. Jones, D.A., L.V. McIntire, C.W. Smith, and L.J. Picker. 1994. A 2-step adhesion cascade for T-cell endothelial-cell interactions under flow conditions. *Journal of Clinical Investigation 94*:2443.
16. Dougherty, G.J., S. Murdoch, and N. Hogg. 1988. The function of human intercellular adhesion molecule-1 (ICAM-1) in the generation of an immune response. *Eur.J.Immunol. 18*:35.
17. Carpen, O.C., P. Pallai, D.E. Staunton, and T.A. Springer. 1992. Association of ICAM-1 with actin-containing cytskeleton and alpha actinin. *J.Cell Biol. 118*:1223.
18. del Pozo, M.A., P. Sanchez-Mateos, and F. Sanchez-Madrid. 1996. Cellular polarization induced by chemokines: a mechanism for leukocyte recruitment? *Immunol.Today 17*:127.
19. Springer, T.A. 1994. Traffic signals for lymphocyte recirculation and leukocyte emigration: the multistep paradigm. *Cell 76*:301.
20. Butcher, E.C. and L.J. Picker. 1996. Lymphocyte homing and homeostasis. *Science 272*:60.
21. Taub, D.D., A.R. Lloyd, J.M. Wang, J.J. Oppenheim, and D.J. Kelvin. 1993. The effects of human recombinant MIP-1 alpha, MIP-1 beta, and RANTES on the chemotaxis and adhesion of T cell subsets. *Adv.Exp.Med.Biol. 351:139-46.*
22. Taub, D.D., K. Conlon, A.R. Lloyd, J.J. Oppenheim, and D.J. Kelvin. 1993. Preferential migration of activated CD4+ and CD8+ T cells in response to MIP-1 alpha and MIP-1 beta. *Science 260*:355.
23. Lloyd, A.R., J.J. Oppenheim, D.J. Kelvin, and D.D. Taub. 1996. Chemokines regulate t-cell adherence to recombinant adhesion molecules and extracellular-matrix proteins. *Journal of Immunology 156*:932.
24. Campbell, J.J., J. Hedrick, A. Zlotnick, M.A. Siani, D.A. Thompson, and E.C. Butcher. 1998. Chemokines and the arrest of lymphocytes rolling under flow conditions. *Science 279*:381.
25. Fong, A.M., L.A. Robinson, D.A. Steeber, T.F. Tedder, O. Yoshie, T. Imai, and D.D. Patel. 1998. Fractalkine and CX3CR1 mediate a novel mechanism of leukocyte capture, firm adhesion, and activation under physiologic flow. *J Exp Med 188(8):1413-9.*

26. Campbell, J.J., J. Pan, and E.C. Butcher. 1999. Cutting edge: developmental switches in chemokine responses during T cell maturation *J.Immunol. 163*:2353.
27. Aiuti, A., M. Tavian, A. Cipponi, F. Ficara, E. Zappone, J. Hoxie, B. Peault, and C. Bordignon. 1999. Expression of CXCR4, the receptor for stromal cell-derived factor-1 on fetal and adult human lympho-hematopoietic progenitors. *Eur.J.Immunol. 29*:1823.
28. D'Apuzzo, M., A. Rolink, M. Loetscher, J.A. Hoxie, I. Clark-Lewis, F. Melchers, M. Baggiolini, and B. Moser. 1997. The chemokine SDF-1, stromal cell-derived factor 1, attracts early stage B cell precursors via the chemokine receptor CXCR4. *Eur.J.Immunol. 27*:1788.
29. Nagasawa, T., S. Hirota, K. Tachibana, N. Takakura, S. Nishikawa, Y. Kitamura, N. Yoshida, H. Kikutani, and T. Kishimoto. 1996. Defects of B-cell lymphopoiesis and bone-marrow myelopoiesis in mice lacking the CXC chemokine PBSF/SDF-1. *Nature 382*:635.
30. Goodnow, C.C. and J.G. Cyster. 1997. Lymphocyte homing: the scent of a follicle. *Curr.Biol. 7*:R219.
31. Forster, R., A.E. Mattis, E. Kremmer, E. Wolf, G. Brem, and M. Lipp. 1996. A putative chemokine receptor, BLR1, directs B cell migration to defined lymphoid organs and specific anatomic compartments of the spleen. *Cell 87(6):1037-47.*
32. Campbell, J.J., E.P. Bowman, K. Murphy, K.R. Youngman, M.A. Siani, D.A. Thompson, L. Wu, A. Zlotnik, and E.C. Butcher. 1998. 6-C-kine (SLC), a lymphocyte adhesion-triggering chemokine expressed by high endothelium, is an agonist for the MIP-3beta receptor CCR7. *J.Cell Biol. 141*:1053.
33. Cyster, J.G. 1999. Chemokines and the homing of dendritic cells to the T cell areas of lymphoid organs [comment]. *J.Exp.Med. 189*:447.
34. Nakano, H., T. Tamura, T. Yoshimoto, H. Yagita, M. Miyasaka, E.C. Butcher, H. Nariuchi, T. Kakiuchi, and A. Matsuzawa. 1997. Genetic defect in T lymphocyte-specific homing into peripheral lymph nodes. *Eur.J.Immunol. 27*:215.
35. Nakano, H., S. Mori, H. Yonekawa, H. Nariuchi, A. Matsuzawa, and T. Kakiuchi. 1998. A novel mutant gene involved in T-lymphocyte-specific homing into peripheral lymphoid organs on mouse chromosome 4. *Blood 91*:2886.
36. Gunn, M.D., S. Kyuwa, C. Tam, T. Kakiuchi, A. Matsuzawa, L.T. Williams, and H. Nakano. 1999. Mice lacking expression of secondary lymphoid organ chemokine have defects in lymphocyte homing and dendritic cell localization [see comments]. *J.Exp.Med. 189*:451.
37. Legler, D.F., M. Loetscher, R.S. Roos, I. Clark-Lewis, M. Baggiolini, and B. Moser. 1998. B cell-attracting chemokine 1, a human CXC chemokine expressed in lymphoid tissues, selectively attracts B lymphocytes via BLR1/CXCR5. *J Exp Med 187(4):655-60.*
38. Gunn, M.D., V.N. Ngo, K.M. Ansel, E.H. Ekland, J.G. Cyster, and L.T. Williams. 1998. A B-cell-homing chemokine made in lymphoid follicles activates Burkitt's lymphoma receptor-1. *Nature 391*:799.
39. Ngo, V.N., H.L. Tang, and J.G. Cyster. 1998. Epstein-Barr virus-induced molecule 1 ligand chemokine is expressed by dendritic cells in lymphoid tissues and strongly attracts naive T cells and activated B cells. *J.Exp.Med. 188*:181.
40. Dieu, M.C., B. Vanbervliet, A. Vicari, J.M. Bridon, E. Oldham, S. Ait-Yahia, F. Briere, A. Zlotnik, S. Lebecque, and C. Caux. 1998. Selective recruitment of immature and mature dendritic cells by distinct chemokines expressed in different anatomic sites. *J.Exp.Med. 188*:373.

41. Lin, C.L., R.M. Suri, R.A. Rahdon, J.M. Austyn, and J.A. Roake. 1998. Dendritic cell chemotaxis and transendothelial migration are induced by distinct chemokines and are regulated on maturation. *Eur.J.Immunol. 28*:4114.
42. Sallusto, F., P. Schaerli, P. Loetscher, C. Schaniel, D. Lenig, C.R. Mackay, S. Qin, and A. Lanzavecchia. 1998. Rapid and coordinated switch in chemokine receptor expression during dendritic cell maturation. *Eur.J.Immunol. 28*:2760.
43. Sozzani, S., P. Allavena, G. D'Amico, W. Luini, G. Bianchi, M. Kataura, T. Imai, O. Yoshie, R. Bonecchi, and A. Mantovani. 1998. Differential regulation of chemokine receptors during dendritic cell maturation: a model for their trafficking properties. *J.Immunol. 161*:1083.
44. Yoshida, R., M. Nagira, M. Kitaura, N. Imagawa, T. Imai, and O. Yoshie. 1998. Secondary lymphoid-tissue chemokine is a functional ligand for the CC chemokine receptor CCR7. *J.Biol.Chem. 273*:7118.
45. Power, C.A., D.J. Church, A. Meyer, S. Alouani, A.E. Proudfoot, I. Clark-Lewis, S. Sozzani, A. Mantovani, and T.N. Wells. 1997. Cloning and characterization of a specific receptor for the novel CC chemokine MIP-3alpha from lung dendritic cells. *J.Exp.Med. 186*:825.
46. Delgado, E., V. Finkel, M. Baggiolini, C.R. Mackay, R.M. Steinman, and A. Granelli-Piperno. 1998. Mature dendritic cells respond to SDF-1, but not to several beta- chemokines. *Immunobiology 198*:490.
47. Schaniel, C., E. Pardali, F. Sallusto, M. Speletas, C. Ruedl, T. Shimizu, T. Seidl, J. Andersson, F. Melchers, A.G. Rolink, and P. Sideras. 1998. Activated murine B lymphocytes and dendritic cells produce a novel CC chemokine which acts selectively on activated T cells. *J.Exp.Med. 188*:451.
48. Campbell, J.J., G. Haraldsen, J. Pan, J. Rottman, S. Qin, P. Ponath, D.P. Andrew, R. Warnke, N. Ruffing, N. Kassam, L. Wu, and E.C. Butcher. 1999. The chemokine receptor CCR4 in vascular recognition by cutaneous but not intestinal memory T cells. *Nature 400*:776.
49. Sallusto, F., D. Lenig, R. Forster, M. Lipp, and A. Lanzavecchia. 1999. Two subsets of memory T lymphocytes with distinct homing potentials and effector functions. *Nature 401*:708.
50. Qin, S., J.B. Rottman, P. Myers, N. Kassam, M. Weinblatt, M. Loetscher, A.E. Koch, B. Moser, and C.R. Mackay. 1998. The chemokine receptors CXCR3 and CCR5 mark subsets of T cells associated with certain inflammatory reactions. *J.Clin.Invest. 101*:746.
51. Loetscher, P., M. Uguccioni, L. Bordoli, M. Baggiolini, B. Moser, C. Chizzolini, and J.M. Dayer. 1998. CCR5 is characteristic of Th1 lymphocytes [letter]. *Nature 391*:344.
52. Bleul, C.C., R.C. Fuhlbrigge, J.M. Casasnovas, A. Aiuti, and T.A. Springer. 1996. A highly efficacious lymphocyte chemoattractant, stromal cell-derived factor 1 (SDF-1). *J.Exp.Med. 184*:1101.
53. Godiska, R., D. Chantry, G.N. Dietsch, and P.W. Gray. 1995. Chemokine expression in murine experimental allergic encephalomyelitis. *J.Neuroimmunol. 58*:167.
54. Sallusto, F., E. Kremmer, B. Palermo, A. Hoy, P. Ponath, S. Qin, R. Forster, M. Lipp, and A. Lanzavecchia. 1999. Switch in chemokine receptor expression upon TCR stimulation reveals novel homing potential for recently activated T cells. *Eur.J.Immunol. 29*:2037.
55. Abbas, A.K., K.M. Murphy, and A. Sher. 1996. Functional diversity of helper T lymphocytes. *Nature 383*:787.

56. Mosmann, T.R. and S. Sad. 1996. The expanding universe of T-cell subsets: Th1, Th2 and more. *Immunol.Today 17*:138.
57. Bonecchi, R., G. Bianchi, P.P. Bordignon, D. D'Ambrosio, R. Lang, A. Borsatti, S. Sozzani, P. Allavena, P.A. Gray, A. Mantovani, and F. Sinigaglia. 1998. Differential expression of chemokine receptors and chemotactic responsiveness of type 1 T helper cells (Th1s) and Th2s. *J.Exp.Med. 187*:129.
58. Shields, P.L., C.M. Morland, M. Salmon, S. Qin, S.G. Hubscher, and D.H. Adams. 1999. Chemokine and chemokine receptor interactions provide a mechanism for selective T cell recruitment to specific liver compartments within hepatitis C-infected liver. *J.Immunol. 163*:6236.
59. Rogge, L., L. Barberis-Maino, M. Biffi, N. Passini, D.H. Presky, U. Gubler, and F. Sinigaglia. 1997. Selective expression of an interleukin-12 receptor component by human T helper 1 cells. *J.Exp.Med. 185*:825.
60. D'Ambrosio, D., A. Iellem, R. Bonecchi, D. Mazzeo, S. Sozzani, A. Mantovani, and F. Sinigaglia. 1998. Selective up-regulation of chemokine receptors CCR4 and CCR8 upon activation of polarized human type 2 Th cells. *J.Immunol. 161*:5111.
61. Sallusto, F., C.R. Mackay, and A. Lanzavecchia. 1997. Selective expression of the eotaxin receptor CCR3 by human T helper 2 cells. *Science 277*:2005.
62. Sallusto, F., D. Lenig, C.R. Mackay, and A. Lanzavecchia. 1998. Flexible programs of chemokine receptor expression on human polarized T helper 1 and 2 lymphocytes. *J.Exp.Med. 187*:875.
63. Ponath, P.D., S.X. Qin, D.J. Ringler, I. Clarklewis, J. Wang, N. Kassam, H. Smith, X.J. Shi, J.A. Gonzalo, W. Newman, J.C. Gutierrezramos, and C.R. Mackay. 1996. Cloning of the human eosinophil chemoattractant, eotaxin - expression, receptor-binding, and functional-properties suggest a mechanism for the selective recruitment of eosinophils. *Journal of Clinical Investigation 97*:604.
64. Uguccioni, M., C.R. Mackay, B. Ochensberger, P. Loetscher, S. Rhis, G.J. LaRosa, P. Rao, P.D. Ponath, M. Baggiolini, and C.A. Dahinden. 1997. High expression of the chemokine receptor CCR3 in human blood basophils. Role in activation by eotaxin, MCP-4, and other chemokines. *J.Clin.Invest. 100*:1137.
65. Corrigan, C.J. and A.B. Kay. 1992. T cells and eosinophils in the pathogenesis of asthma. *Immunol.Today 13*:501.
66. Taub, D.D., S.M. Turcovski-Corrales, M.L. Key, D.L. Longo, and W.J. Murphy. 1996. Chemokines and T lymphocyte activation: I. Beta chemokines costimulate human T lymphocyte activation in vitro. *J.Immunol. 156*:2095.
67. Bacon, K.B., B.A. Premack, P. Gardner, and T.J. Schall. 1995. Activation of dual t-cell signaling pathways by the chemokine rantes. *Science 269*:1727.
68. Strieter, R.M., P.J. Polverini, D.A. Arenberg, and S.L. Kunkel. 1995. The role of CXC chemokines as regulators of angiogenesis. *Shock 4*:155.
69. Sharpe, R.J., H.R. Byers, C.F. Scott, S.I. Bauer, and T.E. Maione. 1990. Growth inhibition of murine melanoma and human colon carcinoma by recombinant human platelet factor 4. *J.Natl.Cancer Inst. 82*:848.
70. Strieter, R.M., S.L. Kunkel, V.M. Elner, C.L. Martonyi, A.E. Koch, P.J. Polverini, and S.G. Elner. 1992. Interleukin-8. A corneal factor that induces neovascularization. *Am.J.Pathol. 141*:1279.
71. Koch, A.E., P.J. Polverini, S.L. Kunkel, L.A. Harlow, L.A. DiPietro, V.M. Elner, S.G. Elner, and R.M. Strieter . 1992. Interleukin-8 as a macrophage-derived mediator of angiogenesis. *Science 258*:1798.

72. Strieter, R.M., P.J. Polverini, S.L. Kunkel, D.A. Arenberg, M.D. Burdick, J. Kasper, J. Dzuiba, J. Van Damme, A. Walz, and D. Marriott. 1995. The functional role of the ELR motif in CXC chemokine-mediated angiogenesis. *J.Biol.Chem. 270*:27348.
73. Strieter, R.M., P.J. Polverini, S.L. Kunkel, D.A. Arenberg, M.D. Burdick, J. Kasper, J. Dzuiba, J. Vandamme, A. Walz, D. Marriott, S.Y. Chan, S. Roczniak, and A.B. Shanafelt. 1995. The functional-role of the elr motif in cxc chemokine-mediated angiogenesis. *Journal of Biological Chemistry 270* :27348.
74. Luster, A.D., S.M. Greenberg, and P. Leder. 1995. The ip-10 chemokine binds to a specific cell-surface heparan- sulfate site shared with platelet factor-4 and inhibits endothelial-cell proliferation. *Journal of Experimental Medicine 182*:219.
75. Arenberg, D.A., S.L. Kunkel, P.J. Polverini, M. Glass, M.D. Burdick, and R.M. Strieter. 1996. Inhibition of interleukin-8 reduces tumorigenesis of human non- small-cell lung-cancer in scid mice. *Journal of Clinical Investigation 97*:2792.
76. Angiolillo, A.L., C. Sgadari, D.D. Taub, F. Liao, J.M. Farber, S. Maheshwari, H.K. Kleinman, G.H. Reaman, and G. Tosato. 1995. Human interferon-inducible protein-10 is a potent inhibitor of angiogenesis in-vivo. *Journal of Experimental Medicine 182*:155.
77. Angiolillo, A.L., C. Sgadari, and G. Tosato. 1996. A role for the interferon-inducible protein 10 in inhibition of angiogenesis by interleukin-12. *Ann.N.Y.Acad.Sci. 795:158-67.*
78. Arenberg, D.A., S.L. Kunkel, P.J. Polverini, S.B. Morris, M.D. Burdick, M.C. Glass, D.T. Taub, M.D. Iannettoni, R.I. Whyte, and R.M. Strieter. 1996. Interferon-gamma-inducible protein 10 (IP-10) is an angiostatic factor that inhibits human non-small cell lung cancer (NSCLC) tumorigenesis and spontaneous metastases. *J.Exp.Med. 184*:981.
79. Luster, A.D. and P. Leder. 1993. Ip-10, a -c-x-c- chemokine, elicits a potent thymus-dependent antitumor response in-vivo. *Journal of Experimental Medicine 178*:1057.
80. Jordan, N.J., G. Kolios, S.E. Abbot, M.A. Sinai, D.A. Thompson, K. Petraki, and J. Westwick. 1999. Expression of functional CXCR4 chemokine receptors on human colonic epithelial cells. *J.Clin.Invest. 104*:1061.
81. Lu, B., B.J. Rutledge, L. Gu, J. Fiorillo, N.W. Lukacs, S.L. Kunkel, R. North, C. Gerard, and B.J. Rollins. 1998. Abnormalities in monocyte recruitment and cytokine expression in monocyte chemoattractant protein 1-deficient mice. *J.Exp.Med. 187*:601.
82. Kurihara, T., G. Warr, J. Loy, and R. Bravo. 1997. Defects in macrophage recruitment and host defense in mice lacking the CCR2 chemokine receptor. *J.Exp.Med. 186*:1757.
83. Graham, G.J., E.G. Wright, R. Hewick, S.D. Wolpe, N.M. Wilkie, D. Donaldson, S. Lorimore, and I.B. Pragnell. 1990. Identification and characterization of an inhibitor of haemopoietic stem cell proliferation. *Nature 344*:442.
84. Cook, D.N., M.A. Beck, T.M. Coffman, S.L. Kirby, J.F. Sheridan, I.B. Pragnell, and O. Smithies. 1995. Requirement of MIP-1a for an inflammatory response to viral infection. *Science 269*:1583.
85. Karpus, W.J., N.W. Lukacs, B.L. Mcrae, R.M. Strieter, S.L. Kunkel, and S.D. Miller. 1995. An important role for the chemokine macrophage inflammatory protein- 1-alpha in the pathogenesis of the t-cell-mediated autoimmune- disease, experimental autoimmune encephalomyelitis. *J. Immunol 155*:5003.
86. Gao, J.L., T.A. Wynn, Y. Chang, E.J. Lee, H.E. Broxmeyer, S. Cooper, H.L. Tiffany, H. Westphal, J. Kwon-Chung, and P.M. Murphy. 1997. Impaired host defense, hema-

topoiesis, granulomatous inflammation and type 1-type 2 cytokine balance in mice lacking CC chemokine receptor 1. *J.Exp.Med. 185*:1959.
87. Tachibana, K., S. Hirota, H. Iizasa, H. Yoshida, K. Kawabata, Y. Kataoka, Y. Kitamura, K. Matsushima, N. Yoshida, S. Nishikawa, T. Kishimoto, and T. Nagasawa. 1998. The chemokine receptor CXCR4 is essential for vascularization of the gastrointestinal tract. *Nature 393*:591.
88. Rothenberg, M.E., J.A. MacLean, E. Pearlman, A.D. Luster, and P. Leder. 1997. Targeted disruption of the chemokine eotaxin partially reduces antigen- induced tissue eosinophilia. *J.Exp.Med. 185*:785.
89. Broxmeyer, H.E., S. Cooper, G. Cacalano, N.L. Hague, E. Bailish, and M.W. Moore. 1996. Involvement of Interleukin (IL) 8 receptor in negative regulation of myeloid progenitor cells in vivo: evidence from mice lacking the murine IL-8 receptor homologue. *J.Exp.Med. 184*:1825.
90. Cacalano, G., J. Lee, K. Kikly, A.M. Ryan, S. Pitts-Meek, B. Hultgren, W.I. Wood, and M.W. Moore. 1994. Neutrophil and B cell expansion in mice that lack the murine IL-8 receptor homolog [published erratum appears in Science 1995 Oct 20;270(5235):365]. *Science 265*:682.
91. Chollet-Martin, S., P. Montravers, C. Gibert, C. Elbim, J.M. Desmonts, J.Y. Fagon, and M.A. Gougerot-Pocidalo. 1993. High levels of interleukin-8 in the blood and alveolar spaces of patients with pneumonia and adult respiratory distress syndrome. *Infect.Immun. 61*:4553.
92. Koch, A.E., S.L. Kunkel, M.R. Shah, R. Fu, D.D. Mazarakis, G.K. Haines, M.D. Burdick, R.M. Pope, and R.M. Strieter. 1995. Macrophage inflammatory protein-1-beta - a c-c chemokine in osteoarthritis. *Clinical Immunology and Immunopathology 77*:307.
93. Balashov, K.E., J.B. Rottman, H.L. Weiner, and W.W. Hancock. 1999. CCR5(+) and CXCR3(+) T cells are increased in multiple sclerosis and their ligands MIP-1alpha and IP-10 are expressed in demyelinating brain lesions. *Proc.Natl.Acad.Sci.U.S.A. 96*:6873.
94. Terkeltaub, R., W.A. Boisvert, and L.K. Curtiss. 1998. Chemokines and atherosclerosis. *Curr.Opin.Lipidol. 9*:397.
95. Wang, J.M., S. Su, W. Gong, and J.J. Oppenheim. 1998. Chemokines, receptors, and their role in cardiovascular pathology. *Int.J.Clin.Lab.Res. 28*:83.
96. Stemme, S., L. Rymo, and G.K. Hansson. 1991. Polyclonal origin of T lymphocytes in human atherosclerotic plaques. *Lab.Invest. 65*:654.
97. Frostegard, J., A.K. Ulfgren, P. Nyberg, U. Hedin, J. Swedenborg, U. Andersson, and G.K. Hansson. 1999. Cytokine expression in advanced human atherosclerotic plaques: dominance of pro-inflammatory (Th1) and macrophage-stimulating cytokines [In Process Citation]. *Atherosclerosis 145*:33.
98. Pattison, J.M., P.J. Nelson, P. Huie, R.K. Sibley, and A.M. Krensky. 1996. RANTES chemokine expression in transplant-associated accelerated atherosclerosis. *J.Heart Lung Transplant. 15*:1194.
99. Reape, T.J., K. Rayner, C.D. Manning, A.N. Gee, M.S. Barnette, K.G. Burnand, and P.H. Groot. 1999. Expression and cellular localization of the CC chemokines PARC and ELC in human atherosclerotic plaques. *Am.J.Pathol. 154*:365.
100. Aiello, R.J., P.A. Bourassa, S. Lindsey, W. Weng, E. Natoli, B.J. Rollins, and P.M. Milos. 1999. Monocyte chemoattractant protein-1 accelerates atherosclerosis in apolipoprotein E-deficient mice. *Arterioscler.Thromb.Vasc.Biol. 19*:1518.

101. Gosling, J., S. Slaymaker, L. Gu, S. Tseng, C.H. Zlot, S.G. Young, B.J. Rollins, and I.F. Charo. 1999. MCP-1 deficiency reduces susceptibility to atherosclerosis in mice that overexpress human apolipoprotein B. *J.Clin.Invest. 103*:773.
102. Boring, L., J. Gosling, M. Cleary, and I.F. Charo. 1998. Decreased lesion formation in CCR2-/- mice reveals a role for chemokines in the initiation of atherosclerosis. *Nature 394*:894.
103. Han, K.H., R.K. Tangirala, S.R. Green, and O. Quehenberger. 1998. Chemokine receptor CCR2 expression and monocyte chemoattractant protein- 1-mediated chemotaxis in human monocytes. A regulatory role for plasma LDL. *Arterioscler.Thromb.Vasc.Biol. 18*:1983.
104. Karakurum, M., R. Shreeniwas, J. Chen, D. Pinsky, S.D. Yan, M. Anderson, K. Sunouchi, J. Major, T. X Hamilton, K. Kuwabara, A. Rot, P.R. Nowygrod, and D. Stern. 1994. Hypoxic induction of interleukin-8 gene-expression in human endothelial cells. *Journal of Clinical Investigation 93*:1564.
105. Sekido, N., N. Mukaida, A. Harada, I. Nakanishi, Y. Watanabe, and K. Matsushima. 1993. Prevention of lung reperfusion injury in rabbits by a monoclonal antibody against interleukin-8. *Nature 365*:654.
106. de Winter, R.J., A. Manten, Y.P. de Jong, R. Adams, S.J. van Deventer, and K.I. Lie. 1997. Interleukin 8 released after acute myocardial infarction is mainly bound to erythrocytes. *Heart 78*:598.
107. Baggiolini, M. and C.A. Dahinden. 1994. CC chemokines in allergic inflammation. *Immunol.Today 15*:127.
108. Alam, R., J. York, M. Boyars, S. Stafford, J.A. Grant, J. Lee, P. Forsythe, T. Sim, and N. Ida. 1996. Increased MCP-1, RANTES, and MIP-1alpha in bronchoalveolar lavage fluid of allergic asthmatic patients. *Am.J.Respir.Crit.Care Med. 153*:1398.
109. Lamkhioued, B., P.M. Renzi, S. Abi-Younes, E.A. Garcia-Zepada, Z. Allakhverdi, O. Ghaffar, M.D. Rothenberg, A.D. Luster, and Q. Hamid. 1997. Increased expression of eotaxin in bronchoalveolar lavage and airways of asthmatics contributes to the chemotaxis of eosinophils to the site of inflammation. *J.Immunol. 159*:4593.
110. Ying, S., D.S. Robinson, Q. Meng, J. Rottman, R. Kennedy, D.J. Ringler, C.R. Mackay, B.L. Daugherty, M.S. Springer, S.R. Durham, T.J. Williams, and A.B. Kay. 1997. Enhanced expression of eotaxin and CCR3 mRNA and protein in atopic asthma. Association with airway hyperresponsiveness and predominant co- localization of eotaxin mRNA to bronchial epithelial and endothelial cells. *Eur.J.Immunol. 27*:3507.
111. Gerber, B.O., M.P. Zanni, M. Uguccioni, M. Loetscher, C.R. Mackay, W.J. Pichler, N. Yawalkar, M. Baggiolini, and B. Moser. 1997. Functional expression of the eotaxin receptor CCR3 in T lymphocytes co- localizing with eosinophils. *Curr.Biol. 7*:836.
112. Goebeler, M., A. Toksoy, U. Spandau, E. Engelhardt, E.B. Brocker, and R. Gillitzer. 1998. The C-X-C chemokine Mig is highly expressed in the papillae of psoriatic lesions. *J.Pathol. 184*:89.
113. Boorsma, D.M., J. Flier, S. Sampat, C. Ottevanger, P. de Haan, L. Hooft, R. Willemze, C.P. Tensen, and T.J. Stoof. 1998. Chemokine IP-10 expression in cultured human keratinocytes. *Arch.Dermatol.Res. 290*:335.
114. Raychaudhuri, S.P., W.Y. Jiang, E.M. Farber, T.J. Schall, M.R. Ruff, and C.B. Pert. 1999. Upregulation of RANTES in psoriatic keratinocytes: a possible pathogenic mechanism for psoriasis. *Acta Derm.Venereol. 79*:9.
115. Zheng, M., G. Sun, and U. Mrowietz. 1996. The chemotactic activity of T-lymphocytes in response to interleukin 8 is significantly decreased in patients with psoriasis and atopic dermatitis. *Exp.Dermatol. 5*:334.

116. Gottlieb, A.B., A.D. Luster, D.N. Posnett, and D.M. Carter. 1988. Detection of a gamma interferon-induced protein IP-10 in psoriatic plaques. *J.Exp.Med. 168*:941.
117. Gillitzer, R., U. Ritter, U. Spandau, M. Goebeler, and E.B. Brocker. 1996. Differential expression of GRO-alpha and IL-8 mRNA in psoriasis: a model for neutrophil migration and accumulation in vivo. *J.Invest.Dermatol. 107*:778.
118. MacDermott, R.P., I.R. Sanderson, and H.C. Reinecker. 1998. The central role of chemokines (chemotactic cytokines) in the immunopathogenesis of ulcerative colitis and Crohn's disease. *Inflamm.Bowel.Dis. 4*:54.
119. Sorensen, T.L., M. Tani, J. Jensen, V. Pierce, C. Lucchinetti, V.A. Folcik, S. Qin, J. Rottman, F. Sellebjerg, R.M. Strieter, J.L. Frederiksen, and R.M. Ransohoff. 1999. Expression of specific chemokines and chemokine receptors in the central nervous system of multiple sclerosis patients. *J.Clin.Invest. 103*:807.
120. Van, D., V, J. Tekstra, R.H. Beelen, C.P. Tensen, and C.J. De Groot. 1999. Expression of MCP-1 by reactive astrocytes in demyelinating multiple sclerosis lesions. *Am.J.Pathol. 154*:45.
121. Cocchi, F., A.L. Devico, A. Garzinodemo, S.K. Arya, R.C. Gallo, and P. Lusso. 1995. Identification of rantes, mip-1-alpha, and mip-1-beta as the major hiv-suppressive factors produced by cd8(+) t-cells. *Science 270*:1811.
122. Dragic, T., V. Litwin, G.P. Allaway, S.R. Martin, Y.X. Huang, K.A. Nagashima, C. Cayanan, P.J. Maddon, R.A. Koup, J.P. Moore, and W.A. Paxton. 1996. Hiv-1 entry into cd4(+) cells is mediated by the chemokine receptor cc-ckr-5. *Nature 381*:667.
123. Oberlin, E., A. Amara, F. Bachelerie, C. Bessia, J.L. Virelizier, F. Arenzanaseisdedos, O. Schwartz, J.M. Heard, I. Clarklewis, D.F. Legler, M. Loetscher, M. Baggiolini, and B. Moser. 1996. The CXC chemokine SDF-1 is the ligand for LESTR/fusin and prevents infection by T-cell-line-adapted HIV-1. *Nature 382*:833.
124. Deng, H., R. Liu, W. Ellmeier, S. Choe, D. Unutmaz, M. Burkhart, P. Di Marzio, S. Marmon, R.E. Sutton, C.M. Hill, C.B. Davis, S.C. Peiper, T.J. Schall, D.R. Littman, and N.R. Landau. 1996. Identification of a major co-receptor for primary isolates of HIV-1 [see comments]. *Nature 381*:661.
125. Liu, R., W.A. Paxton, S. Choe, D. Ceradini, S.R. Martin, R. Horuk, M.E. Macdonald, H. Stuhlmann, R.A. Koup, and N.R. Landau. 1996. Homozygous defect in HIV-1 coreceptor accounts for resistance of some multiply-exposed individuals to HIV-1 infection. *Cell 86*:367.
126. Quillent, C., E. Oberlin, J. Braun, D. Rousset, G. Gonzalez-Canali, P. Metais, L. Montagnier, J.L. Virelizier, F. Arenzana-Seisdedos, and A. Beretta. 1998. HIV-1-resistance phenotype conferred by combination of two separate inherited mutations of CCR5 gene [see comments]. *Lancet 351*:14.
127. Connor, R.I., K.E. Sheridan, D. Ceradini, S. Choe, and N.R. Landau. 1997. Change in coreceptor use coreceptor use correlates with disease progression in HIV-1--infected individuals. *J.Exp.Med. 185*:621.
128. Horuk, R. 1994. The interleukin-8-receptor family: from chemokines to malaria. *Immunol.Today 15*:169.
129. Alcami, A. and G.L. Smith. 1995. Cytokine receptors encoded by poxviruses - a lesson in cytokine biology. *Immunol.Today 16*:474.
130. Bais, C., B. Santomasso, O. Coso, L. Arvanitakis, E.G. Raaka, J.S. Gutkind, A.S. Asch, E. Cesarman, M.C. Gershengorn, E.A. Mesri, and M.C. Gerhengorn. 1998. G-protein-coupled receptor of Kaposi's sarcoma-associated herpesvirus is a viral oncogene and angiogenesis activator [published erratum appears in Nature 1998 Mar 12;392(6672):210]. *Nature 391*:86.

131. Arvanitakis, L., E. Geras-Raaka, A. Varma, M.C. Gershengorn, and E. Cesarman. 1997. Human herpesvirus KSHV encodes a constitutively active G-protein- coupled receptor linked to cell proliferation. *Nature 385*:347.

2

Chemokine Receptor Expression and Regulatory Mechanisms

Ricardo M. Richardson, Ralph Snyderman, and Bodduluri Haribabu

Duke University Medical Center, Durham, North Carolina

INTRODUCTION

Chemokines are a family of structurally related peptides of 8-10 kDaltons that regulate inflammation through cell surface G-protein-coupled receptors on leukocytes. These peptides mediate diverse biological and biochemical activities in leukocytes, including adhesion to endothelium, directed migration, and activation of cytotoxic activities (1). Initially, chemoattractive products of lymphocyte transformation were termed lymphocyte-derived chemotactic factors, LDCF (2). Monocyte-derived neutrophil chemotactic factor (MDCNF), the first well characterized chemokine, was renamed Interleukin-8 (IL-8) as its activities are not specific for neutrophils and it is produced by many types of cells (3, 4). Studies have highlighted the importance of chemokines in mononuclear leukocyte accumulation and activation, as well as in lymphocyte recirculation and homing (5, 6). Two recent developments contributed greatly to the enhanced interest and rapid progress in chemokine biology. One was the discovery that some chemokines protect against infection by human immunodeficiency virus (HIV-1) and that the chemokine receptors CCR5 and CXCR4 are the major co-receptors for the viral entry into CD4 positive cells (7). Second, major genome sequencing efforts worldwide led to the identification of a number of novel chemokines based on their structural features (8). In contrast to the rapid expansion of the number of identified chemokines and chemokine receptors, the understanding of their biological activities and regulation remains in infancy. Indeed, much of what is presumed regarding the regulation of chemoattractant receptors is based on studies with the "classical" chemoattractant receptors for formylpeptides (fMLP), a peptide from the fifth component of complement (C5a), and the platelet activating factor (PAF) (5, 9).

The synthesis of specific chemokines and the expression of chemokine receptors on some cells during development or inflammation provide a level of control for the activities of chemokines (10, 11). A second level of control occurs by modulation of the activities of chemokine receptors through mechanisms such as desensitization or priming (9). This review provides a brief description of the chemokine receptor family followed by an outline of different regulatory mechanisms that modulate the activities of these receptors.. The reader is referred to Chapter 1 of this book and to published reviews (12-14) for a comprehensive look at the biological activities of chemokines and their receptors.

CHEMOKINES AND CHEMOKINE RECEPTORS

Chemokines have been classified into four families, C, CC, CXC, and CX3C, based on the number and positions of the N-terminal-conserved cysteine residues. Since the identification of IL-8 nearly 12 years ago, over 40 chemokines have been identified (13). Chemokines bind to and activate seven transmembrane G-protein-coupled receptors (9). The standard nomenclature for chemokine receptors, established at the 1996 Gordon Research Conference on "Chemotactic Cytokines," is used in Table 1, which lists known chemokines, chemokine receptors, and their predominant expression patterns (13-19). A standard nomenclature for chemokines is needed and hopefully will be established soon. The CC chemokines activate many types of leukocytes, including lymphocytes, basophils, eosinophils and monocytes, whereas the CXC chemokines activate neutrophils and monocytes. The CXC and CC chemokines were initially believed to be associated with acute and chronic inflammation, respectively (1, 13). However, this notion is currently being revised as additional receptors are being discovered and shown to have broader (CXCR4) or unique (CXCR3, CXCR5) tissue specificity (20-22). Most chemokines and chemokine receptors are not specific in that many chemokines activate more than one receptor and many receptors are activated by multiple chemokines (Table1). The structural basis and biological significance of these redundancies remain to be determined. Thus far, exceptions include three receptor-ligand pairs with exclusive specificity: CXCR4 and stromal cell derived factor (SDF-1); CXCR5 and B-lymphocyte chemoattractant (BLC); CX_3CR1 and Fractalkine (22-24).

Mice in which the genes for chemokines SDF-1 or MIP1α were deleted displayed, respectively, perinatal lethality and loss of inflammatory response to viral infections (25, 26). Likewise, mice defective in CXCR4 showed many phenotypes similar to SDF-1 deleted mice indicating the specific nature of this ligand receptor pair (27). Mice deficient in the putative B-cell chemokine receptor gene CXCR5 exhibited severe defects in B-cell migration to spleen and Peyer's

Table 1 Chemokine receptors, their chemokine ligands, and the predominant expression pattern of chemokine receptors on leukocytes.

Chemokine Receptor	Former Receptor Names	Chemokine Ligands	Predominant Cells of Receptor Expression
XCR1		Lymphotactin	
CXCR1	IL-8 RA, IL-8 R1	IL-8	Neutrophils
CXCR2	IL-8 RB, IL-8 R2	IL-8, GROα, NAP, ENA-78	Neutrophils
CXCR3		IP-10, Mig	Activated T Lymphocytes
CXCR4	Fusin, Fumstr, Lestr	SDF-1	Widely Expressed
CXCR5	BLR-1	BLC	B Lymphocytes, Memory T Lymphocytes
CCR1	CC CKR1	MIP-1α, RANTES, MCP-3	Monocytes, T Lymphocytes, Eosinophils, Dendritic Cells
CCR2a,b	MCP-1Ra, MCP-1Rb	MCP-1, MCP-2, MCP-4	Monocytes, Basophils, Activated T Lymphocytes
CCR3	CKR-3	Eotaxin, MCP-2, MCP-3, MCP-4, RANTES	Eosinophils, Basophils, Activated T Lymphocytes
CCR4		TARC, MIP-1α, RANTES	Basophils, Activated T Lymphocytes
CCR5	CC CKR5	RANTES, MIP-1α, MIP-1β	Monocytes, T Lymphocytes, Dendritic Cells
CCR6		MIP-3α	Activated T Lymphocytes, B Lymphocytes, Dendritic Cells
CCR7	BLR-2, EBI1	MIP-3β, SLC	B Lymphocytes, Activated T Lymphocytes
CCR8		I 309	Activated T Lymphocytes, Monocytes
CCR9	GPCR 9-6	TECK	T Lymphocytes
CX3CR1	V28	Fractalkine	Monocytes, T Lymphocytes, Natural Killer Cells

patches, but not to mesenteric lymph nodes (28). Naturally occurring mice that were defective in the expression of the SLC and macrophage inflammatory protein (MIP)-3α chemokines showed impaired homing of naive T-cells to secondary lymphoid organs; mice deficient in CCR-7, which is a receptor for these chemokines, also had severe defects in lymphocyte migration to secondary lymphoid organs and in initiating antigen-specific immune response (29,30). Expression of monocyte chemoattractant protein-1 (MCP-1) is upregulated in atherosclerotic plaques. Mice deficient in the MCP-1 receptor, CCR2, and in apolipoprotein E showed a decrease in atheroma formation indicating a direct role for MCP-1 and CCR2 in the development of atherosclerostic lesion (31). These studies provide clear evidence that chemokines and their receptors are involved not only in lymphocyte recirculation, but also in directing many inflammatory responses.

SIGNAL TRANSDUCTION AND REGULATION OF CHEMOKINE RECEPTORS

All chemoattractant receptors expressed in leukocytes mediate signaling through a heterotimeric G-protein composed of α, β, and γ subunits. Upon receptor activation, G-proteins dissociate into Gα and G$\beta\gamma$ to activate effectors such as phospholipase C (PLC). Chemokine receptors couple to Gi family of G-protein which are pertussis toxin (Ptx) sensitive. In addition, some chemokine receptors, particularly when expressed in cell lines, couple to Gq and G16-like G-proteins which are Ptx-insensitive, as well as to Gi proteins (32-34). Chemokine receptors activate PLC resulting in the generation of the intracellular messengers diacylglycerol (DAG) and inositol trisphosphate (IP_3) (Figure 1). While IP_3 mobilizes Ca^{2+}, DAG, along with elevated Ca^{2+} levels, activates protein kinase C (PKC) (35). However, different chemokine receptors have different downstream effects. For example, studies with CXCR1 and CXCR2 showed that both receptors can activate chemotaxis, and calcium mobilization, but only CXCR1 can activate phospholipase D (36). Activation of MAP-kinase, phospholipase A_2 and phosphotidyl inositol -3 kinase (PI3K) by chemokines has also been demonstrated (37, 38). Studies using wortmannin indicated a role for PI3 kinase in chemotaxis, but not in calcium mobilization and exocytosis (39). Recent studies on leukocytes from PI3 kinase γ deficient mice indicated the importance of this pathway in respiratory burst and motility (40). Chemokine receptors can induce multiple signal transduction pathways, and the type of signal transduced depends on the chemokine, the receptor, and the types of coupling proteins present within a given cell type. Nonetheless, chemotaxis itself requires the activation of a Ptx sensitive G-protein, presumably through release of $\beta\gamma$ subunits (41, 42).

Chemokines and chemokine receptors also regulate the activity of adhesion molecules in coordinating leukocyte migration, but the biochemical mechanisms of this action are not well-understood (43). A specific subset of chemokines,

Figure 1 Chemokine receptors activate signaling pathways through Gαi and Gβγ subunits. Motility related activities are mediated exclusively via the Gβγ subunit, whereas both Gαi and Gβγ subunits activate the cytotoxic functions of leukocytes.

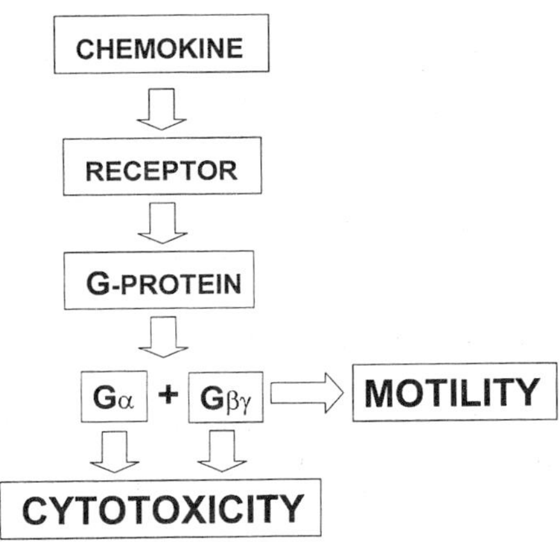

namely SLC, SDF-1, MIP-3α and MIP-3β, can induce the integrin-mediated adhesion of leukocytes to endothelium under physiological flow conditions (44). Further, a study in murine pre-B cells transfected with CXCR1 showed that the small G-protein RhoA is likely involved in this up-regulation of adhesiveness, but the mechanism remain unclear (45). In RBL-2H3 cells transfected with CXCR1, other chemoattractant receptors (fMLPR and C5aR), and L-selectin, activation of chemokine receptors led to rapid phosphorylation of L-selectin on cytoplasmic serine residues, an event associated with increased L-selectin-mediated adhesion (46). Recently, a novel role for chemokines in leukocyte migration has been defined. Interactions of Fractalkine, a transmembrane chemokine/mucin hybrid molecule expressed on TNF-activated endothelium, with its receptor (CX_3CR1) have been shown to mediate the capture, firm adhesion, and activation of leukocytes under physiologic flow conditions in a Ptx-insensitive and integrin-independent manner (47). Thus, chemokines induce the activation and adhesion of circulating leukocytes to endothelium by regulating adhesion molecule function and, in some instances, can themselves act as cell adhesion molecules.

The biological activities of the chemokines described above are subjected to regulation at multiple levels. A well defined method of regulation is the desensitization of the receptor signaling at various sites, including the receptors and downstream components.

CHEMOKINE RECEPTORS DESENSITIZATION BY PHOSPHORYLATION

Desensitization is defined as diminished responsiveness of a signaling system to subsequent stimuli following initial stimulation (48). The mechanism of G-protein-coupled receptor desensitization has been studied in great detail for the visual and adrenergic systems (48, 49). From these studies, two types of desensitization, termed "homologous" and "heterologous," have been described. Homologous desensitization occurs in receptors in the agonist-occupied state and involves phosphorylation by G-protein-coupled receptor kinases. Several of the G-protein-coupled receptor kinases were identified in leukocytes (50). Homologously phosphorylated receptors associate with members of the arrestin family of proteins which results in a decreased affinity of the receptor for G-proteins and in receptor internalization.

Heterologous desensitization occurs when a receptor loses its responsiveness following phosphorylation by second messenger activated kinases [i.e., Protein kinase A (PKA) or protein kinase C (PKC)] which have been activated by different receptors or other signaling processes (48-50). Heterologous desensitization does not require agonist occupancy and does not lead to arrestin-mediated receptor internalization (48-50). Studies with leukocytes have demonstrated an additional level of complexity in receptor desensitization, a form of cross receptor desensitization with selectivity for groups of chemoattractant receptors (9).

Studies with several chemokine receptors expressed in different cell lines have indicated that leukocyte responses to chemokines are regulated by phosphorylation. The receptors for IL-8 (CXCR1 and CXCR2) undergo receptor phosphorylation upon cellular activation by IL-8 or through treatment with phorbol 12-myristate 13-acetate (PMA) which activates protein kinase C (51, 52). Phosphorylation of the receptors has been directly linked to their desensitization. Receptor mutants in which phosphorylation sites have been eliminated by either directed mutagenesis or truncation of the cytoplasmic tail were resistant to desensitization (52, 54). Studies with CXCR4, the SDF1 receptor, expressed in RBL-2H3 cells demonstrated that both SDF-1 and PMA mediated rapid phosphorylation and desensitization, as well as internalization (55). Internalization of the receptor was partially phosphorylation independent since a phosphorylation resistant mutant of the receptor also underwent SDF-1-mediated internalization. It has been shown that internalization of CXCR4 by SDF-1, but not by PMA, was arrestin-dependent (56). In addition to the serine residues 324, 325, 338 and 339, the dileucine motif (Ile-328 and Leu-329) (Table 2) are critical for CXCR4 internalization since mutation of these residues inhibited receptor internalization (56).

Recent studies with CCR5 have also indicated that cellular responses to the receptor are regulated via G-protein-coupled receptor kinase (GRK) dependent and independent mechanisms (57). Serine residues 336, 337, 342, and 349 of the cytoplasmic tail of CCR5 (Figure 2) are important for GRK-mediated phosphorylation and desensitization of the receptor. The strengths of different CC chemokines to mediate cellular responses through CCR5 correlate with their abilities to induce receptor phosphorylation and desensitization. RANTES and aminooxypentane-RANTES (AOP-RANTES), which mediate greater intracellular Ca2+ mobilization than MIP-1α, MIP-1β and methioninylated-RANTES (Met-RANTES), also induce greater receptor phosphorylation (57).

Work performed in human embryonic kidney cells (HEK293) has shown that CCR2b, the receptor for monocyte chemoattractant protein-1 (MCP1), is rapidly phosphorylated and internalized upon MCP-1 activation (58). Alanine substitution of the serine and threonine residues of the cytoplasmic tail of CCR2B blocked MCP-1 mediated receptor phosphorylation, desensitization, and internalization. Co-expression of CCR2b with the β-adrenergic receptor kinase 2 (βARK-2) blocked its activation by MCP1 (58) in Xenopus oocytes. Desensitization of CCR2b mediated intracellular calcium mobilization in Mono Mac 1 cells also correlated with receptor phosphorylation and the rapid translocation of βARK2 and β-arrestin to the membranes, as well as with the formation of a multiprotein complex in the cell membranes (59). These results suggest that βARK-2-mediated phosphorylation is required for desensitization of cellular responses to CCR2.

Richardson et al. (60) have also shown that CCR1 became phosphorylated and desensitized upon activation by RANTES, MIP-1α, or MCP-2. Alanine substitution of specific serine and threonine residues or truncation of the cytoplasmic tail of CCR1 abolished receptor phosphorylation and desensitization of G-protein activation, but did not abolish desensitization of Ca2+ mobilization. The phosphorylation deficient mutants were also resistant to internalization, which suggests that receptor phosphorylation limits some, but not all, CCR1-mediated cellular responses. Overall these studies indicate that receptor phosphorylation upon agonist activation plays an important role in the modulation of chemokine-mediated leukocytes activation. However, receptor phosphorylation independent mechanisms also appear to be important in the regulation and cross-regulation of chemokine receptors.

CROSS-DESENSITIZATION OF CHEMOKINE RECEPTORS

Since multiple chemokines interact with multiple receptors, their responses are likely to be cross-regulated. Although much has been learned about signal transduction and the regulation of single receptors, mechanisms of receptor cross-regulation are only beginning to be unraveled. Early studies (61) showed that pretreatment of neutrophils with C5a diminished the ability of fMLP to induce exocytosis and that pretreatment with fMLP diminished the response to C5a. However, pretreatment of neutrophils with C5a or fMLP had no effect on exocytosis mediated by other agents, such as aggregated immunoglobulin or opsonized zymosan. In contrast to the ability of fMLP and C5a to cross-desensitize these responses, C5a did not cross-desensitize GTPase activity stimulated by fMLP, suggesting that the effect occurred distal to receptor activation (62). Furthermore,

Table 2 Chemoattractant receptor cross-phosphorylation and cross-desensitization.

Receptors	Cross Phosphorylation	Desensitization: Receptor/ G-protein	Desensitization: Ca^{2+} Mobilization
fMLPR → C5aR	+	+	+
C5aR → fMLPR	−	−	+ ←
fMLPR → CXCR1	+	+	+
CXCR1 → fMLPR	−	−	+ ←
fMLPR →M2-CXCR1	−	−	+ ←
M2-CXCR1 →fMLPR	−	−	+ ←
fMLPR → CXCR2	+	+	+
CXCR2 → fMLPR	−	−	−
fMLPR →331T-CXCR2	−	−	+ ←
331T-CXCR2 →fMLPR	−	−	+ ←
C5aR → CXCR2	+	+	+
CXCR2 → C5aR	−	−	−
C5aR →331T-CXCR2	−	−	+ ←
331T-CXCR2 →C5aR	+	+	+
CXCR1 → CCR1	+	+	+
CCR1 → CXCR1	−	−	−
CXCR1 → S3-CCR1	−	−	+ ←
S3-CCR1 → CXCR1	+	+	+
CXCR2 → CCR1	+	+	+
CCR1 → CXCR2	+	+	+
CXCR2 → S3-CCR1	−	−	+ ←
S3-CCR1 → CXCR2	+	+	+

RBL-2H3 cells coexpressing different combinations of chemoattractant receptors were utilized to determine cross-phosphorylation and cross-desensitization patterns. The first and second doses of ligands for the receptors are indicated sequentially. (+) under cross-phosphorylation indicates phosphorylation of the second receptor by the activation of the first receptor. Desensitization was measured by inhibition of GTPase activity (Receptor/G-protein coupling) as well as Ca^{2+} mobilization (+ = inhibition ≥ 30 %; +/− = inhibition 11-29%; − = inhibition ≤10 %). Arrows indicate cross-desensitization of Ca^{2+} mobilization in the absence of receptor cross-phosphorylation and G-protein uncoupling.

Figure 2 Amino acid sequences of the carboxyl-terminal tail of CXCR4 and CCR5. The amino acid residues that are important for receptor phosphorylation and/or internalization are bolded and underlined.

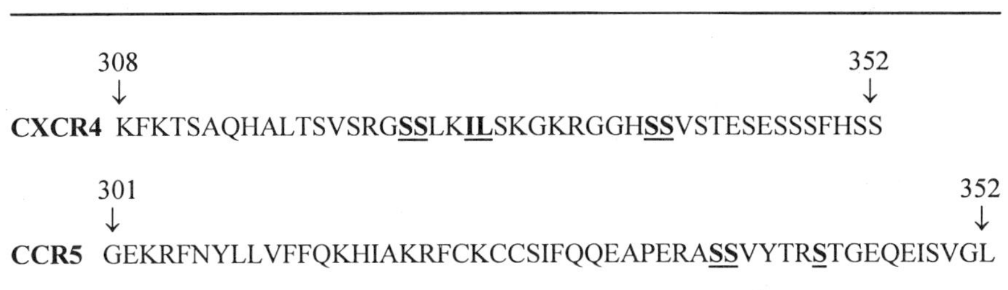

neutrophils that were exposed to fMLP had desensitized IL-8 mediated-Ca^{2+} mobilization and superoxide production, although IL-8 did not affect the responses stimulated by fMLP (63). Didsbury et al. (64) have shown that in HEK293 cells transiently coexpressing receptors for fMLP and C5a activation of one receptor resulted in cross-desensitization of Ca^{2+} mobilization by the other.

Cross-desensitization was specific for the chemoattractant receptors which activate phospholipase C (PLC) via a pertussis toxin (Ptx)-sensitive G-protein. Native α1-Adrenergic receptors, which activate PLC via a Ptx-insensitive G-protein, were not desensitized by fMLP and C5a and vice versa. This discovery led to the extensive characterization of the specificity of this type of cross-regulation in neutrophils (65). For these studies, the chemoattractants fMLP, C5a, IL-8, PAF, and leukotriene B4, as well as the purinoceptor agonist ATPγS, were evaluated for their ability to cross-desensitize each other. It was shown that all receptors undergo effective homologous desensitization. In addition, fMLP, C5a, and IL-8 cross-desensitized Ca^{2+} mobilization to one another as well as to LTB_4 and PAF (65). PAF, LTB_4 or ATPγS did not, however, cross-desensitize the peptide chemoattractant receptors. The strength of receptors to desensitize Ca^{2+} mobilization to one another was ordered such that desensitization by fMLP was greater than C5a which was greater than IL-8. In contrast, the ordered susceptibility of peptide chemoattractant receptors to undergo cross-desensitization was reversed, with IL-8 greater than C5a which was greater than fMLP. The ability of fMLP to desensitize Ca^{2+} mobilization by C5a and IL-8 was correlated with its ability to block C5a and IL-8 stimulated G-protein activation (by preventing receptor-G-protein coupling). Surprisingly, neither C5a nor IL-8 inhibited fMLP-stimulated G protein activation, although both blocked Ca^{2+} mobilization. Based on these studies it was postulated that chemoattractant receptor cross-regulation that resulted in reduced activation of phospholipase C occurred both at the level of receptor-G-protein coupling and at a level distal to G-protein activation.

Recent studies by Blackwood et al., (66) demonstrated that fMLP and C5a cross-regulate both chemotaxis and arachidonic acid release stimulated by each other. Although, IL-8 desensitized chemotaxis stimulated by fMLP and C5a, it was less efficient in blocking arachidonic acid release by these chemoattractants. Campbell et al, (67) however, found that neutrophils displayed normal chemotactic responses to fMLP even after maximal stimulation with IL-8, but activation of neutrophils even with low concentrations of fMLP abrogated these responses to IL-8. Nonetheless, in a murine pre B cell line coexpressing the fMLP receptor (fMLPR) and an IL-8 receptor (CXCR2), both fMLP and IL-8 desensitized each other's chemotactic responses (68). IL-8 was less effective in desensitizing Ca^{2+} mobilization by fMLP than vice versa, consistent with a rank order of potency of chemoattractant receptor cross-regulation for Ca^{2+} mobilization (9). This finding further suggests that cross-regulation of chemoattractant-mediated biological responses, such as adhesion, chemotaxis, and Ca^{2+} mobilization, occurs via the modulation of multiple steps in the signal transduction pathways.

MECHANISM OF CHEMOKINE RECEPTOR CROSS-DESENSITIZATION

Role of Multiple Ligands

Chemokine and chemokine receptors are redundant in their interaction in that a given chemokine may activate several receptors and some chemokine receptors are activated by multiple ligands (Table 1). Since individual receptors mediate multiple and distinct signaling pathways upon activation (1, 69), cross-desensitization among multiple chemokines may be important in limiting their signal redundancy. For example, CCR1 can be activated by several CC chemokines, including RANTES, MIP-1α, MIP-1β, and MCP-2, to mediate cellular responses in neutrophils and transfected cells (60, 70, 71). In human kidney 293 cells expressing CCR1, pretreatment of the cells with MIP-1α abolished Ca^{2+} mobilization to subsequent treatment with either MIP-1α or RANTES, whereas RANTES pretreatment only desensitized the response to RANTES (70). Recent studies in RBL-2H3 cells that express CCR1 showed that RANTES, MIP-1α, and MCP-2 homologously desensitized CCR1-mediated Ca^{2+} mobilization to a second dose of the same chemokine by >90%. These chemokines cross-desensitized Ca^{2+} response to each other to varying degrees (60). RANTES and MIP-1α cross-desensitized responses to a second dose of either chemokine by >90%, whereas MCP-2 blocked the response to both RANTES and MIP-1α by ~50%. Since MCP-2 mediated ~50% of the Ca^{2+} response elicited by RANTES and MIP-1α, its lower rate of cross-desensitization may be due to its character as a partial agonist (60). It was also reported that in CCR5 expressing RBL-2H3 cells, ligands that bind to CCR5 with similar affinities differ in their abilities to induce cellular signaling, receptor phosphorylation and desensitization (57). These data suggest that in the presence of multiple chemokines acting on the same receptor, activation of the receptor by the first chemokine desensitizes the ability of subsequent chemokines to mediate cellular responses. The degree of such desensitization is based on the signal strength of the initial chemokine.

Role of Receptor Cross-Phosphorylation

Studies with RBL cells that co-express different combinations of chemoattractant receptors indicated that one of the sites of cross-desensitization is at the level of receptor-G-protein coupling (Figure 3). This mechanism of cross-desensitization involves cross-phosphorylation of the receptor by a second messenger dependent kinase (likely protein kinase C) followed by the uncoupling of the receptor from its G-protein (9). Chemoattractant receptors expressed in RBL-2H3 cells, including CXCR1, CXCR2, CXCR4, CCR1, and CCR5, undergo homologous and heterologous phosphorylation and desensitization (53, 55, 57, 60, 72). In doubly transfected RBL cells, activation of fMLPR or C5aR cross-phosphorylated CXCR1 and CXCR2, and also cross-desensitized receptor-mediated G-protein activation (72, 73). In RBL-2H3 cells expressing CCR1 and either CXCR1 or CXCR2, both CXCR2 and CCR1 were cross-phosphorylated upon CXCR1 activation. The degree of cross-phosphorylation was correlated with the decrease in receptor-mediated G-protein activation (Table 2) (60). The phosphorylation deficient mutants of CXCR1 (M2-CXCR1), CXCR2 (331T-CCR2) and CCR1 (S3-

Figure 3 Sites for chemokine receptors cross-desensitization and regulation of signal strength. Chemokines activate signaling pathways through the Gαi and Gβγ G protein subunits to activate phospholipase C (PLCβ) and increase second messengers. Second messenger activated kinases (PKC, PKA) phosphorylate susceptible receptors and PLCβ to specifically inhibit Gα and Gβγ mediated PLCβ activation. Potential sites for regulation of signal strength, such as regulators of G-protein signaling (RGS) and modification of Gβγ, are also indicated.

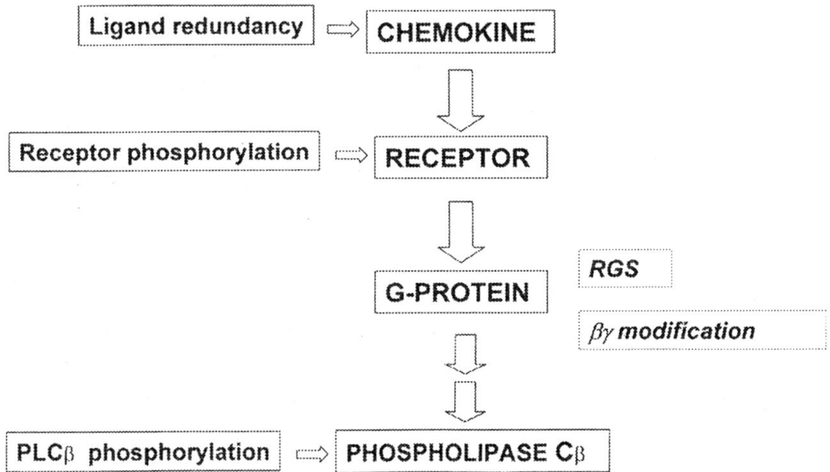

CCR1 and ΔCCR1) were resistant to these processes. These findings indicate that cross-phosphorylation-mediated cross-desensitization plays an important role in limiting chemokine-mediated activation of leukocyte functions. without cross-phosphorylation or suppression of G protein activation (Table 2) (73, 74). CXCR1 and CXCR2 also cross-desensitized Ca2+ mobilization in response to phosphorylation-resistant mutants of CCR1 (60). These findings indicate that the ability of chemoattractant receptors to cross-desensitize Ca^{2+} mobilization to one another is mediated via two processes, PKC-mediated receptor cross-phosphorylation and decreased activation of PLC due to modulation of an unidentified downstream component.

Although this down-stream component has not yet been identified, its modification results in decreased activation of PLCβ as IP_3 production is depressed (72). The finding that PLCβ2 and PLCβ3 are phosphorylated by both PKA and PKC, and that phosphorylation is associated with the inhibition of these enzymes, suggested a role for PLCβ phosphorylation in cross-desensitization (75,76). Purified catalytic subunit of PKA was shown to phosphorylate PLCβ3 immunoprecipitated from RBL cells and preincubation of the cells with fMLP blocked the subsequent *in vitro* phosphorylation of PLCβ3 by PKA (77). These findings are consistent with the hypothesis that receptor-stimulated phosphorylation of PLCβ may play a role in receptor cross-desensitization. Filtz et al (78) have shown that PKC promoted phosphorylation of PLCβ2 from turkey erythrocytes and this action was correlated with a loss of enzymatic activity. However, the phosphorylation-dependent loss of enzymatic activity was not detected in reconstitution assays with purified Gα or Gβγ. These findings suggest that PLCβ phosphorylation may be necessary, but not sufficient, for chemoattractant receptor cross-desensitization at the level of PLCβ activity.

Signal Strength

Studies in neutrophils showed that IL-8 is not only the most susceptible chemoattractant receptor studied to undergo cross-desensitization, but that it also provided the weakest signal for cross-desensitization of other chemoattractant receptors (65). In neutrophils, responses to IL-8 were mediated via the activation of both CXCR1 and CXCR2 (1). While CXCR1 cross-desensitized responses to other peptide chemoattractants, CXCR2 did not (Table 2) (72). The explanation for IL-8 providing the weakest desensitizing signal was the brief length of signaling by its receptors (72). For example, CXCR2, which did not produce a cross-desensitizing signal, was rapidly phosphorylated and internalized upon ligand stimulation so that >95% of the surface receptors were lost within 5 minutes (72). In contrast, its phosphorylation-deficient mutant (331T-CXCR2) was resistant to internalization (<5% internalization after 30 minutes) and generated a signal for cross-desensitization, presumably due to prolonged receptor activation and the level of G-protein mediated signaling (72). Similarly, CXCR1 was resistant to cross-phosphorylation and cross-desensitization by CCR1, but not to phosphorylation deficient mutants (S3-CCR1 and ΔCCR1) which generated greater signals (Table 2) (60). The sustained production of second messengers appears to activate inhibitory pathways to cause both phosphorylation of susceptible receptors and modification of down-stream components to diminish the activation of PLCβ by certain chemokine receptors. Given the multiplicity of chemokine receptors for identical ligands, the evolution of receptors with similar ligand specificity but different signal strength likely plays an important role in modulating chemokine functions.

Other Factors That May Influence Cross-Desensitization

As noted, the strength of a receptor's desensitizing signal appears to depend, at least in part, on the duration of its activation. Since the signal for G_i-coupled-receptors is initially mediated by Gβγ, modification of these proteins may regulate PLCβ activation. Recent studies on isoprenylation and carboxymethylation of the γ subunit of G protein (Gγ) indicate that this type of modification regulates Gβγ-mediated responses in neutrophils and may be a mechanism for cross-desensitization. For example, isoprenylation and carboxymethylation of Gγ allows it to localize to the plasma membrane where it activates effector molecules such as PLCβ (79). *In vitro* reconstitution studies showed that decarboxymethylated Gβγ was 10-fold less effective in activating PLCβ (80). Alternatively, Yasuda et al... (81) showed that phosphorylation of $G\gamma_{12}$ by PKC substantially blocked the ability of the $G\beta_1\gamma_{12}$ to activate effector enzymes. Thus, modification of Gγ by carboxymethylation or phosphorylation could be involved in cross-desensitization.

A newly described family of proteins, known as regulators of G-protein signaling (RGS), reduces the strength of G-protein signaling by enhancing its GTPase activity thus making less Gβγ available (82, 83). Regulation of RGS activity could, therefore, play a role in chemoattractant receptor cross-desensitization by affecting signal strength. In this regard, transient overexpression of RGS1, RGS3 and RGS4, but not RGS2, was found to inhibit chemoattractant receptor-mediated motility in a transfected lymphoid cell line (84). In our studies, expression of RGS4 in RBL-2H3 inhibited phosphoinositide hydrolysis and intracellular Ca^{2+} mobilization to PAFR, but not to fMLPR or CXCR1 (85). In contrast, expression of RGS1 blocked fMLPR-, but not PAFR-mediated Ca^{2+} mobilization (85). These findings lend evidence to the notion that groups of receptors may be regulated separately by specific subtypes of RGS.

CHEMOKINE RECEPTOR SIGNALING AND HIV-INFECTION

Initial studies using mutant and chimeric receptors demonstrated that signaling through G-proteins is neither required nor sufficient for viral membrane fusion of M-tropic strains using CCR5 (86, 87). However, recent experiments indicated that the role of G-protein-coupled receptor signaling in HIV-1 infection is a more complex issue. Envelope glycoproteins of M-tropic viruses induced a calcium signal and chemotaxis through CCR5 in cell lines as well as in primary cells (88). Other studies indicated that envelope glycoproteins of both M- and T-tropic viruses induced tyrosine phosphorylation of Pyk-2, a kinase implicated in a multitude of signaling events (89). Both of these responses are Pertussis toxin sensitive. Since HIV infection is Ptx-insensitive it is not clear how these activities relate to HIV-1 infection. While these activities may not be required for *in vitro* infection they may play a role *in vivo* either by chemoattracting or activating susceptible cells. Other studies demonstrated that internalization of chemokine receptors was not a factor in membrane fusion, but mutants defective in internalization showed a significant loss of protection by β chemokines (90, 91). The fact that CXCR4 and CCR5 (as well as all the newly identified HIV coreceptors) exhibit very limited sequence homology indicates that some non-structural biological activity of these receptors may be required for productive infection. Indeed, as yet undiscovered biological activities of the chemokine receptors may play a role in HIV-1 infection. Further studies on chemokine receptor signaling and regulation are likely to yield important insights regarding membrane fusion and HIV-1 infection.

REFERENCES

1. Baggiolini, M., Dewald, B, and Moser, B. (1997). Human Chemokines - An Update. *Annual Review of Immunology*, **15**, 675-705.
2. Altman, L. C., Snyderman, R.,Oppenheim, J.J. and Mergenhagen, S. E. (1973). A human mononuclear leukocyte chemotactic factor: characterization, specificity and kinetics of production by homologous leukocytes. *J Immunol.* **110**, 801-810.
3. Yoshimura, T., Matsushima, K., Tanaka, S., Robinson, E. A., Appella, E., Oppenheim, J. J. and Leonard, E. J. (1987). Purification of a human monocyte-derived neutrophil chemotactic factor that has peptide sequence similarity to other host defense cytokines. *Proc Natl Acad Sci U S A.* **84**, 9233-9237.
4. Samanta, A. K., Oppenheim, J. J. and Matsushima, K. (1989). Identification and characterization of specific receptors for monocyte-derived neutrophil chemotactic factor (MDNCF) on human neutrophils. *J Exp Med.* **169**, 1185-1189.
5. Murphy, P.M. (1996). Chemokine Receptors: Structure, Function And Role In Microbial Pathogenesis. *Cytokine Growth Factor Rev*, **7**, 47-64
6. Cyster, J. G. (1999). Chemokines and cell migration in secondary lymphoid organs. *Science.* **286**, 2098-2102.
7. Dimitrov, D. S., Xiao, X., Chabot, D. J. and Broder, C. C. (1998). HIV Coreceptors. *Journal of Membrane Biology.* **166**, 75-90.
8. Wells, T.N.C. and Peitsch, M. C. (1997). The Chemokine Information Source - Identification And Characterization Of Novel Chemokines Using The Worldwideweb And Expressed Sequence Tag Databases. *Journal of Leukocyte Biology*, **61**, 545-550.
9. Ali, H., Richardson, R. M., Haribabu, B., and Snyderman, R. (1999). Chemoattractant receptor cross-desensitization. *Journal of Biological Chemistry.* **274**, 6027-6030.
10. Sozzani, S., Allavena, P., Vecchi, A., and Mantovani, A. (1999). The role of chemokines in the regulation of dendritic cell trafficking. *J Leukoc Biol.* **66**, 1-9.

11. Locati, M., and Murphy, P. M. (1999). Chemokines and chemokine receptors: Biology and clinical relevance in inflammation and AIDS. *Annual Review of Medicine*. **50**, 425-440.
12. Mackay, C. R., Lanzavecchia, A. and Sallusto, F. (1999). Chemoattractant receptors and immune responses. *Immunologist*. **7**, 112-118.
13. Zlotnik, A., Morales, J. and Hedrick, J. A. (1999) Recent advances in chemokines and chemokine receptors. *Critical Reviews in Immunology*. **19**, 1-47.
14. Kelner, G.S., Kennedy, J., Bacon, K.B., Kleyensteuber, S., Largaespada, D.A., Jenkins, N.A., Copeland, N.G., Bazan, J.F., Moore, K.W., Schall, T.J., and et al., (1994). Lymphotactin: A Cytokine That Represents A New Class Of Chemokine. *Science*, **266**,1395-1399.
15. Bazan, J.F., Bacon, K. B., Hardiman, G., Wang, W., Soo, K., Rossi, D., Greaves, D.R., Zlotnik, A. and Schall, T. J. (1997). A New Class of Membrane-Bound Chemokine With a CX3C- Motif. *Nature*, **385**, 640-644.
16. Baba, M., T. Imai, T., Nishimura, M., Kakizaki, M., Takagi, S., Hieshima, K., Nomiyama, H and Yoshie, O. (1997). Identification of CCR-6, the Specific Receptor For a Novel Lymphocyte-Directed CC Chemokine LARC. *Journal of Biological Chemistry*, **272**, 14893-14898.
17. Yoshida, R., Imai, T., Hieshima, K., Kusuda, J., Baba, M., Kitaura, M., Nishimura, M., Kakizaki, M., Nomiyama, H. and Yoshie, O. (1997). Molecular cloning of a novel human CC chemokine EBI-1-ligand chemokine that is a specific functional ligand for EBI-1, CCR-7. *Journal of Biological Chemistry*, **272**, 13803-13809.
18. Roos, R.S., Loetscher, M., Legler, D. F., Clarklewis, I., Baggiolini, M. and Moser, B. (1997). Identification of CCR-8, the Receptor For the Human CC-Chemokine I-309. *Journal of Biological Chemistry*, **272**, 17251-17254.
19. Zabel, B. A., Agace, W. W., Campbell, J. J., Heath, H. M., Parent, D., Roberts, A. I., Ebert, E. C., Kassam, N., Qin, S. X., Zovko, M., LaRosa, G. J., Yang, L. L., Soler, D., Butcher, E. C., Ponath, P. D., Parker, C. M. and Andrew, D. P. (1999). Human G protein-coupled receptor GPR-9-G/CC chemokine receptor 9 is selectively expressed on intestinal homing T lymphocytes, mucosal lymphocytes, and thymocytes and is required for thymus-expressed chemokine-mediated chemotaxis. *Journal of Experimental Medicine*. **190**, 1241-1255.
20. Loetscher, M., T. Geiser, O.R. Zwahlen, T. R., Baggiolini, M. and Moser, B. (1994). Cloning Of A Human Seven-Transmembrane Domain Receptor, LESTR, That Is Highly Expressed In Leukocytes. *Journal of Biological Chemistry*, **269**, 232-237.
21. Loetscher, M., Gerber, B., Loetscher, P., Jones, S. A., Piali, L., Clarklewis, I., Baggiolini, M. and Moser. B. (1996) Chemokine Receptor Specific For IP-10 and Mig - Structure, Function, and Expression in Activated T-Lymphocytes. *Journal of Experimental Medicine* **184**, 963-969.
22. Gunn, M.D., Ngo, V.N., Ansel, K.M., Ekland, E.H., Cyster, J.G. and Williams, L.T. (1998) A B-Cell-Homing Chemokine Made in Lymphoid Follicles Activates Burkitts-Lymphoma Receptor-1. *Nature*, **391** 799-803.
23. Oberlin, E., Amara, A., Bachelerie, F., Bessia, C., Virelizier, J. L., Arenzanaseisdedos, F., Schwartz, O., Heard, J. M., Clarklewis, I., Legler, D. F. Loetscher, M., Baggiolini, M. and Moser, B. (1996). The CXC chemokine SDF-1 is the ligand for Lestr/Fusin and prevents infection by T-cell-line-adapted HIV-1. *Nature*, **382**, 833-835.
24. Oberlin, E., Amara, A., Bachelerie, F., Bessia, C., Virelizier, J. L., Arenzanaseisdedos, F., Schwartz, O., Heard, J. M., Clarklewis, I., Legler, D. F. Loetscher, M., Baggiolini,

M. and Moser, B. (1996). The CXC chemokine SDF-1 is the ligand for Lestr/Fusin and prevents infection by T-cell-line-adapted HIV-1. *Nature*, **382**, 833-835.

25. Imai, T., Hieshima, K., Haskell, C., Baba, M., Nagira, M., Nishimura, M. Kakizaki, M., Takagi, S., Nomiyama, H., Schall, T.J., and Yoshie, O. (1997). Identification and Molecular Characterization of Fractalkine Receptor CX(3)CR1, Which Mediates Both Leukocyte Migration and Adhesion. *Cell*, **91**, 521-530.
26. Nagasawa, T., Hirota, S., Tachibana, K., Takakura, N., Nishikawa, S., Kitamura, Y., Yoshida, N., Kikutani, H. and Kishimoto, T. (1996). Defects of B-Cell Lymphopoiesis and Bone-Marrow Myelopoiesis in Mice Lacking the CXC- Chemokine PBSF/SDF-1. *Nature*. **382**, 635-638.
27. Zou, Y. R., Kottmann, A. H., Kuroda, M., Taniuchi, I. and Littman, D. R. (1998) Function of the chemokine receptor CXCR4 in haematopoiesis and in cerebellar development. *Nature*, **393**, 595-599.
28. Cook, D.N., Beck, M.A., Coffman, T.M., Kirby, S.L., Sheridan, J.F., Pragnell, I.B., and Smithies, O., (1995). Requirement Of MIP-1 Alpha For An Inflammatory Response To Viral Infection. *Science*, **269**,1583-1585.
29. Gunn, M. D., Kyuwa, S., Tam, C., Kakiuchi, T., Matsuzawa, A., Williams, L. T. and Nakano, H. (1999). Mice lacking expression of secondary lymphoid organ chemokine have defects in lymphocyte homing and dendritic cell localization. *J Exp Med*, **189**, 451-60.
30. Forster, R., Mattis, A.E., Kremmer, E., Wolf, E., Brem, G. and Lipp, M. (1996). A Putative Chemokine Receptor, BLR1, Directs B Cell Migration to Defined Lymphoid Organs and Specific Anatomic Compartments of the Spleen. *Cell*, **87**, 1037-1047.
31. Boring, L., J. Gosling, M. Cleary, and I. F. Charo. Decreased Lesion Formation in Ccr2(-/-) Mice Reveals a Role For Chemokines in the Initiation of Atherosclerosis. *Nature*. (1998) **394**, 894-897.
32. Wu, D., G.J. LaRosa, and M.I. Simon, G Protein-Coupled Signal Transduction Pathways For Interleukin-8. *Science*, (1993) **261**, 101-103.
33. Kuang, Y.N., Y.P. Wu, H.P. Jiang, and D.Q. Wu, Selective G Protein Coupling By C-C Chemokine Receptors. *Journal of Biological Chemistry*, (1996) **271**, 3975-3978.
34. Arai, H. and I.F. Charo, Differential Regulation Of G-Protein-Mediated Signaling By Chemokine Receptors. *J Biol Chem*, (1996) **271**, 21814-21819.
35. Smith, C.D., Cox, C.C. and Snyderman R. (1986). Receptor-Coupled Activation Of Phosphoinositide-Specific Phospholipase C By An N Protein. *Science*, **232**, 97-100.
36. Jones, S.A., Wolf, M. Qin, S.X. Mackay, C.R. and Baggiolini, M. (1996). Different Functions For the Interleukin 8 Receptors (IL-8R) of Human Neutrophil Leukocytes - NADPH Oxidase and Phospholipase D Are Activated Through IL-8R1 But Not IL-8R2. *Proceedings of the National Academy of Sciences of the United States of America*, **93**, 6682-6686.
37. Jones, S.A., Moser, B. and Thelen, M. (1995). A Comparison Of Post-Receptor Signal Transduction Events In Jurkat Cells Transfected With Either IL-8R1 Or IL-8R2. Chemokine Mediated Activation Of P42/P44 MAP-Kinase (ERK-2). *FEBS Lett*, **364**, 211-214.
38. Turner, L., Ward, S.G. and Westwick, J. (1995). RANTES-Activated Human T Lymphocytes. A Role For Phosphoinositide 3-Kinase. *J. Immunol*, **155**, 2437-44.
39. Haribabu, B., Zhelev, D.V., Pridgen, B., Richardson, R.M., Ali, H., and Snyderman. R. (1999). Chemoattractant Receptors Activate Distinct Pathways for Chemotaxis and Secretion: Role of G-Protein Usage. *Journal of Biological Chemistry* **274**, 37087-37092.

40. Hirsch, E., Katanaev, V.L., Garlanda, C., Azzolino, O., Pirola, L., Silengo, L., Sozzani, S., Mantovani, A., Altruda, F. and Wyman, M.P. (2000). Central role for the G-Protein Coupled Phosphoinositide-3 Kinase γ in Inflammation. *Science*, **287**, 1049-53.
41. Arai, H., Tsou, C.L. and Charo, I.F. (1997) Chemotaxis in a Lymphocyte Cell Line Transfected With C-C Chemokine Receptor 2b - Evidence That Directed Migration Is Mediated By Beta-Gamma Dimers Released By Activation of G(Alpha-I)-Coupled Receptors. *Proceedings of the National Academy of Sciences of the United States of America*, **94**, 14495-14499.
42. Neptune, E.R. and Bourne, H. R. (1997). Receptors Induce Chemotaxis By Releasing the Beta-Gamma Subunit of G(I), Not By Activating G(Q) or G(S). *Proceedings of the National Academy of Sciences of the United States of America*, **94**, 14489-14494.
43. Springer, T.A. (1994). Traffic Signals For Lymphocyte Recirculation And Leukocyte Emigration: The Multistep Paradigm. *Cell*, **76,** 301-314
44. Campbell, J.J., Hedrick, J., Zlotnik, A., Siani, M.A., Thompson, D.A. and Butcher, E.C. (1998). Chemokines and the Arrest of Lymphocytes Rolling Under Flow Conditions. *Science*, **279**, 381-384.
45. Laudanna, C., Campbell, J.J. and Butcher, E.C. (1996). Role of Rho in Chemoattractant-Activated Leukocyte Adhesion Through Integrins. *Science*, **271**, 981-983.
46. Haribabu, B., Steeber, D.A., Ali, H., Richardson, R.M., Snyderman, R. and Tedder, T.F. (1997). Chemoattractant Receptor Induced Phosphorylation of L-selectin. *Journal of Biological Chemistry*, **272,** 13961-13965.
47. Fong, A.M., Robinson, L.A., Steeber, D.A., Tedder, T.F., Yoshie, O., Imai, T. and Patel, D.D. (1998). Fractalkine and CX3CR1 Mediate a Single-step Mechanism of Leukocyte Capture, Firm Adhesion and Activation under Physiologic Flow. *J. Exp. Med.***188**, 1413-1419.
48. Hausdorff, W.P., Caron M.G. and Lefkowitz, R.J. (1990). Turning off the signal: desensitization of beta-adrenergic receptor function. *FASEB J.* **4,** 2881-2889.
49. Liggett, S. B., and Lefkowitz, R. J. (1994). in *Regulation of Cellular Signal transduction Pathways by desensitization and Amplification* (Siblley, D. R., and Houslay, M. D., eds) Vol. 3, pp. 71-97, John Wiley & Sons Ltd., New York
50. Haribabu, B., and Snyderman, R. (1993) Identification of additional members of human G protein–coupled receptor kinase multigene family. *Proc Natl Acad Sci U S A.* **90,** 9398-9402.
51. Mueller, S.G., Schraw, W.P.and Richmond, P. (1994). Melanoma growth stimulatory activity enhances the phosphorylation of the class II interleukin-8 receptor in non-hematopoietic cells. *Journal of Biological Chemistry* **269**, 1973-1980.
52. Mueller, S.G., Schraw, W.P.and Richmond, P. (1995). Activation of protein kinase C enhances the phosphorylation of the type B Interleukin-8 receptor and stimulates its degradation in non-hematopoietic cells. *Journal of Biological Chemistry* 270, 10439-10448.
53. Richardson, R. M., DuBose, R. A., Ali, H., Tomhave, E. D., Haribabu, B., and Snyderman, R. (1995). Regulation of human interleukin-8 receptor A: Identification of a phosphorylation site involved in modulating receptor functions. *Biochemistry* 34, 14193-14201.
54. Mueller, S.G., White, J.R., Schraw, W.P., Lam, V., and Richmond, A. (1997). Ligand-induced desensitization of the human CXC chemokine receptor-2 Is modulated by multiple serine residues in the carboxyl-terminal domain of the receptor . *Journal of Biological Chemistry* 272, 8207-8214.

55. Haribabu, B., Richardson, R. M., Fisher, I., Sozzani, S., Peiper, S. C., Horuk, R., Ali, H. and Ralph Snyderman (1997) Regulation of human chemokine receptors CXCR4. role of phosphorylation in desensitization and internalization . *Journal of Biological Chemistry* 272, 28726-28731.
56. Orsini, M. J., Parent, J-L., Mundell, S. J., and Benovic, J. L. (1999) Trafficking of the HIV coreceptor CXCR4. Role of arrestins and identification of residues in the C-terminal tail that mediate receptor internalization. *Journal of Biological Chemistry* 274, 31076-31086.
57. Oppermann, M., Mack, M., Proudfoot, A. E. I. and Olbrich, H. (1999) Differential effects of CC chemokines on CC chemokine receptor 5 (CCR5) phosphorylation and identification of phosphorylation sites on the CCR5 carboxyl terminus. *Journal of Biological Chemistry* 274, 8875-8885.
58. Franci, C., Gosling, J., Tsou, C-L., Coughlin, S. R. and Israel Charo, F. (1996). Phosphorylation by a G Protein-Coupled Kinase Inhibits Signaling and Promotes Internalization of the Monocyte Chemoattractant Protein-1 Receptor: Critical Role of Carboxyl-Tail Serines/Threonines in Receptor Function. *J Immunol* 157, 5606-5612.
59. Aragay, A. M., Mellado, M., Frade, J. M. R., Martin, A. M., Jimenez-Sainz, M. C., Martinez-A, C. and Mayor, Jr. F. (1998) Monocyte chemoattractant protein-1-induced CCR2B receptor desensitization mediated by the G protein-coupled receptor kinase 2. *Proc Natl Acad Sci U S A,* 95, 2985-2990.
60. Richardson, R. M., Pridgen, B. C., Haribabu, B., and Snyderman, R. (2000) Regulation of the human chemokine receptor CCR1: cross-regulation by CXCR1 and CXCR2. *Journal of Biological Chemistry*, 275:9201-8.
61. Henson, P. M., Schwartzman, N. A., and Zanolari, B. (1981) Intracellular control of human neutrophil secretion. II. Stimulus specificity of desensitization induced by six different soluble and particulate stimuli. *J. Immunol* 127, 754-759.
62. Wilde, M. W., Carlson, K. E., Manning, D. R., and Zigmond, S. H. (1989). Chemoattractant-stimulated GTPase activity is decreased on membranes from polymorphonuclear leukocytes incubated in chemoattractant. *Journal of Biological Chemistry* **264**, 190-196.
63. Moser, B., Schumacher, C., von Tscharner, V., Clark-Lewis, I., and Baggiolini, M. (1991). Neutrophil-activating peptide 2 and gro/melanoma growth-stimulatory activity interact with neutrophil-activating peptide 1/interleukin 8 receptors on human neutrophils. *J Biol Chem* 266, 10666-10671.
64. Didsbury, J. R., Uhing, R. J., Tomhave, E., Gerard, C., Gerard, N., and Snyderman, R. (1991). Receptor class desensitization of leukocyte chemoattractant receptor. *Proc Natl Acad Sci U S A* 88, 11564-11568.
65. Tomhave, E. D., Richardson, R. M., Didsbury, J. R., Menard, L., Snyderman, R., and Ali, H. (1994). Cross-desensitization of receptors for peptide chemoattractants: characterization of a new form of leukocyte regulation. *J Immunol* 153, 3267-3275.
66. Blackwood, R. A., Hartiala, K. T., Kwoh, E. E., Transue, A. T., and Brower, R. C. (1996). Unidirectional heterologous receptor desensitization between both the fMLP and C5a receptor and the IL-8 receptor. *J Leukoc Biol* 60, 88-93.
67. Campbell, J. J., Foxman, E. F., and Butcher, E. C. (1997). Chemoattractant receptor cross talk as a regulatory mechanism in leukocyte adhesion and migration. *Eur J Immunol* **27,** 2571-2578.
68. Foxman, E. F., Campbell, J. J., and Butcher, E. C. (1997). Multistep navigation and the combinatorial control of leukocyte chemotaxis. *J Cell Biol* **139**, 1349-1360.

69. Bacon, K. B., Greaves, D. R., Dairaghi, D. J. and Schall, T. J. (1998). The expanding universe of C, CX3C and CC chemokines. The cytokine handbook, 3rd ed. (Academic Press) pp 753-775.
70. Neote, K., DiGregorio, D., Mak, J. Y., Horuk, R., and Schall, T. J. (1993). Molecular cloning, functional expression, and signaling characteristics of a C-C chemokine receptor. *Cell.* **72**, 415-425.
71. Gao, J., Douglas, D. B., Tiffany, H. L., McDermott, D., Li, X., Francke, U., and Murphy, P. M. (1993). Structure and functional expression of the human macrophage inflammatory protein 1 alpha/RANTES receptor. *J. Exp. Med.* **177**, 1421-1427.
72. Richardson, R. M., Ali, H., Tomhave, E. D., Haribabu, B., and Snyderman, R. Cross-desensitization of Chemoattractant Receptors Occurs at Multiple Levels (1995). *Journal of Biological Chemistry* **270**, 27829-27833.
73. Richardson, R. M., Pridgen, B. C., Haribabu, B., Ali, H., and Snyderman, R. (1998). Differential Cross-regulation of the Human Chemokine Receptors CXCR1 and CXCR2: Evidence for time-dependent signal generation. *Journal of Biological Chemistry* **273**, 23830-23836.
74. Richardson, R. M., Ali, H., Pridgen, B. C., Haribabu, B., and Snyderman, R. (1998). Multiple Signaling Pathways of Human Interleukin-8 Receptor A. Independent regulation by phosphorylation. *Journal of Biological Chemistry* **273,** 10690-10695.
75. Liu, M., and Simon, M. I. (1996). *Nature* **382**, 83-87.
76. Ali, H., Fisher, I., Haribabu, B., Richardson, R. M. and Snyderman, R. (1997). Role of Phospholipase Cβ3 Phosphorylation in the Desensitization of Cellular Responses to Platelet-activating Factor. *Journal of Biological Chemistry* **272**, 11706-11709.
77. Ali, H., Sozzani, S., Fisher, I., Barr, A. J., Richardson, R. M., Haribabu, B., and Snyderman, R. (1998). Differential Regulation of Formyl Peptide and Platelet-activating Factor Receptors: Role of phospholipase Cβ3 phosphorylation by protein kinase A . *Journal of Biological Chemistry* **273**, 11012-11016.
78. Filtz, T. M. Cunningngham, M. L., Staning, K. J., Paterson, A. and Harden, T. K. (1999). Phosphorylation by protein kinase C decreases catalytic activity of avian phospholipase C-beta. *Biochem. J.* **338**, 257-264.
79. Casey, P. J. (1995). Protein lipidation in cell signaling. *Science* **268**, 221-225.
80. Parish, C. A., Smrcka, A. V., and Rando, R. R. (1995). Functional significance of beta gamma-subunit carboxymethylation for the activation of phospholipase C and phosphoinositide 3-kinase. *Biochemistry* **34**, 7722-7727.
81. Yasuda, H., Lindorfer, M. A., Myung, C. S., and Garrison, J. C. (1998). Phosphorylation of the G Protein 12 Subunit Regulates Effector Specificity. *Journal of Biological Chemistry* **273**, 21958-21965.
82. Dohlman, H. G., and Thorner, J. (1997). RGS Proteins and Signaling by Heterotrimeric G Proteins. *Journal of Biological Chemistry* **272**, 3871-3874.
83. Berman D. M. and Gilman, A. G. (1998). Mammalian RGS Proteins: Barbarians at the Gate. *J. Biol. Chem.* **273**,1269-1272.
84. Bowman, E. P., Campbell, J. J., Druey, K. M., Scheschonka, A., Kehrl, J. H., and Butcher, E. C. (1998). Regulation of Chemotactic and Proadhesive Responses to Chemoattractant Receptors by RGS (Regulator of G-protein Signaling) Family Members. *Journal of Biological Chemistry* **273**, 28040-28048.
85. Richardson, R. M. and Snyderman, R. (2000) Selective Inhibition of PAFR-mediated Cellular Responses by RGS4 Requires the Cytoplasmic Tail of the Receptor. *Journal of Biological Chemistry (submitted).*

86. Farzan, M., H. Choe, K. A. Martin, Y. Sun, M. Sidelko, C. R. Mackay, N. P. Gerard, J. Sodroski, C. Gerard. (1997). HIV-1 Entry and Macrophage Inflammatory Protein-1-Beta-Mediated Signaling Are Independent Functions of the Chemokine Receptor CCR5. *Journal of Biological Chemistry,* **272**, 6854-6857.
87. Atchison, R. E., Gosling, J., Monteclaro, F. S., Franci, C., Digilio, L., Charo, I. F., Goldsmith, M. A. (1996). Multiple Extracellular Elements of CCR5 and Hiv-1 Entry-Dissociation From Response to Chemokines. *Science*, **274**, 1924-1926.
88. Weissman, D., Rabin, R. L., Arthos, J., Rubbert, A., Dybul, M., Swofford, R., Venkatesan, S., Farber, J. M., Fauci, A. S. (1997). Macrophage-Tropic HIV and SIV Envelope Proteins Induce a Signal Through the CCR5 Chemokine Receptor. *Nature,* **389**, 981-985.
89. Davis, C. B., Dikic, I., Unutmaz, D., Hill, C. M., Arthos, J., Siani, M. A., Thompson, D. A., Schlessinger, J., Littman, D. R. (1997). Signal Transduction Due to HIV-1 Envelope Interactions With Chemokine Receptors CXCR4 or CCR5. *Journal of Experimental Medicine.* **186**, 1793-1798.
90. Alkhatib, G., Locati, M., Kennedy, P. E., Murphy, P. M., Berger, E. A. (1997). HIV-1 Coreceptor Activity of Ccr5 and Its Inhibition By Chemokines - Independence From G Protein Signaling and Importance of Coreceptor Downmodulation. *Virology,* **234,** 340-348.
91. Amara, A., Legall, S., Schwartz, O., Salamero, J., Montes, M., Loetscher, P., Baggiolini, M., Virelizier, J. L., Arenzanaseisdedos, F. (1997). HIV Coreceptor Downregulation As Antiviral Principle - SDF-1-Alpha-Dependent Internalization of the Chemokine Receptor CXCR4 Contributes to Inhibition of HIV Replication. *Journal of Experimental Medicine.* **186**, 139-146.1

3

Pathogenesis of HIV-1 Infection

G. Paolo Rizzardi and Giuseppe Pantaleo
Centre Hospitalier Universitaire Vaudois, University of Lausanne, Lausanne, Switzerland

This chapter will examine the immunologic and virologic mechanisms involved in the pathogenesis of human immunodeficiency virus type 1 (HIV-1) infection, and the interaction between the virus and the host. Both the increasing use of highly active antiretroviral combination therapy (HAART) and recent advances in our understanding of the immunopathogenesis of the infection have contributed to the identification of potential alternative therapeutic approaches that are presently needed to induce long-term control of the virus.

DIVERSITY IN THE NATURAL HISTORY OF HIV-1 INFECTION

The natural history of HIV-1 infection varies considerably in terms of the pattern and rate of disease progression. The typical course of the infection is defined by three phases occurring over an 8- to 12-year period of time (1, 2). These phases are: a) primary HIV-1 infection, during which most of the events that determine the outcome of the infection in the patient occur; b) chronic asymptomatic infection, lasting on average about 10 to 11 years, which is characterized by the absence of clinically relevant signs and symptoms of disease; and c) and overt AIDS, which is associated with the development of opportunistic infections, certain malignancies, and other HIV-1-associated conditions. In the absence of effective treatment, AIDS invariably causes the death of the subject within several years.

Primary HIV-1 infection is a transient condition lasting 2 to 4 weeks in most cases (see next section and Figure 1), although it can persist for more than 10

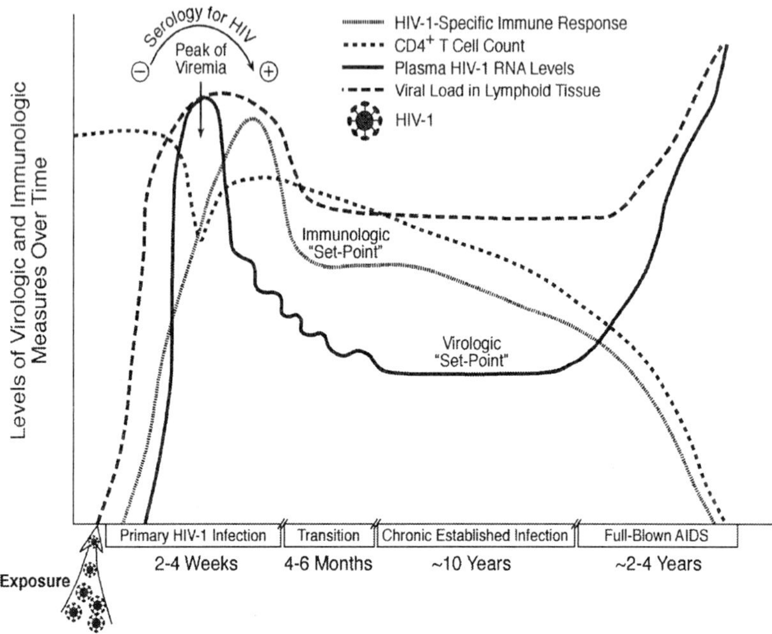

Figure 1 Schematic representation of the kinetics of viral load and immune responses from exposure to HIV-1 throughout the course of the infection.

weeks. This phase is symptomatic in about 70% of subjects (3). The systemic dissemination of HIV-1 coincides with the rapid increase in the levels of HIV-1 RNA in the plasma. These levels generally exceed 1 million RNA copies/ml and may reach several million copies. Increasing viral replication is accompanied by a marked decrease in $CD4^+$ T cell counts and an increase in $CD8^+$ T cell counts. Levels of plasma HIV-1 RNA then achieve a zenith, which defines the peak of plasma viremia. This phase, usually occurring 2 to 4 weeks after exposure, is important for several reasons. First, signs and symptoms of the acute retroviral syndrome usually worsen as the plasma viremia increases and then resolve when levels of HIV-1 RNA decrease due to the appearance of virus-specific host immune responses that play an important role in down-regulating plasma HIV-1 RNA (4-8). Second, the peak of viremia coincides with the appearance of antibodies against HIV-1 proteins (seroconversion). Third, as discussed below, this phase is likely the most beneficial moment to initiate antiretroviral therapy (1, 9) (Figure 1). In fact, primary HIV-1 infection might be defined as a medical emergency because the rapidity of intervention can have a major impact on the subsequent course of the infection, particularly the rate of disease progression. As a

Table 1 Signs and symptoms of primary HIV-1 infection.

Sign or Symptom	% of Patients
Fever	80-90
Fatigue	70-90
Rash	40-80
Headache	32-70
Lymphadenopathy	40-70
Pharyngitis	50-70
Arthralgia	50-70
Myalgia	50-70
Night sweats	50
Gastrointestinal symptoms	30-60
Aseptic meningitis	24
Oral and genital ulcers	5-20

consequence, early identification of primary HIV-1 infection is very important. Unfortunately, this diagnosis can be challenging because the acute retroviral syndrome is nonspecific and may mimic other causes of acute febrile illness, such as acute mononucleosis and toxoplasmosis (Table 1) (1, 3).

Primary HIV-1 infection should always be considered in the differential diagnosis of an acute febrile illness, especially in the presence of recent risks of virus exposure. The syndrome usually lasts less than 2-3 weeks, though this period ranges between a few days and several weeks. Diagnosis of primary HIV-1 infection is based on blood tests in the presence of a consistent medical history and clinical signs of possible exposure. During the symptomatic phase, which usually coincides with the peak of plasma HIV-1 RNA, HIV-1 antibody tests are negative, but p24 antigen and HIV-1 RNA are detectable in the plasma. After the peak viremia, plasma HIV-1 RNA levels tend to decrease and the clinical syndrome resolves, and chronic HIV-1 infection is progressively established (see next section and Figure 1). Following primary HIV-1 infection, the virus invariably establishes the chronic asymptomatic phase of the disease, which lasts for a median period of 10 to 11 years. This phase then leads to overt AIDS, characterized by low $CD4^+$ T cell counts (<200 cells/μl) and the development of opportunistic infections and other HIV-associated diseases.

This pattern of disease progression identifies most (60 to 70%) subjects with HIV-1 infection, so-called "typical progressors". However, some 10 to 20% of subjects develop AIDS in less than 5 years ("rapid progressors"), whereas 5 to 15% of subjects progress to AIDS more slowly (slow progressors). Less than 1% of subjects show no disease progression for at least 8-10 years, while maintaining high $CD4^+$ T cell counts (>500 cells/μl) and (usually) low (500-5,000 copies/ml) to very low (below 50 copies/ml) levels of HIV-1 RNA in the plasma. These subjects, so-called "long-term nonprogressors" (LTNP), represent the natural example of long-term control of HIV-1 infection.

The different patterns of disease progression are associated with varying profiles of CD4 T cell counts and plasma HIV-1 RNA levels over time (Figure 2). This diversity in the natural history of HIV-1 infection is likely due to the heterogeneity of genetic, immunologic, and virologic factors that determe the evolutionary pattern of the infection in a single patient (10). Of special importance are events that occur during the primary infection and the mechanisms that the virus puts in motion to escape the immune response (1, 2, 10, 11). These topics will be discussed in detail below.

FROM EXPOSURE TO ESTABLISHMENT OF HIV-1 INFECTION

Transmission of HIV-1 occurs by several different routes, including sexual contact, blood-to-blood contamination (i.e., via blood and blood-derived product transfusion or needle sharing among injection-drug users), and maternal-infant transmission. The most common route of infection is sexual transmission (12). Despite the variability in the natural history, the exposure to a sufficient virus inoculum is usually followed by the establishment of chronic HIV-1 infection.

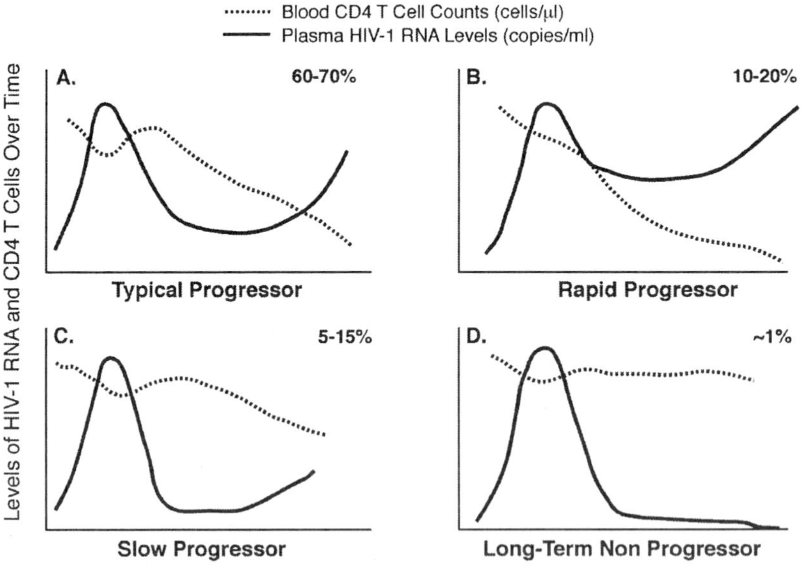

Figure 2 HIV-1 RNA levels and $CD4^+$ T cell counts vary with the pattern of HIV-1 infection progression: typical progressors (panel A); rapid progressors (panel B); slow progressors (panel C); and long-term nonprogressors (LTNP, panel D).

Immediate Pathogenic Events Following HIV-1 Exposure

The experimental infection of rhesus monkeys with the simian immunodeficiency virus (SIV) via the vaginal mucosa has produced insights into the sexual transmission of retroviruses (Figure 3). The first target cells for virus are tissue dendritic cells (DC) (i.e., Langherans' cells in the lamina propria beneath the vaginal epithelium) (13), which are highly developed antigen presenting cells (APC). DC are able to prime naïve T cells and to induce the cell surface expression of major histocompatibility complex (MHC) class I and class II molecules, as well as co-stimulatory molecules (including high levels of chemokines) (14). An effective immune response against acute infection by a microorganism involves the presentation of the antigen in lymph nodes (3). DC play a crucial role in capturing HIV-1, stimulating the initial priming of T cells, and carrying the virus to the nearest lymph node site. The migration of these infected DC to regional lymph nodes and the recruitment of activated virus-specific T cells represent the immediate pathogenic events of HIV-1 infection. Interestingly, these early events confer some advantages to HIV-1. First, effective infection occurs via the preferential transmission of R5 HIV-1 strains (15, 16) i.e., virus strains that utilize CC-chemokine receptor 5 (CCR5) as a co-receptor (discussed below and in Chapter 4). In terms of the rate of disease progression, R5 strains are less pathogenic than X4 strains, which use CXCR4 as co-receptors. This favored transmission of R5 strains can be explained by the facts that DC preferentially express CCR5 (17) and that only R5 HIV-1 envelopes have the ability to activate $CD4^+$ T cells and to recruit them by chemotaxis (18). These two factors, the co-receptor expression on the initial target cell and the signaling ability of R5 HIV-1 envelopes, may explain why 95% of sexually transmitted HIV-1 infections are mediated by R5 virus strains (15, 16). Second, the initial interaction between the virus and the host induces a rapid recruitment of many activated $CD4^+$ T cells to the lymphoid organs where the virus is carried, ensuring that a large number of target cells are available to HIV-1 prior to the appearance of effective virus-specific immune responses.

In fact, about 48 hours after the initial exposure, HIV-1 can be found in regional lymph nodes and disseminating throughout the lymph nodal system. In less than 5 days, virus replication can be detected in the peripheral blood. The transmission of HIV-1 in humans follows the same pathway; the estimated time from initial exposure to detection of virus replication in the bloodstream varies between 4 and 11 days (Figure 3). This model is valid not only for genital-genital transmission, but also for the genital-oral route, because DC are present in the nasopharyngeal tonsils and adenoid tissue. Finally, conditions that decrease the protective role of the mucosal barrier, including concomitant infections, tissue damage, and inflammatory processes in general, may increase the effective size of the initial inoculum and, thereby, increase the risk of infection (1, 3).

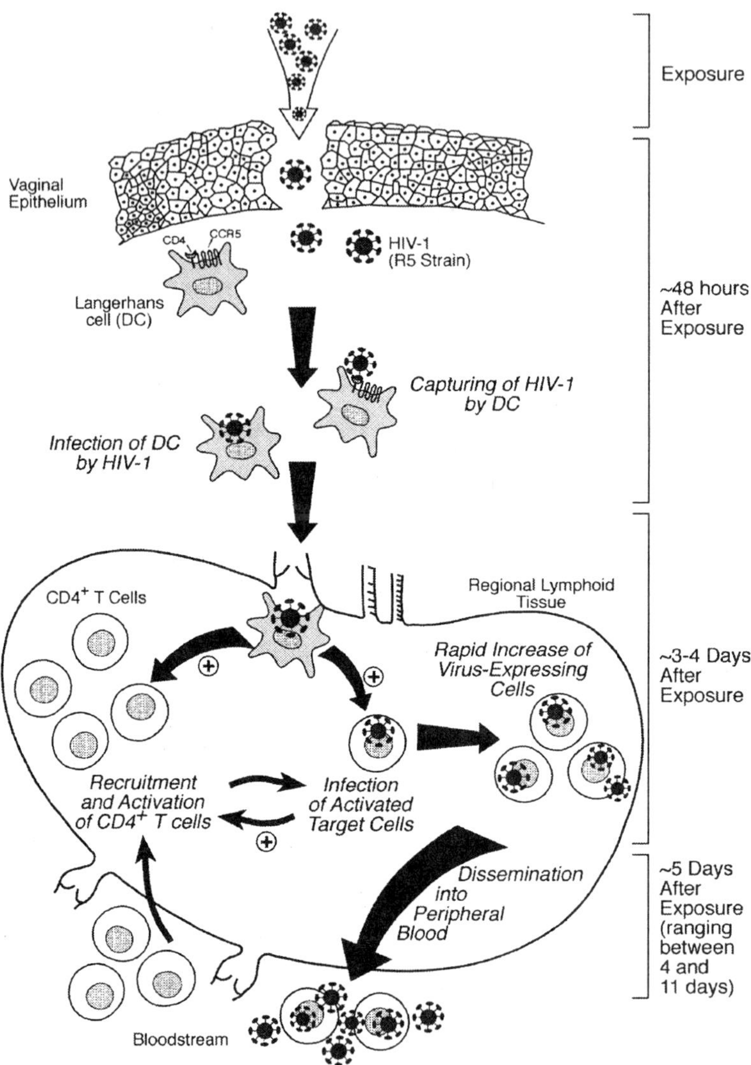

Figure 3 Schematic representation of pathogenic events occurring after sexual exposure to HIV-1. Tissue dendritic cells (DC) are the first cells to become infected with HIV-1. DC carry HIV-1 to regional lymphoid tissue, where they prime, recruit, and activate $CD4^+$ T cells. The infection of activated target cells rapidly increases the number of virus-expressing cells in the lymph node, and leads to the dissemination of HIV-1 into the bloodstream.

HIV-1 Has A Lymph Nodal Tropism

The lymphoid tissue plays a crucial role, not only in the very early steps of the infection, but throughout the course of the disease, including the asymptomatic phase when the infection is actually progressive (19, 20). The analysis of viral distribution in both rhesus monkey and human lymph nodes has shown that during primary infection, virus is mostly present in the form of numerous individual cells expressing viral RNA (21, 22). The number of cells increases in the early phases of infection and immediately precedes the spread of virus into the bloodstream, likely because virus production exceeds the ability of lymphoid structure to contain the infection (Figure 3). In the transition from primary to early chronic infection, virus is present not only in the form of virus expressing cells, but also as free virus trapped by the follicular dendritic cell (FDC) network of lymph node germinal centers (21, 22). This form of virus becomes dominant in the chronic phase of the disease, and follows, at least in part, the emergence of the HIV-1-specific humoral response. In fact, HIV-1 virions can be complexed with immunoglobulins (Ig) and complement (C'), and the binding of these complexes on the extracellular surface of FDC occurs through C' receptors expressed on FDC. The transition between primary and early chronic infection is accompanied by a marked decrease in the levels of virus detected in the peripheral blood. This reduction results from the emergence of virus-specific cytotoxic T lymphocytes (CTL) mediating the elimination of productively infected cells (8), and likely to the appearance of virus in the trapped form that can contribute to the down-regulation of the levels of plasma virus replication. To this extent, virus-specific immune responses may also significantly affect the virus distribution in this phase of the infection (1, 23). However, cross-sectional studies on human lymph node biopsies have indicated that the number of virus expressing cells does not vary significantly between primary and early chronic infection. This finding suggests that the control of virus replication and spread by the virus-specific immune response is only partial, even after the reduction of plasma levels of virus replication (19, 21).

Furthermore, recent studies of lymph node biopsies from subjects with chronic asymptomatic HIV-1 infection have demonstrated that the number of cells in lymphoid tissue that express HIV-1 RNA is strongly correlated with the level of plasma HIV-1 RNA. Both lymphoid tissue HIV-1 RNA expression and plasma HIV-1 RNA levels predict the duration of HAART needed to efficiently suppress HIV-1 replication (24). These results suggest that constant infection of new target cells in lymphoid tissue is a major contributor to the level of plasma HIV-1 RNA (24, 25). Altogether, these findings indicate that lymph nodes (which are the primary anatomic site for HIV-1 replication, viral spread, and establishment of chronic infection) (21, 22) play a fundamental role throughout the course of the disease.

DETERMINANTS CONTRIBUTING TO THE HETEROGENEITY IN THE NATURAL HISTORY OF HIV-1 INFECTION

Studies carried out in subjects with primary HIV-1 infection, LTNP, and HIV-1 negative subjects at high risk of exposure to the virus have identified host factors that determine the course of HIV-1 infection. Such studies have also shown that interactions between the host and the virus significantly affect the rate of disease progression. In this context, genetic, immunologic and virologic factors modulate both the biologic susceptibility to HIV-1 and the host immune response against the virus, and, therefore, explain the heterogeneity in the natural course of the infection (Table 2) (1, 10, 23).

Table 2 Genetic, immunologic, and virologic determinants that may affect the natural history of HIV-1 infection.

Genetic	Immunologic	Virologic
Human leucocyte antigen haplotypes	Events occurring during primary HIV-1 infection contribute to the "immunologic set-point" (see Figure 1)	The extent of HIV-1 replication, genetic determinant variability, and the immunologic "set-point" contribute to the "virologic set-point" (see Figure 1)
Genetic variability affecting chemokine receptor expression	Qualitative differences in the virus-specific immune response (T cell receptor diversity, and degree of clonality of CD8-mediated cytotoxic responses)	Variability in the viral phenotype (NSI or SI) mediated by R5 and X4 HIV-1 strains
Genetic variability affecting the levels of chemokine receptor ligands	Deletion of virus-specific cytotoxic T cell clones	Extent of virus replication and of target cell infection in the lymphoid tissue
	Persistence of HIV-1-specific $CD4^+$ and $CD8^+$ T cell responses	Extent of HIV-1 reservoirs and virus latency
	Degree of persistent immune activation	
	Extent of virus-specific immune responses in the lymphoid tissue	

Genetic Determinants

In recent years, the role of genetic determinants in modulating the course of HIV-1 infection has been increasingly elucidated. Some genetic factors, such as certain human leukocyte antigen (HLA) haplotypes (26-29), may render the host more or less able to elicit broad HIV-1-specific immune responses, thereby, affecting the host immune system's control of the virus and the rate of disease progression. Other genetic factors affect the molecular mechanisms through which HIV-1 infects the host. In this context, the understanding of how HIV-1 can infect its major target cell (i.e., the $CD4^+$ T cell) has been essential. The CD4 molecule is the major receptor that HIV-1 uses to enter the target cell (30-32). However, although the CD4 molecule is necessary for HIV-1 entry, it is not sufficient to enable fusion between target cell membrane and HIV-1 envelope. This observation suggested the presence of viral co-receptors (33, 34). Research reported during 1995 and 1996 identified chemokine receptors as HIV-1 entry co-receptors (35-46) and genetic polymorphisms in chemokine receptors have a two-fold role. As discussed in chapter 7, these polymorphisms can affect the susceptibility to infection by HIV-1 and the rate of disease progression after infection (i.e., the rate of HIV-1-associated morbidity and mortality).

Furthermore, this genetic variability may not only affect chemokine receptor expression, but also the production and release of the chemokines (i.e., the soluble factors that are the natural ligands of chemokine receptors) themselves. In fact, it has been suggested that chemokines may modulate HIV-1 infectivity and that their varying levels may be associated with varying rates of disease progression. This effect might be, at least in part, because high circulating levels of chemokines can down-regulate the cognate receptors, thus rendering the cell less prone to HIV-1 infection, mimicking what happens in the case of the genetically determined deficiency of co-receptor expression (47).

The association between genetic variability and modulation of the natural course of the disease emphasizes the complexity of the interactions between the host and the virus that may affect the risk of progression of an individual patient. A clear definition of how to use genetic markers in clinical decision-making is still lacking, particularly regarding when to start antiretroviral therapy (48). Furthermore, the increasing knowledge of the role of genetic variability provides support for the identification and design of novel strategies, including new classes of drugs that might be active against HIV-1. These strategies are discussed in detail in chapter 12 of this book.

Immunologic Determinants

As discussed above, the immediate interactions between the virus and the host confer a significant advantage to the virus that is not cleared and that can thus establish a chronic infection. However, the immune response of the individual subject with HIV-1 infection plays a primary role in determining the course of the disease. In particular, events occurring during primary and early chronic phases significantly contribute to the variability of the natural history of infection (1, 2, 10). These events are particularly important because they affect the efficiency of the mechanisms that the virus puts in motion to escape the immune response (see below) (11). Altogether, immunologic determinants contribute to the establishment of an immunologic set point, that is characteristic of the individual subject with HIV-1 infection and associated with the rate of disease progression (1, 49).

Qualitative differences in the virus-specific immune response influence the rate of progression of the disease by affecting the extent of immune control on HIV-1 replication. In particular, numerous studies of T cell receptor (TCR) diversity have demonstrated that different degrees of clonality of the CD8-mediated CTL responses are associated with varying rates of disease progression (6, 49). During primary infection, the mobilization of a very restricted (mono- or oligoclonal) TCR repertoire is associated with a rapid progression of HIV-1 disease, whereas the stimulation of multiple virus-specific CTL clones induced by a broader TCR repertoire is correlated with a slower rate of disease progression. This variability may be explained by the deletion of virus-specific CTL clones by constant antigen stimulation. Conceivably, deletion of CTL clones occurs more rapidly in the case of a restricted mobilization of the TCR repertoire, thus severely impairing the control of virus replication over time. The demonstration that HIV-1-specific $CD8^+$ CTL responses effectively reduce the levels of plasma viral RNA provides further support for this hypothesis. Furthermore, the analysis of the TCR repertoire patterns in several subjects with primary HIV-1 infection has shown that there is a certain degree of variability in the CTL clonal expansions, corresponding to either restricted or broader, more diverse, TCR repertoire mobilizations. Most importantly, these varying patterns of CTL response are clearly associated with disease progression (i.e., the broader the TCR repertoire, the slower course of HIV-1 infection) (6, 49). These qualitative differences in the primary immune response likely contribute to the establishment of a certain virologic set point in the individual subject with HIV-1 infection. The virologic set point (see below) is defined as the level of plasma HIV-1 RNA reached after the transition from primary to chronic HIV-1 infection and it varies from one individual to another. Thus, the mobilization of a restricted TCR repertoire during primary HIV-1 infection contributes to the immunologic set point and is associated with a higher virologic set point during the asymptomatic chronic phase of the infection.

Data on patients receiving antiretroviral therapy provide further support for this hypothesis. Among subjects with primary HIV-1 infection, perturbations in the TCR repertoire differ over time between untreated patients and those receiving antiretroviral therapy. Stabilization of the TCR repertoire was more consistently observed in treated patients, and the extent and rapidity of stabilization were also significantly more pronounced in those receiving therapy. Furthermore, among patients taking antiretroviral therapy, the repertoire stabilization was positively correlated with the decay slope of HIV-1 RNA in the plasma, suggesting a relationship between repertoire stabilization and virologic response to therapy. Finally, antiretroviral therapy also induced a global reduction of $CD8^+$ T cell oligoclonality, significantly modulating the mobilization of HIV-1-specific CTL during primary HIV-1 infection (50).

Altogether, these data indicate that there is a close relationship between the immunologic set point and the levels of plasma HIV-1 RNA. However, unlike the immunologic set point, it is worth noting that RNA levels measured during primary HIV-1 infection are not a good predictor of progression (51). Therefore, the immunologic set point is likely an earlier prognosticator of disease progression than the virologic set point, and contributes to the establishment of a certain virologic set point in the individual subject with HIV-1 infection (Figure 1) (11, 49). This conclusion is consistent with the fact that persistent HIV-1-specific $CD8^+$ CTL responses during the chronic asymptomatic phase of the disease are correlated with long-term control of virus replication, as it has been observed in LTNP (29). These responses are likely associated with the elimination of productively infected cells. Therefore, this immunologic set point (i.e., the persistence of virus-specific $CD8^+$ CTL responses during the chronic phase of HIV-1 infection) modulates the course of the disease and may be considered a correlate of protective immunity (1, 29).

It is, however, important to emphasize that the complexities in the differences in the virus-specific immune responses have not been completely dissected. In particular, the recent identification of the CCR7 molecule as an important cell surface marker of T cells (CCR7 defines distinct subsets of naïve and memory T lymphocytes with different homing and effector capacities) (52-54) has greatly stimulated the study of the phenotype distribution changes over time of $CD4^+$ and $CD8^+$ T cells in HIV-1 infection. The analysis of these changes during primary and chronic phases of the disease, and of the role of HAART on these phenotype changes, will likely help to further characterize the immunologic set point. Most importantly, these studies will help to define effective protective virus-specific immune responses and may explain how the host immune system recovers following appropriate therapy.

Finally, the degree of immune activation might be associated with the rate of disease progression. During primary HIV-1 infection, the persistence of systemic manifestations (e.g., fever) for more than 14 days, the involvement of the central nervous system (CNS), and the high levels of inflammatory cytokines (e.g., tumor necrosis factor (TNF)-α and TNF-related molecules), all predict more rapid disease progression (1, 55). These findings suggest that the prolongation of a heightened state of activation is correlated with a faster progression of the infection.

Virologic Determinants

As discussed above, the interaction amongst genetic and immunologic determinants of the host contributes to the establishment of a virologic set point during the early chronic phase of HIV-1 infection (56, 57). The levels of plasma HIV-1 RNA tend to be stable in the established chronic HIV-1 infection, and this stable value defines the virologic set point. This set point accurately predicts disease progression such that a certain level of plasma HIV-1 RNA carries a corresponding risk of progression to AIDS or death. The power of the virologic set point in predicting progression is improved by considering the $CD4^+$ T cell count as well (57). Because it is likely that the virologic set point is the consequence of events occurring during primary HIV-1 infection, it is conceivable that appropriate interventions during primary infection, such as HAART or alternative therapeutic approaches, might reduce the virologic set point and consequently induce a slower rate of disease progression.

Virologic determinants that can affect the natural history of HIV-1 infection also include the viral phenotype, defined by either R5 or X4 HIV-1 strains. These correspond to non-syncytium-inducing (NSI) and syncytium-inducing (SI) strains, respectively. SI strains tend to emerge during the late phase of the disease and a shift in viral phenotype from NSI to SI heralds disease progression. As a matter of fact, the NSI viral phenotype is associated with prolonged AIDS-free survival and segregates in LTNP (58).

Events occurring from initial exposure to the establishment of chronic infection and other determinants that contribute to the heterogeneity in the natural history of HIV-1 infection are, collectively, key factors in the pathogenesis of the infection. These factors significantly affect the ability of the virus to escape the host immune response. Two decades of research in HIV-1 infection have identified several mechanisms that the virus may use to escape control by the host immune system.

HOW THE VIRUS ESCAPES THE HOST IMMUNE RESPONSE AND RENDERS HIV-1 INFECTION A CHRONIC AND PROGRESSIVE DISEASE

Vigorous virus-specific immune responses can be detected very early after infection. Although these immune responses contribute to the control of HIV-1 replication (4-7), they cannot clear the infection, even though similar responses can effectively control other viruses, such as Epstein-Barr virus and cytomegalovirus. As a matter of fact, fundamental to the success of HIV-1 is its ability to target and reshape a broad spectrum of effector components of the host antiviral immune response into viral self-defense mechanisms (11). In this context, some virologic and immunologic mechanisms of viral escape have been identified (Table 3).

Virologic Mechanisms

These virologic mechanisms include the formation of a stable pool of latently HIV-1-infected $CD4^+$ T cells containing replication competent virus (59-63), the genetic variability of HIV-1 (64), and the trapping of infectious virions on the surface of FDC (1, 20).

Table 3 HIV-1 targets and reshapes a broad spectrum of effector components of the host antiviral immune response in order to render HIV-1 infection a chronic and progressive disease.

Virologic Mechanisms	Immunologic Mechanisms
Formation of a stable pool of latently virus-infected $CD4^+$ T cells containing replication competent proviral DNA	Deletion of HIV-1-specific $CD4^+$ T cell clones
High degree of genetic variability of HIV-1	Deletion of HIV-1-specific cytotoxic $CD8^+$ T cell clones
Trapping infectious virions on the surface of follicular dendritic cells in lymph nodal germinal centers	CTL-mediated generation of virus escape mutants
	Egress of CTL from lymphoid compartment
	Impairment of antigen presenting cell functions

The rapid formation of a pool of latently infected memory $CD4^+$ T cells containing replication-competent proviral DNA is a key event in the pathogenesis of HIV-1 infection (65, 66). This pool of $CD4^+$ RO^+DR^- T cells is generally detected in both patients receiving HAART and in untreated subjects with HIV-1 infection. In fact, this pool of cells can be detected even in treated subjects in whom an effective and sustained suppression of virus replication has been achieved for three to four years. The estimated frequency of these latently-infected T cells in HAART-treated patients ranges between 0.2 and 32 cells per million resting memory $CD4^+$ T cells, corresponding to a whole body total of between 5×10^4 and 5×10^6 infected cells. This pool probably originates from productively infected T cells at the time of the primary HIV-1 infection, likely prior to the appearance of the host virus-specific immune responses. Of note, initiation of HAART as early as 10 days after the onset of symptoms of primary HIV-1 infection does not prevent the generation of this pool, despite the successful control of levels of plasma HIV-1 RNA shortly after initiation of HAART (67). This observation emphasizes the rapidity with which this cellular reservoir is formed, and that HAART alone is not able to deter this immunopathogenic process. The decay of this pool of cells during treatment with HAART is very slow, such that the estimated time needed to eradicate HIV-1 is more than 70 years, which suggests that HIV-1 eradication is not a feasible clinical target (68). Furthermore, even among patients who adhere to HAART and avoid drug toxicity and virus drug resistance, long-term maintenance of HAART does not lead to continued improvement of the virologic and immunologic responses. For many patients, continued HAART simply preserves the incomplete responses that have been achieved (69). This crucial caveat of antiretroviral therapy has stimulated the search for new therapeutic strategies that, in combination with HAART, might attain the long-term control of virus replication (69-71). Recent data on the adjunction of mycophenolic acid (MMF) to HAART-treated patients with sustained suppression of virus replication are encouraging (72). MMF, broadly used in renal transplantation, is able to selectively inhibit lymphocyte division by interfering with purine synthesis, and thus DNA synthesis, in lymphocytes (73). The adjunction of MMF to HAART exerted an indirect impact on the pool of resting latently infected CD4$^+$ T cells, contributing to their depletion *in vivo*. This represents the first evidence that an immune modulation strategy may interfere with the HIV-1 life cycle by acting on the HIV-1 target cell rather than by interfering with critical viral enzymes (72).

Genetic variability is another efficient mechanism that HIV-1 uses to escape the host immune response. HIV-1 has a pronounced genetic variability because it possesses the intrinsic ability to mutate very rapidly (64, 74). The epitopes recognized by HIV-1-specific CTL undergo frequent mutations during both the primary and chronic phases of the disease. This causes a rapid impairment of both humoral and cell-mediated virus-specific immune responses in controlling virus replication.

Finally, virus trapped in the FDC network in the germinal centers of lymph nodes is the dominant form of virus found in lymphoid tissue during chronic infection. In general, the immune complex formation and capturing of these complexes in the FDC network are mechanisms used to clear a pathogen within the reticuloendothelial system, and to induce and maintain specific immune responses, respectively. However, in the case of HIV-1 infection, these mechanisms lead to the establishment of a stable reservoir of infectious viral particles that can continuously infect activated CD4$^+$ T cells, and to a chronic inflammatory reaction inducing the progressive impairment of lymph node functional activity (19, 21). This represents another mechanism by which HIV-1 takes advantage of the host immune response.

Immunologic Mechanisms

The immunologic mechanisms of viral escape include the deletion of HIV-specific CD4$^+$ (9) and cytotoxic CD8$^+$ T cell clones (75), the CTL-mediated generation of virus escape mutants (11), the egress of CTL from the lymphoid compartment (76), and the impairment of APC function (11).

HIV-1-specific CD4$^+$ T cell responses are often undetectable in patients with chronic asymptomatic HIV-1 infection, but this is not the case in LTNP, as these people maintain detectable HIV-1-specific T-helper responses. T-helper responses likely have a role in the long-term control of the virus, because CD8$^+$ CTL responses require the continuous cognate helper function provided by antigen-specific CD4$^+$ T cells and because the development of HIV-1-specific antibody responses is strictly dependent upon CD4$^+$ antigen-specific T helper cells (11). Therefore, the generation and maintenance of vigorous virus-specific CTL responses and of humoral responses can be compromised over time. Importantly, the institution of HAART in primary HIV-1 infection, particularly during the peak of plasma HIV-1 RNA levels (9), is effective in preserving these responses, and likely leads to the establishment of a lower virologic set point (see above). In contrast, the initiation of HAART during chronic asymptomatic infection may only partially repair these responses in a minority of patients (77). Altogether, these data indicate that HIV-1-specific $CD4^+$ T cell clones may be deleted very soon after infection, and that rescue of these responses is strictly dependent upon the time of initiation of HAART.

Likewise, during primary HIV-1 infection, rapid depletion of certain HIV-1-specific cytotoxic $CD8^+$ T cell clones also may occur (75). In fact, some virus-specific CTL clones undergo a massive clonal expansion during primary HIV-1 infection, and these clones can be deleted via a mechanism of clonal exhaustion, as has been described in mice during acute lymphocytic choriomeningitis virus infection (11). This process, which occurs to a varying extent in different patients, induces the early impairment of the HIV-1-specific CTL response and affects the rate of disease progression. The decrease of plasma HIV-1 RNA levels during primary HIV-1 infection depends on the appearance of virus-specific CTL responses (6, 7, 8, 36). The higher the frequency of HIV-1-specific CTL, the slower is the rate of disease progression (7, 29) and the lower are the levels of circulating viral RNA. Although the clonal exhaustion of HIV-1-specific cytotoxic responses does not necessarily result in a complete loss of virus-specific CTL activity, this is another way that the virus targets and affects host immune responses.

In addition, CTL virus escape mutants are commonly detected both during primary and chronic HIV-1 infection. This is additional evidence of the virus's ability to reshape the host immune response into a self-defense mechanism. In fact, if virus-specific CTL responses may be effective against the virus, the selective pressure exerted by the CTL response itself can favor the rapid emergence of virus mutants, that in turn escape the host immune response (11, 75).

As discussed above, HIV-1 is lymph node tropic and infection of target cells and production of new viral particles occurs throughout the course of the disease (19-21, 24, 78, 79). Thus, to control HIV-1, effective virus-specific CTL responses should be predominant in the lymphoid tissue, in order to kill virus-infected cells. On the contrary, however, activated antigen-specific CTL move from lymphoid tissue into the bloodstream. The early accumulation of HIV-1-specific activated CTL in peripheral blood, conceivably representing the attempt to spread virus-specific effector cells to different anatomic sites, actually redirects the effector response against the virus away from the primary site of virus replication and dissemination (i.e., the lymph node) (11, 76). However, as mentioned above, the nature and the modulation of these responses need to be further characterized. In this context, the study of CCR7 distribution and effector cytolitic activities of CTL will contribute to the dissection of varying pathways of generation and maturation of virus-specific responses.

Along with T-helper and T-cytotoxic responses, the APC function is crucial in the generation of active effector host immune responses. Specialized APC, such as monocytes/macrophages and DC, are affected by HIV-1, which causes their depletion or functional impairment, including interference with the formation of MHC-antigenic peptide complexes. In fact, HIV-1 nef protein may down-regulate the expression of MHC class I molecules on APC, affecting the correct recognition of virus-infected target cells by CTL (80).

AN UNDERSTANDING OF HIV-1 PATHOGENESIS SHOULD DRIVE THE DEVELOPMENT OF EFFECTIVE THERAPEUTIC OPTIONS

Present knowledge of HIV-1 pathogenesis emphasizes the complexity of the interactions between the virus and the host, which contribute to the establishment of the immunologic and virologic set points. Furthermore, ongoing research efforts in this field have defined new therapeutic targets, as well as immune-based strategies, aimed at the eradication or long-term control of the virus (Figure 4) (69-71).

The use of HAART has radically modified the course of HIV-1 infection (81-83), inducing a dramatic decrease of HIV-1-associated morbidity and

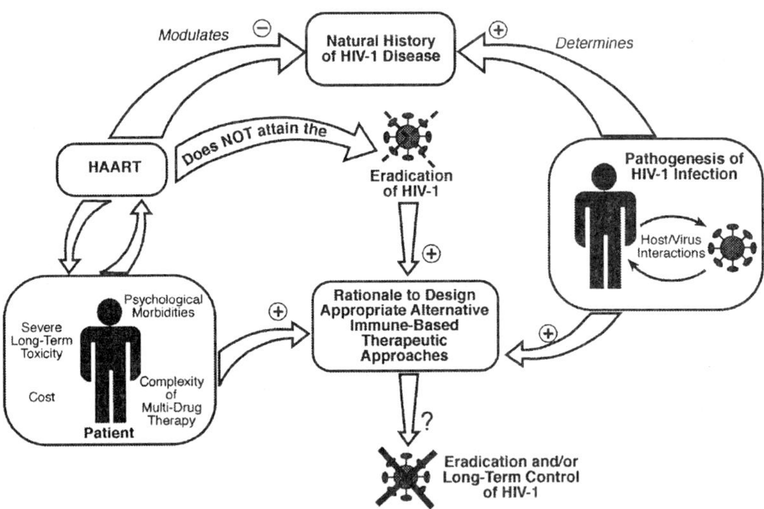

Figure 4 Interactions that determine the course of HIV-1 infection. HAART has dramatically reduced HIV-1-associated morbidity and mortality, but it does not eradicate HIV-1. HAART is associated with various drawbacks, including complex drug regimens, psychological morbidity associated with lifelong therapy, and potential severe long-term toxicities. Alternative therapeutic approaches are required for the treatment of HIV-1 infection.

mortality (84, 85). However, HAART alone will not eradicate the virus and once therapy is discontinued HIV-1 disease renews its progressive course. It is important to emphasize that, although efficacious, HAART is complex and potentially accompanied by various, severe drug-toxicities (86-88). Furthermore, the number of pills comprising a multi-drug regimen, the consequent daily schedule, and the psychological morbidity associated with the commitment to lifelong therapy are critical issues for patients (77). In this context, there has been an increasing effort to design and develop alternative therapeutic strategies based upon the modulation of the immune system. These efforts are aimed at improving host control of infection and purging the virus from its reservoirs (72, 89, 90). The design of such approaches has greatly stimulated the study of both viral and T cell dynamics (91-95). Long-term analysis of changes in T cell production following HAART support the hypothesis that, in addition to T cell destruction, a limited renewal of $CD4^+$ T cells might represent an important mechanism that explains the gradual depletion of $CD4^+$ T cells during HIV-1 infection (93, 95). The inhibition in T cell production might occur at varying levels, interfering with the cell cycle and with the T cell production in the bone marrow (defect in the number of progenitors) and in the thymus (defect in the number ofprecursors). On the basis of recent data, HAART is able to reverse this regeneration block, at least in subjects who had not undergone severe immune system damage prior to the initiation of antiretroviral therapy (95). Overall, the development of effective therapeutic options should take into account these advances in the understanding of HIV-1 pathogenesis. An example is the increasing knowledge of the role of genetic variability that provides support for the identification and design of novel strategies, including new classes of drugs that might be active against the virus (see Chapter 12). Likewise, recent advances in the definition of pathogenetic mechanisms involved in the disease, such as the identification of cellular reservoirs of infection, have to be considered in designing new approaches to treat HIV-1 infection, including novel immune-based therapeutic approaches (69).

In conclusion, because HIV-1 eradication is not achievable with presently available antiretroviral drugs, there is undoubtedly the need to develop other strategies to fight HIV-1. A top priority for HIV-1 researchers is to investigate alternative therapeutic approaches and potential novel classes of antiretroviral drugs that might broaden the therapeutic armamentarium of the future.

REFERENCES

1. Rizzardi, G.P., and G. Pantaleo. 1999. The immunopathogenesis of HIV-1 infection. *In* Infectious Disease. Vol. 2. A. Armstrong, and J. Cohen, editors. Mosby, London. 5.6.1-5.6.12.
2. Pantaleo, G., O. Cohen, C. Graziosi, M. Vaccarezza, S. Paolucci, J.F. Demarest, and A.S. Fauci. 1997. Immunopathogenesis of human immunodeficiency virus infection. *In* AIDS. V.T.J. De Vita, S. Hellman, and S.A. Rosenberg, editors. Lippincott-Raven, Philadelphia. 78-88.

3. Kahn, J.O., and B.D. Walker. 1998. Acute human immunodeficiency virus type I infection. N Engl J Med. 339:33-39.
4. Koup, R.A., J.T. Safrit, Y. Cao, C.A. Andres, G. McLeod, W. Borkowsky, C. Farthing, and D.D. Ho. 1994. Temporal association of cellular immune responses with the initial control of viremia in primary human immunodeficiency virus type 1 syndrome. J Virol. 68:4650-4655.
5. Borrow, P., H. Lewicki, B.H. Hahn, G.M. Shaw, and M.B. Oldstone. 1994. Virus-specific CD8+ cytotoxic T-lymphocyte activity associated with control of viremia in primary human immunodeficiency virus type 1 infection. J Virol. 68:6103-6110.
6. Pantaleo, G., J.F. Demarest, H. Soudeyns, C. Graziosi, F. Denis, J.W. Adelsberger, P. Borrow, M.S. Saag, G.M. Shaw, R.P. Sekaly, and A.S. Fauci. 1994. Major expansion of CD8+ T cells with a predominant Vβ usage during the primary immune response to HIV. Nature. 370:463-467.
7. Musey, L., J. Hughes, T. Schacker, T. Shea, L. Corey, and M.J. McElrath. 1997. Cytotoxic-T-cell responses, viral load, and disease progression in early human immunodeficiency virus type 1. N Engl J Med. 337:1267-1274.
8. Ogg, G.S., X. Jin, S. Bonhoeffer, P.R. Dunbar, M.A. Nowak, S. Monard, J.P. Segal, Y. Cao, S.L. Rowland-Jones, V. Cerundolo, A. Hurley, M. Markowitz, D.D. Ho, D.F. Nixon, and A.J. McMichael. 1998. Quantitation of HIV-1-specific cytotoxic T lymphocytes and plasma load of viral RNA. Science. 279:2103-2106.
9. Rosenberg, E.S., J.M. Billingsley, A.M. Caliendo, S.L. Boswell, P.E. Sax, S.A. Kalams, and B.D. Walker. 1997. Vigorous HIV-1-specific CD4+ T cell responses associated with control of viremia. Science. 278:1447-1450.
10. Fauci, A.S. 1996. Host factors and the pathogenesis of HIV-induced disease. Nature. 384:529-534.
11. Soudeyns, H., and G. Pantaleo. 1999. The moving target: mechanisms of HIV persistence during primary infection. Immunol Today. 20:446-450.
12. Royce, R.A., A. Seña, W.J. Cates, and M.S. Cohen. 1997. Sexual transmission of HIV. N Engl J Med. 336:1072-1078.
13. Spira, A.I., P.A. Marx, B.K. Patterson, J. Mahoney, R.A. Koup, S.M. Wolinsky, and D.D. Ho. 1996. Cellular targets of infection and route of viral dissemination after an intravaginal inoculation of simian immunodeficiency virus into rhesus macaques. J Exp Med. 183:215-225.
14. Cameron, P., M. Pope, A. Granelli-Piperno, and R.M. Steinman. 1996. Dendritic cells and the replication of HIV-1. J Leukocyte Biol. 59:158-171.
15. Zhu, T., H. Mo, N. Wang, D.S. Nam, Y. Cao, R.A. Koup, and D.D. Ho. 1993. Genotypic and phenotypic characterization of HIV-1 patients with primary infection. Science. 261:1179-1181.
16. Zhu, T., N. Wang, A. Carr, D.S. Nam, R. Moor-Jankowski, D.A. Cooper, and D.D. Ho. 1996. Genetic characterization of human immunodeficiency virus type 1 in blood and genital secretions: evidence for viral compartmentalization and selection during sexual transmission. J Virol. 70:3098-3107.
17. Zaitseva, M., A. Blauvelt, S. Lee, C.K. Lapham, V. Klaus-Kovtun, H. Mostowski, J. Manischewitz, and H. Golding. 1997. Expression and function of CCR5 and CXCR4 on human Langerhans cells and macrophages: implications for HIV primary infection. Nat Med. 3:1369-1375.
18. Weissman, D., R.L. Rabin, J. Arthos, A. Rubbert, M. Dybul, R. Swofford, S. Venkatesan, J.M. Farber, and A.S. Fauci. 1997. Macrophage-tropic HIV and SIV envelope proteins induce a signal through the CCR5 chemokine receptor. Nature. 389:981-985.

19. Pantaleo, G., C. Graziosi, J.F. Demarest, L. Butini, M. Montroni, C.H. Fox, J.M. Orenstein, D.P. Kotler, and A.S. Fauci. 1993. HIV infection is active and progressive in lymphoid tissue during the clinically latent stage of disease. Nature. 362:355-358.
20. Pantaleo, G., C. Graziosi, J.F. Demarest, O.J. Cohen, M. Vaccarezza, K. Gantt, C. Muro-Cacho, and A.S. Fauci. 1994. Role of lymphoid organs in the pathogenesis of human immunodeficiency virus (HIV) infection. Immunol Rev. 140:105-130.
21. Pantaleo, G., O.J. Cohen, T. Schacker, M. Vaccarezza, C. Graziosi, G.P. Rizzardi, J. Kahn, C.H. Fox, S.M. Schnittman, D.H. Schwartz, L. Corey, and A.S. Fauci. 1998. Evolutionary pattern of human immunodeficiency virus (HIV) replication and distribution in lymph nodes following primary infection: implications for antiviral therapy. Nat Med. 4:341-345.
22. Chakrabarti, L., P. Isola, M.C. Cumont, M.A. Claessens-Maire, M. Hurtrel, L. Montagnier, and B. Hurtrel. 1994. Early stages of simian immunodeficiency virus infection in lymph nodes. Evidence for high viral load and successive populations of target cells. Am J Pathol. 144:1226-1237.
23. Graziosi, C., H. Soudeyns, G.P. Rizzardi, P.A. Bart, A. Chapuis, and G. Pantaleo. 1998. Immunopathogenesis of HIV infection. AIDS Res Hum Retroviruses. 14 Suppl 2:S135-142.
24. Rizzardi, G.P., R.J. De Boer, S. Hoover, G. Tambussi, A. Chapuis, N. Halkic, P.A. Bart, V. Miller, S. Staszewski, D.W. Notermans, L. Perrin, C.H. Fox, J.M. Lange, A. Lazzarin, and G. Pantaleo. 2000. Predicting the duration of antiviral treatment needed to suppress plasma HIV-1 RNA. J Clin Invest. 105:777-782.
25. Cohen, O.J., and A.S. Fauci. 2000. Benchmarks for antiretroviral therapy. J Clin Invest. 105:709-710.
26. Carrington, M., G.W. Nelson, M.P. Martin, T. Kissner, D. Vlahov, J.J. Goedert, R. Kaslow, S. Buchbinder, K. Hoots, and S.J. O'Brien. 1999. HLA and HIV-1: heterozygote advantage and B*35-Cw*04 disadvantage. Science. 283:1748-1752.
27. Hendel, H., S. Caillat-Zucman, H. Lebuanec, M. Carrington, S. O'Brien, J.M. Andrieu, F. Schachter, D. Zagury, J. Rappaport, C. Winkler, G.W. Nelson, and J.F. Zagury. 1999. New class I and II HLA alleles strongly associated with opposite patterns of progression to AIDS. J Immunol. 162:6942-6946.
28. Kaslow, R.A., and J.M. McNicholl. 1999. Genetic determinants of HIV-1 infection and its manifestations. Proc Assoc Am Physicians. 111:299-307.
29. Haynes, B.F., G. Pantaleo, and A.S. Fauci. 1996. Toward an understanding of the correlates of protective immunity to HIV infection. Science. 271:324-328.
30. Dalgleish, A.G., P.C. Beverley, P.R. Clapham, D.H. Crawford, M.F. Greaves, and R.A. Weiss. 1984. The CD4 (T4) antigen is an essential component of the receptor for the AIDS retrovirus. Nature. 312:763-767.
31. Maddon, P.J., D.R. Littman, M. Godfrey, D.E. Maddon, L. Chess, and R. Axel. 1985. The isolation and nucleotide sequence of a cDNA encoding the T cell surface protein T4: a new member of the immunoglobulin gene family. Cell. 42:93-104.
32. Maddon, P.J., A.G. Dalgleish, J.S. McDougal, P.R. Clapham, R.A. Weiss, and R. Axel. 1986. The T4 gene encodes the AIDS virus receptor and is expressed in the immune system and the brain. Cell. 47:333-348.
33. Ashorn, P.A., E.A. Berger, and B. Moss. 1990. Human immunodeficiency virus envelope glycoprotein/CD4-mediated fusion of nonprimate cells with human cells. J Virol. 64:2149-2156.
34. Page, K.A., N.R. Landau, and D.R. Littman. 1990. Construction and use of a human immunodeficiency virus vector for analysis of virus infectivity. J Virol. 64:5270-5276.

35. Cocchi, F., A.L. DeVico, A. Garzino-Demo, S.K. Arya, R.C. Gallo, and P. Lusso. 1995. Identification of RANTES, MIP-1 alpha, and MIP-1 beta as the major HIV-suppressive factors produced by CD8+ T cells. Science. 270:1811-1815.
36. Cocchi, F., A.L. DeVico, A. Garzino-Demo, A. Cara, R.C. Gallo, and P. Lusso. 1996. The V3 domain of the HIV-1 gp120 envelope glycoprotein is critical for chemokine-mediated blockade of infection. Nat Med. 2:1244-1247.
37. Paxton, W.A., S.R. Martin, D. Tse, T.R. O'Brien, J. Skurnick, N.L. VanDevanter, N. Padian, J.F. Braun, D.P. Kotler, S.M. Wolinsky, and R.A. Koup. 1996. Relative resistance to HIV-1 infection of CD4 lymphocytes from persons who remain uninfected despite multiple high-risk sexual exposure. Nat Med. 2:412-417.
38. Feng, Y., C.C. Broder, P.E. Kennedy, and E.A. Berger. 1996. HIV-1 entry cofactor: functional cDNA cloning of a seven-transmembrane, G protein-coupled receptor. Science. 272:872-877.
39. Samson, M., O. Labbe, C. Mollereau, G. Vassart, and M. Parmentier. 1996. Molecular cloning and functional expression of a new human CC-chemokine receptor gene. Biochemistry. 35:3362-3367.
40. Dragic, T., V. Litwin, G.P. Allaway, S.R. Martin, Y. Huang, K.A. Nagashima, C. Cayanan, P.J. Maddon, R.A. Koup, J.P. Moore, and W.A. Paxton. 1996. HIV-1 entry into $CD4^+$ cells is mediated by the chemokyne receptor CC-CKR-5. Nature. 381:667-673.
41. Deng, H., R. Liu, W. Ellmeier, S. Choe, D. Unutmaz, M. Burkhart, P. Di Marzio, S. Marmon, R.E. Sutton, C.M. Hill, C.B. Davis, S.C. Peiper, T.J. Schall, D.R. Littman, and N.R. Landau. 1996. Identification of a major co-receptor for primary isolates of HIV-1. Nature. 381:661-666.
42. Alkhatib, G., C. Combadiere, C.C. Broder, Y. Feng, P.E. Kennedy, P.M. Murphy, and E.A. Berger. 1996. CC CKR5: a RANTES, MIP-1alpha, MIP-1beta receptor as a fusion cofactor for macrophage-tropic HIV-1. Science. 272:1955-1958.
43. Choe, H., M. Farzan, Y. Sun, N. Sullivan, B. Rollins, P.D. Ponath, L. Wu, C.R. Mackay, G. LaRosa, W. Newman, N. Gerard, C. Gerard, and J. Sodroski. 1996. The beta-chemokine receptors CCR3 and CCR5 facilitate infection by primary HIV-1 isolates. Cell. 85:1135-1148.
44. Doranz, B.J., J. Rucker, Y. Yi, R.J. Smyth, M. Samson, S.C. Peiper, M. Parmentier, R.G. Collman, and R.W. Doms. 1996. A dual-tropic primary HIV-1 isolate that uses fusin and the beta-chemokine receptors CKR-5, CKR-3, and CKR-2b as fusion cofactors. Cell. 85:1149-1158.
45. Samson, M., F. Libert, B.J. Doranz, J. Rucker, C. Liesnard, C.M. Farber, S. Saragosti, C. Lapoumeroulie, J. Cognaux, C. Forceille, G. Muyldermans, C. Verhofstede, G. Burtonboy, M. Georges, T. Imai, S. Rana, Y. Yi, R.J. Smyth, R.G. Collman, R.W. Doms, G. Vassart, and M. Parmentier. 1996. Resistance to HIV-1 infection in caucasian individuals bearing mutant alleles of the CCR-5 chemokine receptor gene. Nature. 382:722-725.
46. Liu, R., W.A. Paxton, S. Choe, D. Ceradini, S.R. Martin, R. Horuk, M.E. MacDonald, H. Stuhlmann, R.A. Koup, and N.R. Landau. 1996. Homozygous defect in HIV-1 coreceptor accounts for resistance of some multiply-exposed individuals to HIV-1 infection. Cell. 86:367-377.
47. Gallo, R.C., A. Garzino-Demo, and A.L. DeVico. 1999. HIV infection and pathogenesis: what about chemokines? J Clin Immunol. 19:293-299.
48. Telenti, A., and G.P. Rizzardi. 2000. Limits to potent antiretroviral therapy. Rev Med Virol. 10: 385-393.

49. Pantaleo, G., J.F. Demarest, T. Schacker, M. Vaccarezza, O.J. Cohen, M. Daucher, C. Graziosi, S.S. Schnittman, T.C. Quinn, G.M. Shaw, L. Perrin, G. Tambussi, A. Lazzarin, R.P. Sekaly, H. Soudeyns, L. Corey, and A.S. Fauci. 1997. The qualitative nature of the primary immune response to HIV infection is a prognosticator of disease progression independent of the initial level of plasma viremia. Proc Natl Acad Sci USA. 94:254-258.
50. Soudeyns, H., G. Campi, G.P. Rizzardi, C. Lenge, J.F. Demarest, G. Tambussi, A. Lazzarin, D. Kaufmann, G. Casorati, L. Corey, and G. Pantaleo. 2000. Initiation of antiretroviral therapy during primary HIV-1 infection induces rapid stabilization of the T-cell receptor beta chain repertoire and reduces the level of T-cell oligoclonality. Blood. 95:1743-1751.
51. Schacker, T.W., J.P. Hughes, T. Shea, R.W. Coombs, and L. Corey. 1998. Biological and virologic characteristics of primary HIV infection. Ann Intern Med. 128:613-620.
52. Butcher, E.C., and L.J. Picker. 1996. Lymphocyte homing and homeostasis. Science. 272:60-66.
53. Sallusto, F., D. Lenig, R. Forster, M. Lipp, and A. Lanzavecchia. 1999. Two subsets of memory T lymphocytes with distinct homing potentials and effector functions. Nature. 401:708-712.
54. Sallusto, F., C.R. Mackay, and A. Lanzavecchia. 2000. The role of chemokine receptors in primary, effector, and memory immune responses. Annu Rev Immunol. 18:593-620.
55. Rizzardi, G.P., W. Barcellini, G. Tambussi, F. Lillo, M. Malnati, L. Perrin, and A. Lazzarin. 1996. Plasma levels of soluble CD30, tumour necrosis factor (TNF)-alpha and TNF receptors during primary HIV-1 infection: correlation with HIV-1 RNA and the clinical outcome. AIDS. 10:F45-F50.
56. Mellors, J.W., C.R. Rinaldo, P. Gupta, R.M. White, J.A. Todd, and L.A. Kingsley. 1996. Prognosis in HIV-1 infection predicted by the quantity of virus in plasma. Science. 272:1167-1170.
57. Mellors, J.W., A. Munoz, J.V. Giorgi, J.B. Margolick, C.J. Tassoni, P. Gupta, L.A. Kingsley, J.A. Todd, A.J. Saah, R. Detels, J.P. Phair, and C.R. Rinaldo, Jr. 1997. Plasma viral load and CD4+ lymphocytes as prognostic markers of HIV-1 infection. Ann Intern Med. 126:946-954.
58. Schuitemaker, H., M. Koot, N.A. Kootstra, M.W. Dercksen, R.E. de Goede, R.P. van Steenwijk, J.M. Lange, J.K. Schattenkerk, F. Miedema, and M. Tersmette. 1992. Biological phenotype of human immunodeficiency virus type 1 clones at different stages of infection: progression of disease is associated with a shift from monocytotropic to T-cell-tropic virus population. J Virol. 66:1354-1360.
59. Chun, T.W., D. Finzi, J. Margolick, K. Chadwick, D. Schwartz, and R.F. Siliciano. 1995. In vivo fate of HIV-1-infected T cells: quantitative analysis of the transition to stable latency. Nat Med. 1:1284-1290.
60. Chun, T.W., L. Carruth, D. Finzi, X. Shen, J.A. DiGiuseppe, H. Taylor, M. Hermankova, K. Chadwick, J. Margolick, T.C. Quinn, Y.H. Kuo, R. Brookmeyer, M.A. Zeiger, P. Barditch-Crovo, and R.F. Siliciano. 1997. Quantification of latent tissue reservoirs and total body viral load in HIV-1 infection. Nature. 387:183-188.
61. Finzi, D., M. Hermankova, T. Pierson, L.M. Carruth, C. Buck, R.E. Chaisson, T.C. Quinn, K. Chadwick, J. Margolick, R. Brookmeyer, J. Gallant, M. Markowitz, D.D. Ho, D.D. Richman, and R.F. Siliciano. 1997. Identification of a reservoir for HIV-1 in patients on highly active antiretroviral therapy. Science. 278:1295-1300.

62. Wong, J.K., M. Hezareh, H.F. Gunthard, D.V. Havlir, C.C. Ignacio, C.A. Spina, and D.D. Richman. 1997. Recovery of replication-competent HIV despite prolonged suppression of plasma viremia. Science. 278:1291-1295.
63. Chun, T.W., L. Stuyver, S.B. Mizell, L.A. Ehler, J.A. Mican, M. Baseler, A.L. Lloyd, M.A. Nowak, and A.S. Fauci. 1997. Presence of an inducible HIV-1 latent reservoir during highly active antiretroviral therapy. Proc Natl Acad Sci USA. 94:13193-13197.
64. Coffin, J.M. 1995. HIV population dynamics in vivo: implications for genetic variation, pathogenesis, and therapy. Science. 267:483-489.
65. Chun, T.W., and A.S. Fauci. 1999. Latent reservoirs of HIV: obstacles to the eradication of virus. Proc Natl Acad Sci U S A. 96:10958-10961.
66. Finzi, D., and R.F. Siliciano. 1998. Viral dynamics in HIV-1 infection. Cell. 93:665-671.
67. Pantaleo, G., and L. Perrin. 1998. Can HIV be eradicated? AIDS. 12:S175-180.
68. Finzi, D., J. Blankson, J.D. Siliciano, J.B. Margolick, K. Chadwick, T. Pierson, K. Smith, J. Lisziewicz, F. Lori, C. Flexner, T.C. Quinn, R.E. Chaisson, E. Rosenberg, B. Walker, S. Gange, J. Gallant, and R.F. Siliciano. 1999. Latent infection of CD4+ T cells provides a mechanism for lifelong persistence of HIV-1, even in patients on effective combination therapy. Nat Med. 5:512-517.
69. Rizzardi, G.P., and G. Pantaleo. 2001. Other approaches to combat HIV-1 infection. *In* HIV Human Virus Guide. Vol. 1. D.D. Richman, editor. International Medical Press, London. In press.
70. Pantaleo, G. 1997. How immune-based interventions can change HIV therapy. Nat Med. 3:483-486.
71. Rizzardi, G.P., and G. Pantaleo. 1999. Therapeutic perspectives in HIV-1 infection from recent advances in HIV- 1 pathogenesis: it is time to move on. J Biol Regul Homeost Agents. 13:151-157.
72. Chapuis, A.G., G.P. Rizzardi, C. D'Agostino, A. Attinger, C. Knabenhans, S. Fleury, H. Acha-Orbea, and G. Pantaleo. 2000. Effects of mycophenolic acid on human immunodeficiency virus infection in vitro and in vivo. Nat Med. 6:762-768.
73. Fulton, B., and A. Markham. 1996. Mycophenolate mofetil. A review of its pharmacodynamic and pharmacokinetic properties and clinical efficacy in renal transplantation. Drugs. 51:278-298.
74. Phillips, R.E., S. Rowland-Jones, D.F. Nixon, F.M. Gotch, J.P. Edwards, A.O. Ogunlesi, J.G. Elvin, J.A. Rothbard, C.R. Bangham, C.R. Rizza, and A.J. McMichael. 1991. Human immunodeficiency virus genetic variation that can escape cytotoxic T cell recognition. Nature. 354:453-459.
75. Pantaleo, G., H. Soudeyns, J.F. Demarest, M. Vaccarezza, C. Graziosi, S. Paolucci, M. Daucher, O.J. Cohen, F. Denis, W. Biddison, R.-P. Sekaly, and A.S. Fauci. 1997. Evidence for rapid disappearance of initially expanded HIV-specific CD8+ T cell clones during primary infection. Proc Natl Acad Sci USA. 94:9848-9853.
76. Pantaleo, G., H. Soudeyns, J.F. Demarest, M. Vaccarezza, C. Graziosi, S. Paolucci, M.B. Daucher, O.J. Cohen, F. Denis, W.E. Biddison, R.P. Sekaly, and A.S. Fauci. 1997. Accumulation of human immunodeficiency virus-specific cytotoxic T lymphocytes away from the predominant site of virus replication during primary infection. Eur J Immunol. 27:3166-3173.
77. Rizzardi, G.P., G. Tambussi, P.A. Bart, A.G. Chapuis, A. Lazzarin, and G. Pantaleo. 2000. Virological and immunological responses to HAART in asymptomatic therapy-naïve HIV-1-infected subjects according to CD4 cell count. AIDS, 14:2257-2263.

78. Haase, A.T., K. Henry, M. Zupancic, G. Sedgewick, R.A. Faust, H. Melroe, W. Cavert, K. Gebhard, K. Staskus, Z.Q. Zhang, P.J. Dailey, H.H. Balfour, Jr., A. Erice, and A.S. Perelson. 1996. Quantitative image analysis of HIV-1 infection in lymphoid tissue. Science. 274:985-989.
79. Cavert, W., D.W. Notermans, K. Staskus, S.W. Wietgrefe, M. Zupancic, K. Gebhard, K. Henry, Z.Q. Zhang, R. Mills, H. McDade, C.M. Schuwirth, J. Goudsmit, S.A. Danner, and A.T. Haase. 1997. Kinetics of response in lymphoid tissues to antiretroviral therapy of HIV-1 infection. Science. 276:960-964.
80. Collins, K.L., B.K. Chen, S.A. Kalams, B.D. Walker, and D. Baltimore. 1998. HIV-1 Nef protein protects infected primary cells against killing by cytotoxic T lymphocytes. Nature. 391:397-401.
81. Deeks, S.G., M. Smith, M. Holodniy, and J.O. Kahn. 1997. HIV-1 protease inhibitors. A review for clinicians. JAMA. 277:145-153.
82. Gulick, R.M., J.W. Mellors, D. Havlir, J.J. Eron, C. Gonzalez, D. McMahon, D.D. Richman, F.T. Valentine, L. Jonas, A. Meibohm, E.A. Emini, and J.A. Chodakewitz. 1997. Treatment with indinavir, zidovudine, and lamivudine in adults with human immunodeficiency virus infection and prior antiretroviral therapy. N Engl J Med. 337:734-739.
83. Hammer, S.M., K.E. Squires, M.D. Hughes, J.M. Grimes, L.M. Demeter, J.S. Currier, J.J. Eron, Jr., J.E. Feinberg, H.H. Balfour, Jr., L.R. Deyton, J.A. Chodakewitz, and M.A. Fischl. 1997. A controlled trial of two nucleoside analogues plus indinavir in persons with human immunodeficiency virus infection and CD4 cell counts of 200 per cubic millimeter or less. ACTG 320 Study Team. N Engl J Med. 337:725-733.
84. Centers for Disease Control and Prevention. 1997. Update: trends in AIDS incidence, deaths, and prevalence--United States, 1996. MMWR Morb Mortal Wkly Rep. 46:165-173.
85. Palella, F.J.J., K.M. Delaney, A.C. Moorman, M.O. Loveless, J. Fuhrer, G.A. Satten, D.J. Aschman, and S.D. Holmberg. 1998. Declining morbidity and mortality among patients with advanced human immunodeficiency virus infection. N Engl J Med. 338:853-860.
86. Brinkman, K., J.A. Smeitink, J.A. Romijn, and P. Reiss. 1999. Mitochondrial toxicity induced by nucleoside-analogue reverse- transcriptase inhibitors is a key factor in the pathogenesis of antiretroviral-therapy-related lipodystrophy. Lancet. 354:1112-1115.
87. Carr, A., K. Samaras, A. Thorisdottir, G.R. Kaufmann, D.J. Chisholm, and D.A. Cooper. 1999. Diagnosis, prediction, and natural course of HIV-1 protease-inhibitor-associated lipodystrophy, hyperlipidaemia, and diabetes mellitus: a cohort study. Lancet. 353:2093-2099.
88. Flexner, C. 1998. HIV-protease inhibitors. N Engl J Med. 338:1281-1292.
89. Chun, T.W., D. Engel, S.B. Mizell, C.W. Hallahan, M. Fischette, S. Park, R.T. Davey, Jr., M. Dybul, J.A. Kovacs, J.A. Metcalf, J.M. Mican, M.M. Berrey, L. Corey, H.C. Lane, and A.S. Fauci. 1999. Effect of interleukin-2 on the pool of latently infected, resting CD4+ T cells in HIV-1-infected patients receiving highly active anti- retroviral therapy. Nat Med. 5:651-655.
90. Fraser, C., N.M. Ferguson, A.C. Ghani, J.M. Prins, J.M. Lange, J. Goudsmit, R.M. Anderson, and F. de Wolf. 2000. Reduction of the HIV-1-infected T-cell reservoir by immune activation treatment is dose-dependent and restricted by the potency of antiretroviral drugs. AIDS. 14:659-669.

91. Perelson, A.S., P. Essunger, Y. Cao, M. Vesanen, A. Hurley, K. Saksela, M. Markowitz, and D.D. Ho. 1997. Decay characteristics of HIV-1-infected compartments during combination therapy. Nature. 387:188-191.
92. Hellerstein, M., M.B. Hanley, D. Cesar, S. Siler, C. Papageorgopoulos, E. Wieder, D. Schmidt, R. Hoh, R. Neese, D. Macallan, S. Deeks, and J.M. McCune. 1999. Directly measured kinetics of circulating T lymphocytes in normal and HIV-1-infected humans. Nat Med. 5:83-89.
93. Fleury, S., R.J. de Boer, G.P. Rizzardi, K.C. Wolthers, S.A. Otto, C.C. Welbon, C. Graziosi, C. Knabenhans, H. Soudeyns, P.A. Bart, S. Gallant, J.M. Corpataux, M. Gillet, P. Meylan, P. Schnyder, J.Y. Meuwly, W. Spreen, M.P. Glauser, F. Miedema, and G. Pantaleo. 1998. Limited CD4+ T-cell renewal in early HIV-1 infection: effect of highly active antiretroviral therapy. Nat Med. 4:794-801.
94. McCune, J.M., M.B. Hanley, D. Cesar, R. Halvorsen, R. Hoh, D. Schmidt, E. Wieder, S. Deeks, S. Siler, R. Neese, and M. Hellerstein. 2000. Factors influencing T-cell turnover in HIV-1-seropositive patients. J Clin Invest. 105:R1-8.
95. Fleury, S., G.P. Rizzardi, A. Chapuis, G. Tambussi, C. Knabenhans, E. Simeoni, J. Meuwly, J. Corpataux, A. Lazzarin, F. Miedema, and G. Pantaleo. 2000. Long-term kinetics of T cell production in HIV-infected subjects treated with highly active antiretroviral therapy. Proc Natl Acad Sci U S A. 97:5393-5398.

4

Chemokine Receptors as HIV-1 Coreceptors

Nelson L. Michael
Walter Reed Army Institute of Research, Rockville, Maryland

THE CURRENT HIV-1 PANDEMIC

The human immunodeficiency virus type 1 (HIV-1) is the etiologic agent of the acquired immunodeficiency syndrome (AIDS). HIV-1 directly targets host defenses by infection of T-lymphocytes, macrophages, and dendritic cells of the immune system and replicates best when those cells are activated. Thus, the series of events that leads to specific immune response to HIV-1 infection ironically exposes the immune system to repeated cycles of activation and subsequent immune cell infection and destruction. Intensive research on the mechanism of HIV-1 entry into, and replication within, susceptible host target cells and the generation of HIV-1 specific immunity has provided the scientific foundation to study viral transmission and disease progression collectively known as 'HIV pathogenesis'.

The number of individuals living with HIV-1 is estimated to be 34 million with another 5 million new infections annually. Fifteen million individuals have already succumbed to this pandemic. Although the most developed countries can support disease delaying therapy, there is no evidence that HIV-1 infection can be truly cured—only managed. The implications of these numbers, especially for sub-Saharan Africa, Southeast Asia, and India where HIV-1 prevalence is extremely high, are uniformly staggering in terms of human, economic, and political costs. After an initial period of economic recovery, Africa currently has lost all modern gains in life expectancy and reduction in infant mortality due largely to HIV-1 infection. One in three people living in Botswana and one in five living in South Africa are infected with HIV-1 and will die in the absence of effective therapeutic intervention. The death toll of this pandemic has already exceeded that for World War II.

A large-scale scientific and political mobilization will be required to develop and deploy effective HIV-1 therapeutics to treat those already infected and vaccines to prevent new infections. Both of these efforts will be greatly strengthened by a firm understanding of each aspect of the viral-host interaction as these will provide the rationale basis for designing interventions. This chapter will focus on the specific portion of the HIV-1 life cycle where virus gains entry into susecptible target cells through engagement of its envelope protein with two major classes of host cell surface molecules. The first, CD4, was recognized as the major receptor for HIV-1 entry in 1986. The second class of molecules, known as entry coreceptors, was discovered in 1996 after a decade of intensive research. These molecules belong to the gene family of chemokine receptors whose normal physiologic role is to bind these chemoattractant proteins, initiate signal cascades, and mediate the movement of cells involved in lymphoid trafficking, lymphoid cell and organ development, tissue inflammatory responses, angiogenesis, wound healing, and metastasis. HIV-1 has subverted this normal physiologic role to gain efficient entry into human host cells.

THE BIOLOGY OF HIV-1 CELLULAR ENTRY

Weiss and colleagues demonstrated in 1984 that monoclonal antibodies to CD4 blocked HIV-1 entry into cells suggesting that CD4 was a critical component of the viral receptor (1). This observation was directly confirmed following the cloning of the gene (2) and demonstration in 1986 that it enabled the infection of CD4 transduced human cells (3). However, it quickly became apparent that, while necessary for HIV-1 entry, CD4 was not sufficient to allow for HIV-1 envelope fusion to the plasma membrane. Human, but not murine, cells transduced with human CD4 were generally susceptible to HIV-1 infection with prototypic HIV-1 laboratory strains that we now know use the broadly expressed HIV-1 entry coreceptor CXCR4. Human CD4 transduced murine cells could bind HIV-1 (4), but would not permit membrane fusion and subsequent viral entry (4, 5). Additional observations suggested that cell surface receptors, with unique host range, were involved in HIV-1 entry. HIV-1 isolates obtained directly from infected patients (primary isolates) could readily infect primary T-cells and macrophages but could only rarely infect T-cell lines. Conversely, HIV-1 adapted to T-cell lines could not infect primary macrophages (6-9). This dichotomy was substantiated by the identification in 1990 of sequences in the HIV-1 envelope gene, to include the V3 loop region, that correlated with cellular tropism (10, 11).

Three critical observations were made in 1995-1996 that led to the identification of the family of chemokine receptors as the elusive HIV-1 entry coreceptors. First, Gallo and colleagues showed in 1995 that the ß-chemokines RANTES, MIP-1α and MIP-1ß inhibited the infection of primary T-cells by

HIV-1 primary isolates but not T-cell line adapted HIV-1 (12) and subsequently mapped the molecular determinant of this phenotype to the V3 loop of the HIV-1 envelope (13). Second, Koup and colleagues showed in 1996 that the T-cells of some individuals who were highly exposed to HIV-1 through repeated risk behaviors were highly resistant to infection with primary, but not T-cell line adapted, HIV-1 and that this resistance correlated with elevated expression of ß-chemokines (14). These two observations greatly increased confidence in the landmark work of Berger and colleagues in 1996 who reported that the CXC chemokine receptor fusin, now called CXCR4, was capable of mediating HIV-1 envelope fusion with the plasma membrane of cells expressing CD4 and CXCR4 if the HIV-1 envelope was derived from a T-cell line adapted virus and not a primary isolate (15). They further showed that antibodies to CXCR4 blocked T-cell line adapted HIV-1 infection of primary human T-cells. Thus, the long search for the second receptor for HIV-1 entry had borne first fruit.

Pre-publication disclosure of Berger's findings triggered a rush for the discovery of the co-receptor responsible for HIV-1 entry of primary isolates which most believed would be a related chemokine receptor. Parmentier and colleagues had just isolated the cDNA for a ß-chemokine known as CKR-5 (16), now called CCR5, whose ligand binding profile precisely matched those that Gallo's group had shown a year earlier blocked infection of primary T-cells with primary HIV-1 isolates—RANTES, MIP-1α and MIP-1ß. Five separate groups raced to demonstrate that CCR5 was the major entry co-receptor for primary HIV-1 isolates (17-21). The first publications confirming this hypothesis appeared only five weeks after the publication of Berger's original manuscript (17, 18). Two of these publications also implicated the chemokine receptors CCR2 (20, 21) and CCR3 (21) as HIV-1 entry coreceptors with much less affinity for HIV-1 envelope than CCR5 and CXCR4. This would begin a period of intense interest in the discovery and understanding of additional, so called "minor", HIV-1 entry coreceptors.

The central role of CCR5 as the major entry co-receptor for primary HIV-1 isolates was elegantly borne out by the discovery of otherwise healthy individuals with homozygous 32 base pair inactivating deletions in the *CCR5* coding sequences whose T-cells were completely resistant to infection with most HIV-1 primary, but not T-cell line adapted, HIV-1 (22, 23). These individuals were also shown to be highly, but not completely, resistant to HIV-1 infection in vivo (see review (24)). This polymorphism, and many others in multiple chemokine and chemokine receptor genes, is extensively reviewed elsewhere (24) and in Chapter 7 of this book.

We now know that cellular entry of HIV-1 requires binding to both CD4 and to one of the seven transmembrane G-protein coupled chemokine receptors which act as coreceptors (15, 17-19, 21, 25-27; Figure 1). HIV-1 strains have previously been characterized by their ability to produce syncytia following infection of neoplastic cell lines (viral phenotype) (28, 29). Syncytium inducing (SI) viruses are frequently found in progressive or late-stage HIV disease while

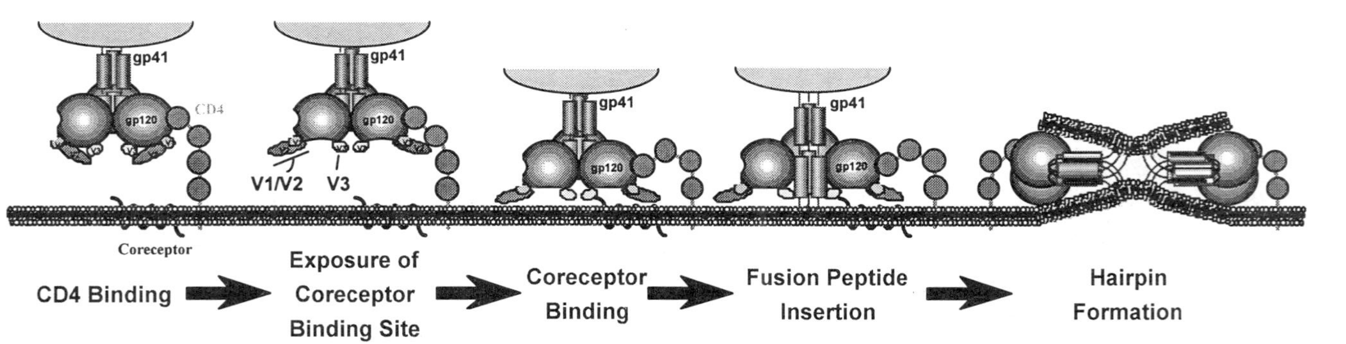

Figure 1 Mechanism of HIV-1 entry into target cells. The HIV-1 virion is shown on the top of the figure with the homotrimeric envelope gp41/gp120 complex engaging the terminal domain of CD4 via the CD4 binding domain on gp120. The three gp41polypeptides are embedded in the virion plasma membrane while the three gp120 polypeptides are non-covalently associated with the gp41 molecules. The CD4 molecule is embedded in the plasma bilayer of a target cell susceptible to HIV-1 infection. CD4-gp120 engagement brings the virion proximal to the cell surface while changing the gp120 conformation exposing residues in the V1, V2, and V3 loop domains of gp120 capable of binding the largely hydrophobic, seven-transmembrane spanning HIV-1 entry co-receptor molecule. Co-receptor binding then occurs via the N-terminal (and second extracellular loop) domain of the co-receptor to the gp120 V3 loop with involvement of the V1 and V2 loop regions. This triggers release of coiled-coil gp41domains such that helical packed distal and N-terminal/proximal domains unpack driving specific N-terminal gp41 polypeptides (fusion peptide) into the target cell surface membrane with subsequent hairpin formation between the gp41 domains, close apposition of the virion and cell plasma membranes, and eventual membrane fusion and virion entry. (Courtesy of Dr. Robert Doms, University of Pennsylvania.)

non-syncytium inducing (NSI) viruses are present throughout disease (28, 29). HIV-1 can also be classified by its ability to infect primary macrophages and CD4+ T cell lines (cell tropism). All HIV-1 isolates can replicate in primary T-cells and many will replicate in primary macrophages. However, T-cell line adapted, SI isolates cannot replicate in macrophages while some, but not all, primary NSI isolates can infect macrophages. This simple paradigm is complicated by the presence of dual-tropic HIV-1 strains containing both SI and NSI constituents capable of infecting both T-cell lines and primary macrophages. Truly dual tropic molecular clones of HIV-1 also have been described (21). Recent evidence suggests that certain HIV-1 envelope sequences are more likely to induce signal transduction in primary macrophages which, in turn, is conducive to subsequent productive infection through a currently undefined post-entry mechanism (30).

MAJOR HIV-1 ENTRY CORECEPTORS: CCR5 AND CXCR4

With the discovery of the chemokine receptor gene family as HIV-1 entry coreceptors, HIV-1 strains can also be classified by co-receptor utilization. Strictly NSI viruses primarily utilize CCR5 and are termed 'R5 HIV-1' while strictly SI viruses primarily utilize the chemokine receptor CXCR4 and are termed 'X4 HIV-1 (31). However, most primary SI isolates use CXCR4 in conjunction with CCR5 (R5X4 HIV-1) (31-33). Not all NSI isolates are capable of infecting macrophages (34) and not all CCR5-using isolates can infect macrophages (33, 35). Thus, the intersection between viral phenotype, cell tropism, and co-receptor utilization is both complex and beyond simple generalization.

MINOR HIV-1 ENTRY CORECEPTORS

Beyond the major HIV-1 coreceptors CCR5 and CXCR4, a panoply of other molecules have been identified as HIV-1 entry coreceptors, albeit with much lower efficiencies than the major coreceptors and based primarily on data from in vitro viral entry and/or membrane fusion studies. The first two such 'minor coreceptors' identified were CCR2B and CCR3 (21, 27, 36). Evidence exists for CCR3 playing a role in HIV-1 infection of microglial cells of the central nervous system (37, 38). CCR3 is also expressed on T-cells which provide help for activation of the humoral immune response (T_H2 cells) (39, 40) although the implications of this observation for HIV pathogenesis are currently unanswered. Little evidence supports an in vivo role for CCR2B in HIV pathogenesis as virtually no primary HIV-1 isolates have been shown to utilize this co-receptor (41, 42). To date, the only lentiviruses known to efficiently utilize CCR2B are SIV isolates naturally found in red-capped macaques (43).

Two seven-transmembrane receptors with extensive sequence homology to CCR5 and CXCR4, Bonzo/STRL33/TYMSTR (44-48) and BOB/GPR15 (45, 46, 49), have been shown to mediate entry of simian immunodeficiency virus (SIV), as well as some M-tropic HIV-1 and HIV-2 strains. However, recent data from Moore's group showing that R5Bonzo and R5X4Bonzo human primary HIV-1 isolates cannot infect primary human T-cells through the use of Bonzo alone (41) questions the physiologic role of Bonzo in HIV pathogenesis. Doms and colleagues have provided evidence in support of the physiologic role of Bonzo/STRL33, although they acknowledge that this entry co-receptor is rarely used by primary HIV-1 (50). Other molecules identified through in vitro studies as HIV-1 entry coreceptors, GPR1 (46, 49), CCR8 (51, 52), US28 (53), V28/CX3CR1 (51), APJ (54, 55), ChemR23 (56), and CMKRL1/leukotriene B4 receptor (57), similarly lack strong in vivo evidence for a clear role in HIV pathogenesis. Recent evidence that genetic polymorphisms in the *CX3CR1* gene are associated with HIV-1 disease progression is likely explained by interactions with the HIV-1 life cycle other than cell entry (58).

CHEMOKINE LIGANDS

The CC chemokines RANTES, MIP-1α, and MIP-1ß are natural ligands for CCR5 (16, 59), and the CXC chemokine stromal cell-derived factor-1 (SDF-1) is the only known natural ligand for CXCR4 (25, 60). Ligand binding to both receptors is associated with G-protein coupled signal transduction and leukocyte chemoattraction (16, 25, 59, 60), as well as partial viral entry antagonism (12, 13, 17-19, 25, 27, 60-62). Viral entry and signal transduction are separable in vitro functions for CCR5 (63-65), but the latter may be relevant to viral pathogenesis as evidence exists for enhancement of post-entry HIV-1 replication through ligation of chemokine receptors with viral envelope (30, 66).

THERAPEUTIC IMPLICATIONS OF HIV-1 ENTRY CO-RECEPTOR STUDIES

The recent observation that simultaneous inhibition of HIV-1 reverse transcriptase and protease does not prevent viral resistance, and will not be sufficient for viral eradication (67), underscores the pressing need for new classes of antiviral drugs. One plausible target for such agents is HIV-1 entry into CD4+ cells, as shown by clinical trials of the fusion inhibitor T20, a peptide that prevents the functioning of the viral gp41 protein (68). Other targets for entry inhibitors include the major cell surface entry coreceptors CCR5 and CXCR4 that, with CD4, mediate virus binding and membrane fusion (69). As CCR5, but not CXCR4, is apparently dispensable for normal health (69), specific inhibition of CCR5 function is an attractive concept. It is, however, one not without potential pitfalls. Concern exists on whether CCR5 inhibitors might select for new, and possibly more pathogenic, viral variants which instead use CXCR4 ("virologic toxicity").

CCR5 is the principal co-receptor for HIV-1 variants transmitted between, and persistent within, the majority of hosts. These viruses, often called "macrophage-tropic" or non-syncytium-inducing (NSI) but now designated R5 (31), are lethal; the majority of individuals who die of AIDS harbor exclusively R5 variants (70). Furthermore, in SIV-infected monkeys, variants emerge over time that are increasingly more virulent but which still use only CCR5, as shown by Overbaugh's group in another recent report (71). However, in approximately 40% of infected humans, viruses arise which can use CXCR4 as well as, or sometimes instead of, CCR5 (69, 72). The appearance of these strains, previously known as "T-cell line-tropic" or syncytium-inducing (SI), now called R5X4 or X4(31), heralds accelerated CD4+ T-cell loss and disease progression (70, 72). Drugs which selected for such variants would clearly be undesirable. Although such virologic toxicity might be circumvented by simultaneous blockade of CCR5 and CXCR4, initial clinical efficacy always has to be established with individual agents.

What factors influence the phenotypic switch from R5 to X4 viruses in vivo? This process typically occurs only after several years, which is surprisingly slow given that changing only 2 or 3 residues in the viral envelope can be sufficient to convert an R5 virus into an R5X4 variant (27, 72). The marked contrast between the slowness of R5X4 and X4 virus emergence in vivo and the exceptionally high rates of HIV-1 replication and mutation (73) implies that a selection pressure specifically suppresses the transition to CXCR4 use. Although R5X4 and X4 viruses are transmissible, can predominate in some hosts shortly after infection, and are associated with rapid disease progression (70), examples of suppression of R5X4 viruses following blood-borne transmission (74, 75) also support the existence of an early, negative selection pressure against such strains. Studies of host humoral and cellular HIV-1 immune responses have not, however, revealed what this selection pressure might be. Antibody-mediated viral neutralization is not dependent on which co-receptor is used (76), and the amino acid changes in the envelope sufficient to generate X4 viruses affect only a very small percentage of available cytotoxic T-cell epitopes. Another possibility is that the natural CXCR4 ligand, stromal-cell derived factor 1 (SDF-1), prevents the replication of X4 viruses by receptor occlusion or internalization in lymphoid organs, where both its concentration and HIV-1 replication are high. Recent evidence supporting this hypothesis was provided by Parker and colleagues in analysis of tissues from the rectum, vagina, endocervix, and small intestine (77). The progressive degradation of lymphoid architecture, and SDF-1 production capacity, caused by prolonged replication of R5 viruses might eventually relax this hypothetical restriction of CXCR4 usage, allowing the emergence of X4 viruses. These strains could then replicate in CXCR4-expressing CD4+ T-cells, cells which are significantly more abundant than CCR5-expressing CD4+ T-cells in peripheral blood and lymphoid tissues (78, 79).

Novel insights into HIV-1 phenotypic evolution have come from recent studies on rare individuals who acquired HIV-1 infection despite being homozygous for the *CCR5* Δ32 allele. The lack of functional CCR5 expression in these individuals is strongly protective against HIV-1 transmission (80). However, 9 infected *CCR5* Δ32 homozygotes have now been identified (see Chapter 11). Virologic and clinical details are limited for several of these cases, but a general theme is now emerging.

Firstly, the infecting strains exclusively utilize CXCR4 (81, 82), questioning the physiological relevance of other identified HIV-1 coreceptors (41). Secondly, the rate of CD4+ T-cell decline in these subjects is rapid, reminiscent of R5X4 viral infection in individuals who have wild-type *CCR5* alleles (70, 81, 82), and consistent with viral propagation occurring through a large and available population of CD4+ CXCR4+ T-cell targets. Thirdly, and surprisingly, this rapid CD4+ T-cell decline is not accompanied by high levels of plasma viremia or an acceleration of disease progression (81, 82). One explanation would be that the relatively abundant CXCR4+ CCR5- CD4+ T-cells each produce, on average, less virus than the scarcer CXCR4+ CCR5+ CD4+ T-cells, an idea supported by observations that viral loads tend to be high in *CCR5* wild-type individuals infected with R5X4 viruses even if their CD4+ T-cell counts are low (82). Although the sequellae of early and persistent replication of X4 viruses in *CCR5* 32 homozygotes may imperfectly predict what happens in *CCR5*-wild type individuals treated with a CCR5 inhibitor, it is intriguing that X4 tropism per se does not uniformly portend rapid clinical disease progression. Furthermore, the frequency with which X4 viruses emerge in individuals who are heterozygous for the *CCR5* Δ32 allele is no greater than in wild-type individuals (83), despite the reduced CCR5 expression associated with the *CCR5* Δ32 heterozygous genotype (61). A reduction in CCR5 availability, whether naturally occurring or inhibitor-created, is not, therefore, certain to drive the rapid emergence of X4 viruses, especially in the presence of the selection pressure that may normally suppress these viruses.

Recent evidence that X4 variants can sometimes evolve in R5 HIV-1-infected SCID-hu mice treated with derivatives of the chemokine CCR5-ligand RANTES may not be predictive for clinical therapeutics with plausible CCR5 inhibitors (84). Firstly, human immune system engraftment in these animals was limited to peripheral lymphocytes and not lymphoid tissues; secondly, RANTES can positively enhance the replication of X4 viruses through mechanisms unique to that molecule (85). More relevant information may come from primate studies and carefully monitored human clinical trials. In practice, any HIV-1 entry inhibitor, whether co-receptor targeted or otherwise, would be combined with existing reverse transcriptase and protease inhibitors. The greater the overall suppression of HIV-1 replication, the slower is the rate of emergence of phenotypic variants or other escape mutants.

Co-receptor inhibitors would interdict a previously undisturbed segment of the viral life cycle. Given recent demonstrations of both viral resistance and persistent provirus in the face of currently employed antiretroviral drug regimens, the careful clinical assessment of HIV-1 entry inhibitors is urgently needed (68). However, the ultimate challenge of slowing and then eradicating HIV-1 infection worldwide will only be feasible once an effective and low-cost HIV-1 preventive vaccine is developed. Targeting the specific mechanism of HIV-1 entry into host cells via CD4 and the chemokine receptors that serve as coreceptors is an attractive approach that has shown early promise for both therapeutic and vaccine development (86-90).

ACKNOWLEDGMENTS

The views and opinions expressed herein are those of the authors and do not purport to reflect the official policy or position of the U.S. Army or the Department of Defense.

REFERENCES

1. Dalgleish, A. G., P. C. Beverley, P. R. Clapham, D. H. Crawford, M. F. Greaves, and R. A. Weiss. 1984. The CD4 (T4) antigen is an essential component of the receptor for the AIDS retrovirus. Nature. 312:763-767.
2. Maddon, P. J., D. R. Littman, M. Godfrey, D. E. Maddon, L. Chess, and R. Axel. 1985. The isolation and nucleotide sequence of a cDNA encoding the T cell surface protein T4: a new member of the immunoglobulin gene family. Cell. 42:93-104.
3. Maddon, P. J., A. G. Dalgleish, J. S. McDougal, P. R. Clapham, R. A. Weiss, and R. Axel. 1986. The T4 gene encodes the AIDS virus receptor and is expressed in the immune system and the brain. Cell. 47:333-348.
4. Ashorn, P. A., E. A. Berger, and B. Moss. 1990. Human immunodeficiency virus envelope glycoprotein/CD4-mediated fusion of nonprimate cells with human cells. J Virol. 64:p2149-56.
5. Page, K. A., N. R. Landau, and D. R. Littman. 1990. Construction and use of a human immunodeficiency virus vector for analysis of virus infectivity. J Virol. 64:p5270-6.
6. Fisher, A. G., B. Ensoli, D. Looney, A. Rose, R. C. Gallo, M. S. Saag, G. M. Shaw, B. H. Hahn, and F. Wong-Staal. 1988. Biologically diverse molecular variants within a single HIV-1 isolate. Nature. 334:p444-7.
7. Cheng-Mayer, C., C. Weiss, D. Seto, and J. A. Levy. 1989. Isolates of human immunodeficiency virus type 1 from the brain may constitute a special group of the AIDS virus. Proc Natl Acad Sci U S A. 86:p8575-9.
8. Koyanagi, Y., S. Miles, R. T. Mitsuyasu, J. E. Merrill, H. V. Vinters, and I. S. Chen. 1987. Dual infection of the central nervous system by AIDS viruses with distinct cellular tropisms. Science. 236:819-22.
9. Gartner, S., P. Markovits, D. M. Markovitz, M. H. Kaplan, R. C. Gallo, and M. Popovic. 1986. The role of mononuclear phagocytes in HTLV-III/LAV infection. Science. 233:215-219.
10. Liu, Z. Q., C. Wood, J. A. Levy, and C. Cheng-Mayer. 1990. The viral envelope gene is involved in macrophage tropism of a human immunodeficiency virus type 1 strain isolated from brain tissue. J Virol. 64:p6148-53.
11. O'Brien, W. A., Y. Koyanagi, A. Namazie, J. Q. Zhao, A. Diagne, K. Idler, J. A. Zack, and I. S. Chen. 1990. HIV-1 tropism for mononuclear phagocytes can be determined by regions of gp120 outside the CD4-binding domain. Nature. 348:69-73.
12. Cocchi, F., A. L. De Vico, A. Garzino-Demo, S. K. Arya, R. C. Gallo, and P. Lusso. 1995. Identification of RANTES, MIP-1 alpha, and MIP-1 beta as the major HIV-suppressive factors produced by CD8+ T cells. Science. 270:1811-5.

13. Cocchi, F., A. L. De Vico, A. Garzino-Demo, A. Cara, R. C. Gallo, and P. Lusso. 1996. The V3 domain of the HIV-1 gp120 envelope glycoprotein is critical for chemokine-mediated blockade of infection. Nature Medicine. 2:1244-7.
14. Paxton, W. A., S. R. Martin, D. Tse, T. R. O'Brien, J. Skurnick, N. L. VanDevanter, N. Padian, J. F. Braun, D. P. Kotler, S. M. Wolinsky, and R. A. Koup. 1996. Relative resistance to HIV-1infection of CD4 lymphocytes from persons who remain uninfected despite multiple high risk exposures. Nature Medicine. 2:412-417.
15. Feng, Y., C. Broder, P. E. Kennedy, and E. A. Berger. 1996. HIV-1 entry cofactor: functional cDNA cloning of a seven-transmembrane G protein-coupled receptor. Science. 272:872-877.
16. Sampson, M., O. Labbe, C. Mollereau, G. Vassart, and M. Parmentier. 1996. Molecular cloning and functional expression of a new human CC-chemokine receptor gene. Biochemistry. 35:3362-3367.
17. Dragic, T., V. Litwin, G. P. Allaway, S. R. Martin, Y. Huang, K. A. Nagashima, C. Cayanan, P. J. Maddon, R. A. Koup, J. P. Moore, and W. A. Paxton. 1996. HIV-1 entry in to CD4+ cells is mediated by the chemokine receptor CC-CKR-5. Nature. 381:667-673.
18. Deng, H., R. Liu, W. Ellmeier, S. Choe, D. Unutmaz, M. Burkhart, P. Di Marzio, S. Marmon, R. E. Sutton, C. M. Hill, C. B. Davis, S. C. Peiper, T. J. Schall, D. R. Littman, and N. R. Landau. 1996. Identification of a major co-receptor for primary isolates of HIV-1. Nature. 381:661-666.
19. Alkhatib, G., C. Combadiere, C. C. Broder, Y. Feng, P. E. Kennedy, P. M. Murphy, and E. A. Berger. 1996. CC CKR5: A RANTES, MIP-1a, MIP-1ß receptor as a fusion cofactor for macrophage-tropic HIV-1. Science. 272:1955-1958.
20. Choe, H., M. Farzan, Y. Sun, N. Sullivan, B. Rollins, P. D. Ponath, L. Wu, C. R. Mackay, G. LaRosa, W. Newman, N. Gerard, C. Gerard, and J. Sodroski. 1996. The beta-chemokine receptors CCR3 and CCR5 facilitate infection by primary HIV-1 isolates. Cell. 85:1135-48.
21. Doranz, B. J., J. Rucker, Y. Yi, R. J. Smyth, M. Samson, S. C. Peiper, M. Parmentier, R. G. Collman, and R. W. Doms. 1996. A dual-tropic primary HIV-1 isolate that uses fusin and the beta-chemokine receptors CKR-5, CKR-3, and CKR-2b as fusion cofactors. Cell. 85:1149-58.
22. Sampson, M., F. Libert, B. L. Doranz, J. Rucker, C. Liesnard, C.-M. Farber, S. Saragosti, C. Lapoumeroulie, J. Cognaux, C. Forceille, G. Muyldermans, C. Verhofstede, G. Burtonboy, M. George, T. Imai, S. Rana, Y. Yi, R. J. Smyth, R. G. Collman, R. W. Doms, G. Vassart, and M. Parmentier. 1996. Resistance to HIV-1 infection in caucasian individuals bearing mutant alleles of the CCR-5 chemokine receptor gene. Nature. 382:722-725.
23. Liu, R., W. A. Paxton, S. Choe, D. Ceradini, S. R. Martin, R. Horuk, M. E. MacDonald, H. Stuhlmann, R. A. Koup, and N. R. Landau. 1996. Homozygous defect in HIV-1 coreceptor accounts for resistance of some multiply-exposed individuals to HIV-1 infection. Cell. 86:367-377.
24. Michael, N. L. 1999. Host genetic influences on HIV-1 pathogenesis. Curr Opin Immunol. 11:p466-74.
25. Bleul, C. C., M. Farzan, H. Choe, C. Parolin, I. Clark-Lewis, J. Sodroski, and T. A. Springer. 1996. The lymphocyte chemoattractant SDF-1 is a ligand for LESTER/fusin and blocks HIV-1 entry. Nature. 382:829-832.

26. Berson, J. F., D. Long, G. J. Doranz, J. Rucker, F. R. Jirik, and R. W. Doms. 1996. A seven-transmembrane domain receptor involved in fusion and entry of T-cell-tropic human immunodeficiency virus type 1 strains. J. Virol. 70:6288-6295.
27. Choe, H., M. Farzan, Y. Sun, N. Sullivan, B. Rollins, P. D. Ponath, L. Wu, C. R. Mackay, G. LaRosa, W. Newman, N. Gerard, C. Gerard, and J. Sodroski. 1996. The ß-chemokine receptors CCR3 and CCR5 facilitate infection by primary HIV-1 isolates. Cell. 85:1135-1148.
28. Fenyo, E. M., M. L. Morfeldt, F. Chiodi, B. Lind, A. von Gegerfelt, J. Albert, E. Olausson, and B. Asjo. 1988. Distinct replicative and cytopathic characteristics of human immunodeficiency virus isolation. J Virol. 62:4414-4419.
29. Tersmette, M., J. M. A. Lang, R. E. Y. de Goede, F. de Wolf, J. K. Eeftink-Schattenkerk, P. T. Schellekens, R. A. Coutinho, J. G. Huisman, J. Goudsmit, and F. Miedema. 1989. Association between biological properties of human immunodeficiency virus variants and risk for AIDS and AIDS mortality. Lancet. 1:983-985.
30. Arthos, J., A. Rubbert, R. L. Rabin, C. Cicala, E. Machado, K. Wildt, M. Hanbach, T. D. Steenbeke, R. Swofford, J. M. Farber, and A. S. Fauci. 2000. CCR5 signal transduction in macrophages by human immunodeficiency virus and simian immunodeficiency virus envelopes. [In Process Citation]. J Virol. 74:p6418-6424.
31. Berger, E. A., R. W. Doms, E.-M. Fenyo, B. T. M. Korber, D. R. Littman, J. P. Moore, Q. J. Sattentau, H. Schuitemaker, J. Sodroski, and R. A. Weiss. 1998. A new classification for HIV-1. Nature. 391.
32. Connor, R. I., K. E. Sheridan, D. Ceradini, S. Choe, and N. R. Landau. 1997. Change in coreceptor use correlates with disease progression in HIV-1 infected individuals. J. Exp. Med. 185:621-628.
33. Dittmar, M. T., A. McKnight, G. Simmons, P. R. Clapham, R. A. Weiss, and P. Simmonds. 1997. HIV-1 tropism and co-receptor use [letter]. Nature. 385:495-6.
34. Chesebro, B., K. Wehrly, J. Nishio, and S. Perryman. 1996. Mapping of independent V3 envelope determinants of human immunodeficiency virus type 1 macrophage tropism and syncytium formation in lymphocytes. J Virol. 70:9055-9.
35. Cheng-Mayer, C., R. Liu, N. R. Landau, and L. Stamatatos. 1997. Macrophage tropism of human immunodeficiency virus type 1 and utilization of the CC-CKR5 coreceptor. J Virol. 71:1657-61.
36. Rana, S., G. Besson, D. G. Cook, J. Rucker, R. J. Smyth, Y. Yi, J. D. Turner, H.-H. Guo, J.-G. Du, S. C. Peiper, E. Lavi, M. Samson, F. Libert, C. Liesnard, G. Vassart, R. W. Doms, M. Parmentier, and R. G. Collman. 1997. Role of CCR5 in infection of primary macrophages and lymphocytes by M-tropic strains of HIV: resistance to patient-derived and prototype isolates resulting from the ccr5 mutation. J. Virol. 71:3219-3227.
37. He, J., Y. Chen, M. Farzan, H. Choe, A. Ohagen, S. Gartner, J. Busciglio, X. Yang, W. Hofmann, W. Newman, C. R. Mackay, J. Sodroski, and D. Gabuzda. 1997. CCR3 and CCR5 are coreceptors for HIV-1 infection of microglia. Nature. 385:645-9.
38. Albright, A. V., J. T. Shieh, T. Itoh, B. Lee, D. Pleasure, M. J. O'Connor, R. W. Doms, and F. Gonzalez-Scarano. 1999. Microglia express CCR5, CXCR4, and CCR3, but of these, CCR5 is the principal coreceptor for human immunodeficiency virus type 1 dementia isolates. J Virol. 73:p205-13.
39. Sallusto, F., C. R. Mackay, and A. Lanzavecchia. 1997. Selective expression of the eotaxin receptor CCR3 by human T helper 2 cells. Science. 277:p2005-7.

40. Gerber, B. O., M. P. Zanni, M. Uguccioni, M. Loetscher, C. R. Mackay, W. J. Pichler, N. Yawalkar, M. Baggiolini, and B. Moser. 1997. Functional expression of the eotaxin receptor CCR3 in T lymphocytes co-localizing with eosinophils. Curr Biol. 7:p836-43.
41. Zhang, Y., and J. P. Moore. 1999. Will multiple coreceptors need to be targeted by inhibitors of human immunodeficiency virus type 1 entry? J. Virol. 73:3443-3448.
42. Zhang, Y. J., T. Dragic, Y. Cao, L. Kostrikis, D. S. Kwon, D. R. Littman, V. N. Kewal Ramani, and J. P. Moore. 1998. Use of coreceptors other than CCR5 by non-syncytium-inducing adult and pediatric isolates of human immunodeficiency virus type 1 is rare in vitro. J Virol. 72:p9337-44.
43. Chen, Z., D. Kwon, Z. Jin, S. Monard, P. Telfer, M. S. Jones, C. Y. Lu, R. F. Aguilar, D. D. Ho, and P. A. Marx. 1998. Natural infection of a homozygous delta24 CCR5 red-capped mangabey with an R2b-tropic simian immunodeficiency virus. J Exp Med. 188:p2057-65.
44. Alkhatib, G., F. Liao, E. A. Berger, J. M. Farber, and K. W. C. Peden. 1997. A new SIV co-receptor, STRL33. Nature. 388:238.
45. Deng, H., D. Unutmaz, V. N. KewalRamani, and D. R. Littman. 1997. Expression cloning of new receptors used by simian and human immunodeficiency viruses. Nature. 388:296-300.
46. Edinger, A. L., T. L. Hoffman, M. Sharron, B. Lee, B. O'Dowd, and R. W. Doms. 1998. Use of GPR1, GPR15, and STRL33 as coreceptors by diverse human immunodeficiency virus type 1 and simian immunodeficiency virus envelope proteins. Virology. 249:p367-78.
47. Loetscher, M., A. Amara, E. Oberlin, N. Brass, D. Legler, P. Loetscher, M. D'Apuzzo, E. Meese, D. Rousset, J. L. Virelizier, M. Baggiolini, F. Arenzana-Seisdedos, and B. Moser. 1997. TYMSTR, a putative chemokine receptor selectively expressed in activated T cells, exhibits HIV-1 coreceptor function. Curr Biol. 7:p652-60.
48. Liao, F., G. Alkhatib, K. W. Peden, G. Sharma, E. A. Berger, and J. M. Farber. 1997. STRL33, A novel chemokine receptor-like protein, functions as a fusion cofactor for both macrophage-tropic and T cell line-tropic HIV-1. J Exp Med. 185:p2015-23.
49. Farzan, M., H. Choe, K. Martin, L. Marcon, W. Hofmann, G. Karlsson, Y. Sun, P. Barrett, N. Marchand, N. Sullivan, N. Gerard, C. Gerard, and J. Sodroski. 1997. Two orphan seven-transmembrane segment receptors which are expressed in CD4-positive cells support simian immunodeficiency virus infection. J Exp Med. 186:p405-11.
50. Sharron, M., S. Pöhlmann, K. Price, L. E, M. Tsang, F. Kirchhoff, R. Doms, and B. Lee. 2000. Expression and coreceptor activity of STRL33/Bonzo on primary peripheral blood lymphocytes. Blood. 96:41-49.
51. Rucker, J., A. L. Edinger, M. Sharron, M. Samson, B. Lee, J. F. Berson, Y. Yi, B. Margulies, R. G. Collman, B. J. Doranz, M. Parmentier, and R. W. Doms. 1997. Utilization of chemokine receptors, orphan receptors, and herpesvirus-encoded receptors by diverse human and simian immunodeficiency viruses. J Virol. 71:p8999-9007.
52. Horuk, R., J. Hesselgesser, Y. Zhou, D. Faulds, M. Halks-Miller, S. Harvey, D. Taub, M. Samson, M. Parmentier, J. Rucker, B. J. Doranz, and R. W. Doms. 1998. The CC chemokine I-309 inhibits CCR8-dependent infection by diverse HIV-1 strains. J Biol Chem. 273:p386-91.
53. Pleskoff, O., C. Treboute, and M. Alizon. 1998. The cytomegalovirus-encoded chemokine receptor US28 can enhance cell-cell fusion mediated by different viral proteins. J Virol. 72:p6389-97.
54. Choe, H., M. Farzan, M. Konkel, K. Martin, Y. Sun, L. Marcon, M. Cayabyab, M. Berman, M. E. Dorf, N. Gerard, C. Gerard, and J. Sodroski. 1998. The orphan seven-

transmembrane receptor apj supports the entry of primary T-cell-line-tropic and dual-tropic human immunodeficiency virus type 1. J Virol. 72:p6113-8.
55. Edinger, A. L., T. L. Hoffman, M. Sharron, B. Lee, Y. Yi, W. Choe, D. L. Kolson, B. Mitrovic, Y. Zhou, D. Faulds, R. G. Collman, J. Hesselgesser, R. Horuk, and R. W. Doms. 1998. An orphan seven-transmembrane domain receptor expressed widely in the brain functions as a coreceptor for human immunodeficiency virus type 1 and simian immunodeficiency virus. J Virol. 72:p7934-40.
56. Samson, M., A. L. Edinger, P. Stordeur, J. Rucker, V. Verhasselt, M. Sharron, C. Govaerts, C. Mollereau, G. Vassart, R. W. Doms, and M. Parmentier. 1998. ChemR23, a putative chemoattractant receptor, is expressed in monocyte-derived dendritic cells and macrophages and is a coreceptor for SIV and some primary HIV-1 strains. Eur J Immunol. 28:p1689-700.
57. Owman, C., A. Garzino-Demo, F. Cocchi, M. Popovic, A. Sabirsh, and R. C. Gallo. 1998. The leukotriene B4 receptor functions as a novel type of coreceptor mediating entry of primary HIV-1 isolates into CD4-positive cells. Proc Natl Acad Sci U S A. 95:p9530-4.
58. Faure, S., L. Meyer, D. Costagliola, C. Vaneensberghe, E. Genin, B. Autran, J. F. Delfraissy, D. H. McDermott, P. M. Murphy, P. Debre, I. Theodorou, and C. Combadiere. 2000. Rapid progression to AIDS in HIV+ individuals with a structural variant of the chemokine receptor CX3CR1. Science. 287:p2274-7.
59. Raport, C. J., J. Gosling, V. L. Schweickart, P. W. Gray, and I. F. Charo. 1996. Molecular cloning and functional characterization of a novel human CC chemokine receptor (CCR5) for RANTES, MIP-1beta, and MIP-1alpha. J Biol Chem. 271:17161-6.
60. Oberlin, E., A. Amara, F. Bachelerie, C. Bessia, J.-L. Virelizier, F. Arenzana-Seisdedos, O. Schwartz, J.-M. Heard, I. Clark-Lewis, D. F. Legier, M. Loetscher, M. Baggiolini, and B. Moser. 1996. The CXC chemokine SDF-1 is the ligand for LESTR/fusin and prevents infection by T-cell-line-adapted HIV-1. Nature. 382:833-835.
61. Wu, L., W. A. Paxton, N. Kassam, N. Ruffing, J. B. Rottman, N. Sullivan, H. Choe, J. Sodroski, W. Newman, R. A. Koup, and C. R. Mackay. 1997. CCR5 levels and expression pattern correlate with infectability by macrophage-tropic HIV-1, in vitro. J. Exp. Med. 185:1681-1691.
62. Jansson, M., M. Popovic, A. Karlsson, F. Cocchi, P. Rossi, J. Albert, and H. Wigzell. 1996. Sensitivity to inhibition by beta-chemokines correlates with biological phenotypes of primary HIV-1 isolates. Proc Natl Acad Sci U S A. 93:15382-7.
63. Farzan, M., H. Choe, K. A. Martin, Y. Sun, M. Sidelko, C. R. Mackay, N. P. Gerard, J. Sodroski, and C. Gerard. 1997. HIV-1 entry and macrophage inflammatory protein-1beta-mediated signaling are independent functions of the chemokine receptor CCR5. J Biol Chem. 272:6854-7.
64. Gosling, J., F. S. Monteclaro, R. E. Atchinson, H. Arai, C.-L. Tsou, M. A. Goldsmith, and I. F. Charo. 1997. Molecular uncoupling of C-C chemokine receptor 5-induced chemotaxis and signal transduction from HIV-1 coreceptor activity. Proc. Natl. Acad. Sci. (USA). 94:5061-5066.
65. Atchison, R. E., J. Gosling, F. S. Monteclaro, C. Franci, L. Digilio, I. F. Charo, and M. A. Goldsmith. 1996. Multiple extracellular elements of CCR5 and HIV-1 entry: dissociation from response to chemokines. Science. 274:1924-6.
66. Kinter, A., A. Catanzaro, J. Monaco, M. Ruiz, J. Justement, S. Moir, J. Arthos, A. Oliva, L. Ehler, S. Mizell, R. Jackson, M. Ostrowski, J. Hoxie, R. Offord, and A. S.

Fauci. 1998. CC-chemokines enhance the replication of T-tropic strains of HIV-1 in CD4+ T cells: Role of signal transduction. Proc.Natl.Acad.Sci.USA. 95:11880-11885.
67. Finzi, D., J. Blankson, J. D. Siliciano, J. B. Margolick, K. Chadwick, T. Pierson, K. Smith, J. Lisziewicz, F. Lori, C. Flexner, T. C. Quinn, R. E. Chaisson, E. Rosenberg, B. Walker, S. Gange, J. Gallant, and R. F. Siliciano. 1999. Latent infection of CD4+ T-cells provides a mechanism for lifelong persistence of HIV-1, even in patients on effective combination therapy. Nature Medicine. 5:512-517.
68. Kilby, J. M., S. Hopkins, T. M. Venetta, B. Di Massimo, G. A. Cloud, J. Y. Lee, L. Alldredge, E. Hunter, D. Lambert, D. Bolognesi, T. Matthews, M. R. Johnson, M. A. Nowak, G. M. Shaw, and M. S. Saag. 1998. Potent suppression of HIV-1 replication in humans by T-20, a peptide inhibitor of gp41-mediated virus entry. Nat Med. 4:p1302-7.
69. Berger, E. A. 1997. HIV entry and tropism: the chemokine receptor connection. AIDS. 11:S3-16.
70. Richman, D. D., and S. A. Bozzette. 1994. The impact of the syncytium-inducing phenotype of human immunodeficiency virus on disease progression. J Infect Dis. 169:p968-74.
71. Kimata, J. T., L. Kuller, D. B. Anderson, P. Dailey, and J. Overbaugh. 1999. Emerging cytopathic and antigenic simian immunodeficiency virus variants influence AIDS progression. Nature Medicine. 5:535-541.
72. Simmons, G., D. Wilkinson, J. D. Reeves, M. T. Dittmar, S. Beddows, J. Weber, G. Carnegie, U. Desselberger, P. W. Gray, R. A. Weiss, and P. R. Clapham. 1996. Primary, syncytium-inducing human immunodeficiency virus type 1 isolates are dual-tropic and most can use either Lestr or CCR5 as coreceptors for virus entry. J Virol. 70:p8355-60.
73. Perelson, A. S., A. U. Neumann, M. Markowitz, J. M. Leonard, and D. D. Ho. 1996. HIV-1 dynamics in vivo: virion clearance rate, infected cell life-span, and viral generation time. Science. 271:1582-6.
74. Cornelissen, M., G. Mulder-Kampinga, J. Veenstra, F. Zorgdrager, C. Kuiken, S. Hartman, J. Dekker, L. van der Hoek, C. Sol, R. Coutinho, and et al. 1995. Syncytium-inducing (SI) phenotype suppression at seroconversion after intramuscular inoculation of a non-syncytium-inducing/SI phenotypically mixed human immunodeficiency virus population. J Virol. 69:p1810-8.
75. Lathey, J. L., R. D. Pratt, and S. A. Spector. 1997. Appearance of autologous neutralizing antibody correlates with reduction in virus load and phenotype switch during primary infection with human immunodeficiency virus type 1 [letter; comment]. J Infect Dis. 175:p231-2.
76. Trkola, A., T. Ketas, V. N. Kewalramani, F. Endorf, J. M. Binley, H. Katinger, J. Robinson, D. R. Littman, and J. P. Moore. 1998. Neutralization sensitivity of human immunodeficiency virus type 1 primary isolates to antibodies and CD4-based reagents is independent of coreceptor usage. J Virol. 72:p1876-85.
77. Agace, W. W., A. Amara, A. I. Roberts, J. L. Pablos, S. Thelen, M. Uguccioni, X. Y. Li, J. Marsal, F. Arenzana-Seisdedos, T. Delaunay, E. C. Ebert, B. Moser, and C. M. Parker. 2000. Constitutive expression of stromal derived factor-1 by mucosal epithelia and its role in HIV transmission and propagation. Curr Biol. 10:p325-8.
78. Bleul, C. C., L. Wu, J. A. Hoxie, T. A. Springer, and C. R. Mackay. 1997. The HIV coreceptors CXCR4 and CCR5 are differentially expressed and regulated on human T lymphocytes. Proc Natl Acad Sci U S A. 94:1925-30.

79. Grivel, J., and L. B. Margolis. 1999. CCR5- and CXCR4-tropic HIV-1 are equally cytopathic for their T-cell targets in human lymphoid tissue. Nature Medicine. 3:344-346.
80. Dean, M., M. Carrington, C. Winkler, G. A. Huttley, M. W. Smith, R. Allikmets, J. J. Goedert, S. P. Buchbinder, E. Vittinghoff, E. Gomperts, S. Donfield, D. Vlahov, R. Kaslow, A. Saah, C. Rinaldo, R. Detels, Hemophilia Growth and. Development Study, Multicenter AIDS Cohort Study, Multicenter Hemophilia Cohort Study, San Francisco City Cohort, ALIVE Study, and S. J. O'Brien. 1996. Genetic restriction of HIV-1 infection and progression to AIDS by a deletion allele of the CKR5 structural gene. Science. 273:1856-1862.
81. Michael, N. L., J. A. Nelson, V. N. Kewal Ramani, G. Chang, S. J. O'Brien, J. R. Mascola, B. Volsky, M. Louder, G. C. White, 2nd, D. R. Littman, R. Swanstrom, and T. R. O'Brien. 1998. Exclusive and persistent use of the entry coreceptor CXCR4 by human immunodeficiency virus type 1 from a subject homozygous for CCR5 delta32. J Virol. 72:6040-7.
82. Sheppard, H. W., C. Celum, N. L. Michael, S. A. O'Brien, D. Dondero, and S. Buchbinder. HIV-1 infection in two individuals homozygous for the 32 bp CCR5 defect: Acquisition of SI virus at seroconversion. J Acquir Immune Defic Syndr:submitted.
83. Michael, N. L., G. Chang, L. G. Louie, J. R. Mascola, D. Dondero, D. L. Birx, and H. W. Sheppard. 1997. The role of viral phenotype and CCR-5 gene defects in HIV-1 transmission and disease progression. Nature Med. 3:338-40.
84. Mosier, D. E., G. R. Picchio, R. J. Guliza, R. Sabbe, P. Poignard, L. Picard, R. E. Offord, D. A. Thompson, and J. Wilken. 1999. Highly potent RANTES analogues either prevent CCR5-using human immunodeficiency virus type 1 infection in vivo or rapidly select for CXCR4-using variants. J. Virol. 73:3544-3550.
85. Gordon, C. J., M. A. Muesing, A. E. I. Proudfoot, C. A. Power, J. P. Moore, and A. Trkola. 1999. Enhancement of human immunodeficiency virus type 1 infection by the CC-chemokine RANTES Is independent of the mechanism of virus-cell fusion. J. Virol. 73:684-694.
86. Kwong, P. D., R. Wyatt, J. Robinson, R. W. Sweet, J. Sodroski, and W. A. Hendrickson. 1998. Structure of an HIV gp120 envelope glycoprotein in complex with the CD4 receptor and a neutralizing human antibody. Nature. 393:p648-59.
87. Rizzuto, C. D., R. Wyatt, N. Hernandez-Ramos, Y. Sun, P. D. Kwong, W. A. Hendrickson, and J. Sodroski. 1998. A conserved HIV gp120 glycoprotein structure involved in chemokine receptor binding. Science. 280:p1949-53.
88. Zhang, W., G. Canziani, C. Plugariu, R. Wyatt, J. Sodroski, R. Sweet, P. Kwong, W. Hendrickson, and I. Chaiken. 1999. Conformational changes of gp120 in epitopes near the CCR5 binding site are induced by CD4 and a CD4 miniprotein mimetic. Biochemistry. 38:p9405-16.
89. Mirzabekov, T., H. Kontos, M. Farzan, W. Marasco, and J. Sodroski. 2000. Paramagnetic proteoliposomes containing a pure, native, and oriented seven-transmembrane segment protein, CCR5. [In Process Citation]. Nat Biotechnol. 18:p649-654.
90. La Casse, R. A., K. E. Follis, M. Trahey, J. D. Scarborough, D. R. Littman, and J. H. Nunberg. 1999. Fusion-competent vaccines: broad neutralization of primary isolates of HIV. Science. 283:p357-62.

5

Strategies for Gene Discovery

Michael Dean
National Cancer Institute, Frederick, Maryland

COMPLEX DISEASES OVERVIEW

Nearly all diseases are believed to have a genetic component, even those caused by infectious agents or other environmental elements. The host genome may influence disease susceptibility, the rate of disease progression, the risk of specific outcomes, or the response to therapy. Identifying the genes responsible for these traits is a difficult challenge because several host genes can be involved, there may be variability in the environmental (infectious agent) exposure, and many infectious agents themselves have considerable genetic heterogeneity. Thus, determination of the role of host genetics in complex diseases requires a different strategy from that for simple inherited diseases.

The strategies used to identify genes that influence complex diseases have included sibling pair studies, twin studies, and candidate gene analysis. Sib pair studies are advantageous in that they can employ highly polymorphic microsatellite markers that are spaced evenly across the genome, and in that no knowledge of the nature of the modifying gene is required. Using this approach, loci associated with insulin dependent diabetes mellitus and other complex diseases have been identified (1). However, the sib pair approach requires the identification of at least 100-200 pairs of siblings in which one or both sibs are affected with the disease of interest (2). In addition, an individual gene must exert a fairly strong influence on the disease outcome for its linkage to the disease to be identified using the sib pair approach. Once a linked region of the genome is identified, positional cloning can isolate the causative gene and its variants. While positional cloning is usually straightforward in a simply inherited disorder, it is quite difficult in a complex disease.

Most genes involved in complex diseases have been identified as candidate genes in case control studies. In this approach variations in genes believed to play a role in the disease are tested in affected patients and in unaffected controls. Success of the candidate gene approach depends on identifying either the variant in the gene of interest that affects the phenotype (the functional variant) or an allele that is associated with the functional variant through linkage disequilibrium. Many successful association studies have been carried out using variants in the human histocompatibility (HLA) locus. Since the genes in the HLA locus are involved in multiple functions of the immune response, these genes are candidates for nearly all infectious diseases. The HLA complex has the advantage of including a large number of genes that have a high degree of polymorphism and a high degree of linkage disequilibrium.

The identification of a large number of single nucleotide polymorphisms (SNPs) across the genome, and the development of technology capable of typing large number of markers, has opened the possibility of performing genome wide scans with SNPs (3). While a genome scan for a mendelian disorder can be accomplished with 300 microsatellites (small arrays of short tandemly repeated DNA sequences) or 600 SNPs (4), it is unclear how many microsatellites and SNPs are required to conduct a linkage disequilibrium based scan for a complex disease. While some regions of the genome display linkage disequilibrium over several million base pairs of DNA, others display very little linkage disequilibrium over distances as short as 10-50 kilobases (kb) (Figure 1). A collection of 60,000 SNPs would provide an average coverage across the genome of one SNP per each 50 kb; 300,000 SNPs would provide a density of one SNP per 10 kb. Simulations of the extent of linkage disequilibrium suggest that there should be little linkage disequilibrium over regions greater than 3 kb (4). The problem with predicting the result of SNP scans, however, is that the genetic history of genomic segments varies widely, both across regions of the genome and across populations. Linkage disequilibrium tends to decay over time through recombination, but can be increased by selection, population contraction, and population admixture (mating between individuals with different genetic backgrounds). Analysis of SNP haplotypes and SNP-microsatellite haplotypes offers greatly increased power for detecting association. The HLA loci provide the most complete data, and extensive and complex patterns of linkage disequilibrium are seen over large distances (>2000 kb) in this region of chromosome 6. Because extensive selection has occurred for these polymorphisms, this region is not representative of the entire genome. However, Huttley et al. (5) have found several other regions that contain extensive linkage disequilibrium between microsatellite loci. For frequent SNPs, that tend to be old variants, there is little recurrent mutation and often less linkage disequilibrium, particularly in large outbred populations.

The genome SNP scan strategy depends on linkage disequilibrium associations between phenotype-causing variants and flanking markers. Prevailing thought is that most variants that contribute to common diseases will have a low

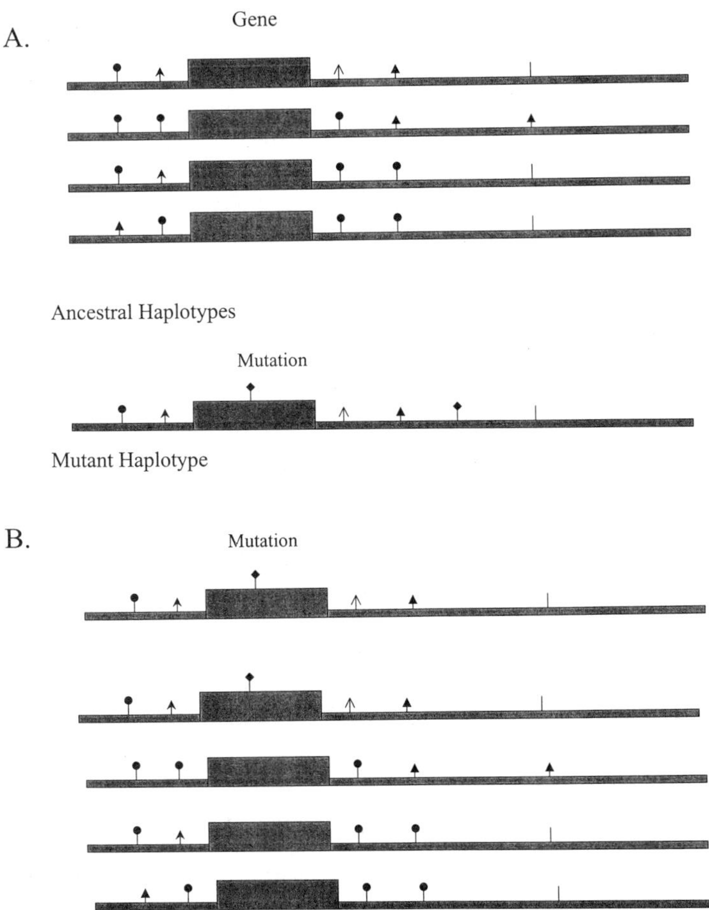

Figure 1 Linkage disequilibrium and gene mutation. Panel (A) illustrates a situation in which a recent mutation on a particular haplotype results in a perfect association between that mutation and the flanking variable sites (represented by different symbols). This association decays over time due to recombination between the mutant site and the flanking sites, and due to new mutations at the flanking variable sites. In (B) an older variant is present on a gene in a population. This variant is found on multiple haplotypes if mutation or recombination occurred after the variant arose.

relative risk and will be frequent in the population. There is certainly precedent for this theory in alleles that are already known to be associated with common disorders (Table 1). It is likely that many common alleles that cause diseases will be included in genome wide SNP searches, and if these loci are tested against the proper phenotypes, associations will be found. Alleles with frequencies greater than 0.10 and genotype relative risk (GRR) greater than 2.0 can be detected in case control studies with 700 or fewer cases (2). However, rarer alleles may potentially contribute a significant fraction of the incidence of a common disease. For example, for a disease with a population prevalence of 1%, an allele with a GRR=4 and an allele frequency of 0.01 will account for 8% of the affected individuals. Over 1000 cases would be required to find such an allele in a case control study. However, rare alleles are relatively unlikely to be found in SNP searches and many will not be used in genotyping. Thus, a very strong disequilibrium with flanking SNP alleles or haplotypes will be required to detect such alleles.

Table 1 Some alleles associated with common disorders or phenotypes.

Gene	Allele	Common Disorder	Frequency [a]	Relative Risk	Population
APOE	E4	Alzheimer's progression	0.40	3.0[b]	Caucasian
Factor V	Leiden	Deep vein thrombosis	0.02	3.3	Caucasian
HBB	HbS	P. falciparum resistance	0.15	3.0	African
FY	$FY*^{Anull}$	P. vivax resistance	0.02	2.1	Melanesia[c]
HLA	DR3, DR4	Insulin dependent diabetes	0.66	9.5	Caucasian[d]
HLA	Cw*0602	Psoriasis	0.27	8.0	Caucasian
HLA	B*27	Ankylosing spondylitis	0.10	>100	Caucasian
HLA	DR4	Rheumatoid arthritis	0.30	3-5	Caucasian, Asian
CFTR	ΔF_{508}	Pancreatitis	0.03	2.7	Caucasian
ADH2	ADH2*2	Alcoholism resistance	0.31	0.19	Asian
ALDH2	ALDH2*2	Alcoholism resistance	0.17	0.33	Asian

[a] Phenotype frequencies are presented for HLA; allele frequencies are presented for other genes.
[b] RR of homozygotes has been reported to be between 5-30.
[c] The FY[a-B-] allele is nearly fixed in many regions of Africa and *P. vivax* is not present in these areas.
[d] Several protective alleles with RR= 0.1-0.2 have been described.

DIRECT GENE ANALYSIS

Direct gene analysis is an approach that is well suited for finding rare alleles that cause diseases. In this approach DNA from affected individuals is scanned for variations in functional candidate genes. Alleles that are very rare in the population and rare even in the disease group can be detected by direct gene analysis. For instance, the sequencing of the *leptin* gene in obese individuals has identified a few subjects with a mutated *leptin* gene (6). *Leptin* was first identified as the mouse *obese* locus and thus was immediately an obvious candidate gene for human obesity. However, if *leptin* had not been found in this manner, it would have been discovered eventually through expressed sequence tag (EST) or genomic sequencing efforts. Because the leptin protein is a ligand for the receptor encoded by the mouse *diabetes* and rat *fatty* mutations (7), *leptin* would have been considered a candidate gene for obesity. Direct gene analysis would reveal mutations in the gene in a few obese individuals, and mouse knockout studies would have confirmed the gene's role in weight control.

Direct gene analysis can be considered an extension of the standard approach for identifying genes involved in mendelian disorders (Figure 2A). For simple inherited diseases, linkage analysis is used to identify a region of the genome linked to the disease locus. That region of the genome is cloned, and genes in the area become candidate genes. The candidate genes are scanned for mutations by a series of methods and the alterations identified are tested for association with the disease. In contrast, direct gene analysis (Figure 2B) begins with a candidate gene that is selected based on its potential functional relevance to the disease. Direct gene analysis is complicated by the many genes and alleles that can be tested for a given disease. One must be concerned with interpreting the statistical significance of results if multiple comparisons have been made. In addition, because human populations are sometimes complex mixtures of many subpopulations, unrecognized population differences between cases and controls that can lead to spurious associations.

The transmission disequilibrium test (TDT) (8) eliminates the problem of population substructure. The TDT uses the genetic data from parents of the affected individual to determine which allele was transmitted to the affected individual and which was not. Only parents who are heterozygous for the locus of interest are included in the analysis. The null hypothesis is that there will be an equal probability for transmission of each allele. Variants on the TDT test allow the use of siblings or other relatives instead (in addition to) of the parents (9). The disadvantage of the TDT is, of course, the need to collect specimens from relatives of the patients.

HIV RESPONSE GENES

In infectious disease epidemics, there are nearly always individual differences in the response to the pathogen. These differences may involve resistance to infection with the agent or a different disease outcome after infection (e.g., a decreased chance of survival). Epidemiologic analyses have shown that inherited factors play a significant role in the risk of mortality due to infectious agents (10). Over 30 million individuals worldwide have become infected in the HIV-1 pandemic, and although AIDS has dropped out of the top 15 causes of death in the United States,

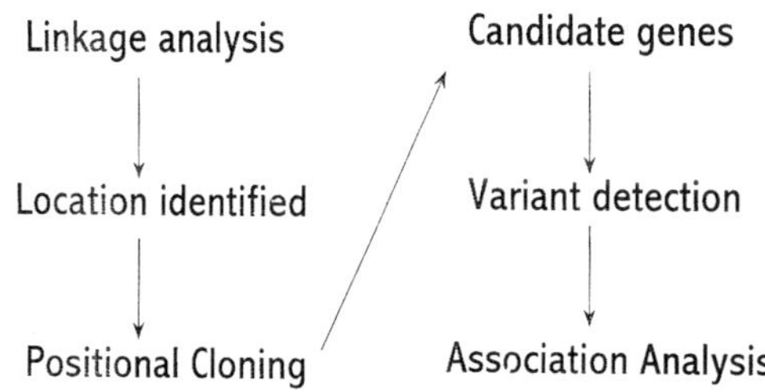

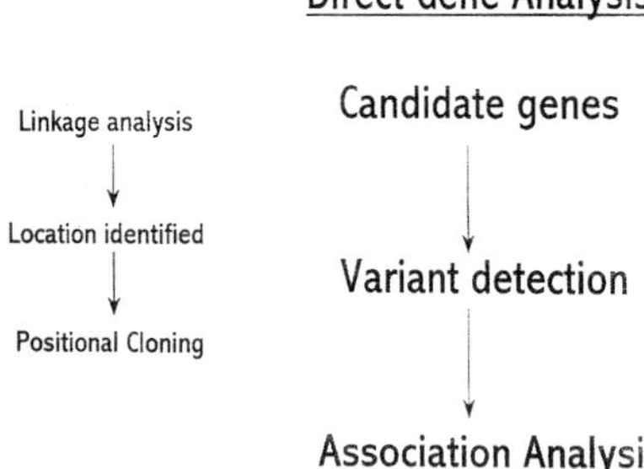

Figure 2 Gene identification. (A) The process of positional cloning is diagramed starting from linkage analysis and the identification of a locus, cloning/identifying the genes in the region (these become candidate genes), mutation detection, and association of variants with the disease. (B) In the direct gene analysis approach, functional candidate genes are tested directly for variation. It should be noted that direct gene analysis is in fact the last few steps of the positional cloning process.

the rate of infection has not dramatically declined. There is considerable heterogeneity in the response of individuals to HIV-1 (11, 12). This variation includes susceptibility to infection, progression from infection to AIDS, and the types of AIDS-defining illnesses seen in each patient. This variation suggests that differences in host genetic background may play a role in the outcome of infection, although HIV-1 shows extensive genetic variation and a rapid rate of evolution (13-15).

The demonstration that the chemokines RANTES, MIP1α, and MIP1β act as inhibitors of HIV-1 infection (16) and the discovery that chemokine receptors function as critical HIV coreceptors (reviewed in reference 17) led to intense investigation of these genes. Dragic et al. (18) observed that T lymphocytes from some HIV-1 exposed, but uninfected individuals are highly resistant to infection.

To investigate the role of alterations in the *CCR5* gene in HIV infection we amplified portions of the coding region and analyzed them by a combined single-stranded conformation polymorphism/heteroduplex analysis approach (19,20). DNA from several groups of subjects (healthy controls; people at high risk for HIV-1 who had remained uninfected; HIV-1 infected patients who had not developed AIDS; AIDS patients) were studied and several molecular genetic variants were identified. The most common alteration was a 32 bp deletion (*CCR5-Δ32*) that results in a frame-shift at amino acid 185 (21). Liu et al. (22) and Samson et al. (23) also identified the same mutation. The *CCR5-Δ32* allele results in a truncated protein that is defective both as a chemokine receptor and an HIV-1 co-receptor (24).

DNA from over 3400 participants in six cohort studies of AIDS high-risk groups (Table 2) was genotyped for this mutation. The genotype distribution of this mutation is significantly different between HIV-1-infected and uninfected subjects (OR=0.03, P<0.0001). There were 30 homozygotes for *CCR5-Δ32* observed among the individuals tested, and all but two of these were HIV-1-antibody negative individuals. As described in chapter 11, the exceptions were individuals whose earliest isolated virus exclusively utilized CXCR4 as a coreceptor, rather than CCR5 (25,26). Therefore, the *CCR5-Δ32* allele is associated with resistance to HIV-1 infection.

Survival analyses were performed for the combined cohorts comparing the *CCR5* genotypes (+/+ and +/Δ32). The results demonstrated that +/Δ32 heterozygotes have a delayed progression to AIDS compared to *CCR5* +/+ homozygotes (21,27,28). These data suggest that the *CCR5-Δ32* allele delays the progression of AIDS in HIV-infected patients, and that therapies that block CCR5 may have therapeutic benefits (29). A variant in the *CCR2* gene (*CCR2-V64I*) is also associated with delayed progression to AIDS (30,31). While the mechanism of this effect is not known, it may involve an interaction between the CCR2 and CXCR4 proteins (32). In addition, alleles in the *CCR5* promoter region are associated with more rapid progression to AIDS (33,34). Current models suggest that these alleles are associated with a higher level of CCR5 protein expression, and provide for a

Table 2 Genotype distribution for *CCR5-Δ32* in HIV uninfected and infected subjects.

	CCR5 Genotype		
	+/+	+/Δ32	Δ32/Δ32
HIV-	793 (0.80)	174 (0.17)	29 (0.03)
HIV+	1988 (0.82)	440 (0.18)	2 (0.0008)

OR=0.03, P<0.0001

Numbers of patients and frequencies, in parenthesis, are shown for homozygous normal (+/+), heterozygous, and homozygous *CCR5-Δ32* subjects. The HIV- subjects represent individuals from HIV high-risk groups (hemophiliac, homosexual, intravenous drug use), however the degree of exposure is not precisely known (adapted from ref. 21).

more rapid viral spread, but this theory has not yet been confirmed by *in vitro* studies.

FUTURE PROSPECTS

A great deal of effort in biology and biotechnology is rightly focused on common multifactorial diseases. The genetic influence on disorders such as asthma, obesity, schizophrenia, and infectious diseases has been largely unapproachable by previous technology. With the rapid advance of human genome sequencing, the characterization of large collections of SNPs, and the ongoing development of mass genotyping technology, there is much hope that the genetic basis of these disorders can be more readily understood.

Common Diseases and Rare Alleles

Most common mendelian disorders are the combined result of large numbers of rare alleles. In principle there is no reason why similar allelic heterogeneity should not contribute to multifactorial disease as well (Figure 3). If the combined RR of all alleles of a gene is 5, but no one allele has a RR of greater that 1.5, this locus may be hard to detect with flanking SNPs. For example heterozygotes for severe cystic fibrosis gene (*CFTR*) alleles are at increased risk for pancreatitis. In Northern Europeans the major *CFTR* allele (*ΔF508*) is found at a frequency of 1.5% and accounts for 70% of CF alleles. In the Ashkenazi Jewish population the frequency of *ΔF508* is lower and represents only 30% of alleles. Thus, a locus that is difficult to detect in Northern Europeans would be even harder to detect in an Ashkenazi sample.

If a disorder displays both locus heterogeneity and allelic heterogeneity then no single approach will find all of the alleles that contribute to that disease. Risch and Meritangas demonstrated that association studies are more powerful in identifying the most common and potent alleles (2). In regions where there is extensive linkage disequilibrium, less dense SNP maps will be required. However, linkage disequilibrium can make it more difficult to find the functional allele. For example, many genes are associated with HLA loci, but few are understood at the molecular level.

Whole Genome Re-sequencing

The logical extension of direct gene analysis is whole genome resequencing. Once the genome sequence is complete and the most common SNPs identified, shotgun sequencing of 5-10 affected individuals could yield a number of candidate alleles for a disease. While impractical at today's cost, sequencing technologies 100 times cheaper would make such an approach feasible.

Table 3 shows the costs of various size studies designed to identify complex disease genes, including smaller scale efforts achievable today and larger studies that will be practical in the near future. Assuming that today's lowest cost is $1 per genotype, then genotyping 1000 subjects with 10-1000 markers currently would cost $10,000 - $1,000,000. If the cost falls to $0.10 per genotype, as has been promised for the near future by several companies, a project involving 2000 subjects each typed for 5000 SNPs could be performed for $100,000. Genotyping costs need to reach the $0.01 level to make 100,000 SNP experiments conceivable. For candidate gene scanning, hundreds of genes can be scanned at today's cost, and 100-fold improvements will permit more grandiose studies. Pooling strategies in which samples are analyzed in groups of 100 or more will allow a greater

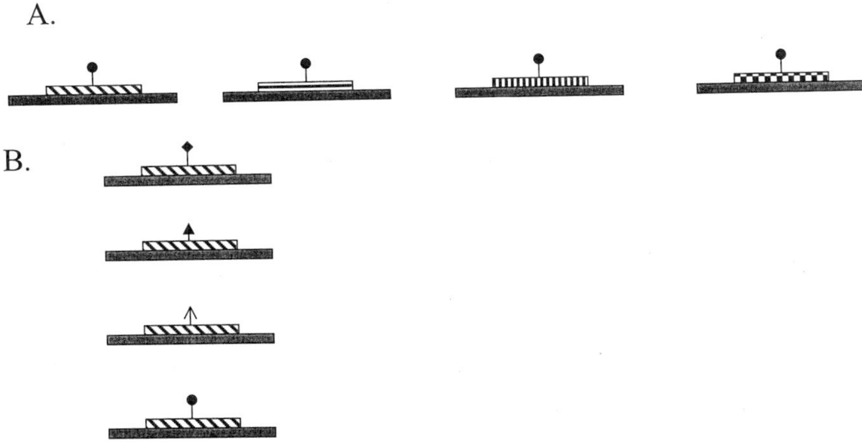

Figure 3 Locus heterogeneity and allelic heterogeneity. (A) Locus heterogeneity, variants in several genes (represented by different shading) contribute to the incidence of a complex phenotype. The frequency of these alleles, and their penetrance determines the fraction of the phenotype contributed by any one locus. (B) Allelic heterogeneity, multiple variants in the same locus contribute to a phenotype. Allelic heterogeneity is common in Mendelian disorders, and may be more common than suspected in complex disorders.

efficiency in this process and permit studies to be performed that would otherwise be impractical.

The good news is that both SNP and scanning studies that are likely to be productive are feasible at current costs. Modest projects are within the reach of academic labs and the costs of larger efforts are in line with current expenditures on positional cloning studies. Reductions in the cost of genotyping are being aggressively pursued through mass spectroscopy, microfluidics, non-PCR-based methods, and other approaches. Similar efforts for scanning, such as universal resequencing chips, multiplex DHPLC, and low cost sequencing, should keep pace with the Human Genome Project. In parallel, biology-based efforts such as non-mammalian models, rodent mutants, whole-genome expression analysis, and protein interaction technologies should improve our ability to pick the best candidate genes to screen. As with the linkage studies of the last 15-20 years, collecting properly phenotyped samples will be the most important ingredient for success in these studies.

Table 3 Costs of studies that use single nucleotide polymorphisms (SNPs) to scan the genome for association.

Sample Size	Number of SNPs	Number of Genotypes	Cost per Genotype	Total Cost
1000	10	10,000	$1.00	$10,000
1000	100	100,000	$1.00	$100,000
2000	5000	1,000,000	$1.00	$1,000,000
2000	5000	1,000,000	$0.10	$100,000
2000	100,000	200,000,000	$0.01	$2,000,000
2000	100,000	200,000,000	$0.001	$200,000

Table 4 Comparative cost of direct gene analysis and whole genome resequencing.

Sample Size	Number of Genes	Kilobases Scanned	Cost/Kilobase	Cost
100	10	3000	$7.00	$21,000
100	1000	300,000	$7.00	$2,100,000
100	1000	300,000	$1.00	$300,000
100	40,000	4,000,000	$0.10	$400,000
10	whole genome	30,000,000	$0.10	$3,000,000

CONCLUSIONS

An understanding of the biological basis for complex diseases leads to the identification of genes that can be hypothesized to play a role in a disorder. Common alleles of candidate genes (e.g., *CCR5-Δ32*) can be screened for in general population samples and rare alleles can be screened for in patient samples. This direct gene analysis approach has many advantages over pedigree-based approaches. The involvement of specific genes and variants can be tested in relatively small number of cases and controls or in disease cohorts. The direct gene analysis approach can be applied to disorders in which pedigrees are difficult to collect, such as infectious diseases (e.g., HIV infection), as well as in late-onset disorders (e.g., Alzheimer's disease, heart failure) and diseases with low penetrance (nearly all complex disorders).

Direct gene analysis may reveal rare alterations in candidate genes that provide insight into these diseases. Identification of such genes increases our understanding of the molecular basis of disease, provides further insights into the disease process, and opens up new avenues for therapy. As an example, the identification of the *CCR5-Δ32*allele as important in HIV infection and disease progression, and the finding that individuals with this allele are generally healthy has led a number of research labs and companies to begin to develop new anti-viral therapies that target this protein (see Chapter 12).

Identification of all of the genes in the human genome, and characterization of the genetic variations in those genes, provides the tools to dissect even very complex phenotypes, traits and diseases. The further development of methods for identifying and genotyping genetic variants will allow direct gene analysis to be applied to the whole human genome in the near future.

ACKNOWLEDGMENTS

The author thanks Mary Carrington for helpful discussions. The content of this publication does not necessarily reflect the views or policies of the Department of Health and Human Services, nor does mention of trade names, commercial products, or organizations imply endorsement by the U.S. government.

REFERENCES

1. Todd JA. From genome to aetiology in a multifactorial disease, type 1 diabetes. Bioessays 1999; 21:164-74.
2. Risch N, Merikangas K. The future of genetic studies of complex human diseases. Science 1996; 273:1516-1517.
3. Collins FS, Guyer MS, Charkravarti A. Variations on a theme: cataloging human DNA sequence variation. Science 1997; 278:1580-1581.

4. Kruglyak L. Prospects for whole-genome linkage disequilibrium mapping of common disease genes. Nat Genet 1999; 22:139-44.
5. Huttley GA, Smith MW, Carrington M, O'Brien SJ. A scan for linkage disequilibrium across the human genome. Genetics 1999; 152:1711-1722.
6. Ozata M, Ozdemir IC, Licinio J. Human leptin deficiency caused by a missense mutation: multiple endocrine defects, decreased sympathetic tone, and immune system dysfunction indicate new targets for leptin action, greater central than peripheral resistance to the effects of leptin, and spontaneous correction of leptin-mediated defects. J Clin Endocrinol Metab 1999; 84:3686-95.
7. Chua SC, Jr., Chung WK, Wu-Peng XS, et al. Phenotypes of mouse diabetes and rat fatty due to mutations in the OB (leptin) receptor. Science 1996; 271:994-996.
8. Spielman RS, McGinnis RE, Ewens WJ. Transmission test for linkage disequilibrium: the insulin gene region and insulin-dependent diabetes mellitus (IDDM). Am J Hum Genet 1993; 52:506-516.
9. Spielman RS, Ewens WJ. A sibship test for linkage in the presence of association: the sib transmission/disequilibrium test. Am J Hum Genet 1998; 62:450-458.
10. Sorensen TI, Nielsen GG, Anderson PK, Teasdale TW. Genetic and environmental influences on premature death in adult adoptees. New England Journal of Medicine 1988; 318:727-732.
11. Detels R. Recent scientific contributions to understanding HIV/AIDS from the Multicenter AIDS Cohort Study. J. Epidemiol 1992; 2:S11-S19.
12. Goedert JJ, Kessler DM, Aledort LM, et al. A prospective study of human immunodeficiency virus type 1 infection and the development of AIDS in subjects with hemophilia. New England Journal of Medicine 1989; 321:1141-1148.
13. Delwart EL, Shpaer EG, Louwagie J, et al. Genetic relationships determined by a DNA heteroduplex mobility assay: analysis of HIV-1 env genes. Science 1993; 262:1257-61.
14. Coffin JM. HIV population dynamics in vivo: implications for genetic variation, pathogenesis, and therapy. Science 1995; 267:483-489.
15. Wain-Hobson S. The fastest genome evolution ever described: HIV variation in situ. Curr Opin Genet Dev 1993; 3:878-83.
16. Cocchi F, DeVico AL, Garzino-Demo A, Arya SK, Gallo RC, Lusso P. Identification of RANTES, MIP-1(alpha), and MIP-1(beta) as the major HIV-suppressive factors produced by CD8+T cells. *Science* 1995; 270:1811-1815.
17. Berger EA, Murphy PM, Farber JM. Chemokine receptors as HIV-1 coreceptors: roles in viral entry, tropism, and disease. Annu Rev Immunol 1999; 17:657-700.
18. Dragic T, Litwin V, Allaway GP, et al. HIV-1 entry into CD4+ cells is mediated by the chemokine receptor CC-CKR-5. *Nature* 1996; 381:667-673.
19. White MB, Carvalho M, Derse D, O'Brien SJ, Dean M. Detecting single base substitutions as heteroduplex polymorphisms. *Genomics* 1992; 12:301-306.
20. Orita M, Suzuki Y, Sekiya T, Hayashi K. Rapid and sensitive detection of point mutations and DNA polymorphisms using the polymerase chain reaction. *Genomics* 1989; 5:874-879.
21. Dean M, Carrington M, Winkler C, et al. Genetic restriction of HIV-1 infection and progression to AIDS by a deletion allele of the CKR5 structural gene. Science 1996; 273:1856-1862.
22. Liu R, Paxton WA, Choe S, et al. Homozygous defect in HIV-1 coreceptor accounts for resistance of some multiply-exposed individuals to HIV-1 infection. *Cell* 1996; 86:367-377.

23. Samson M, Libert F, Doranz BJ, et al. Resistance to HIV-1 infection in caucasian individuals bearing mutant alleles of the CCR-5 chemokine receptor gene. *Nature* 1996; 382:722-725.
24. Benkirane M, Jin D-Y, Chun RF, Koup RA, Jeang K-T. Mechanism of Transdominant Inhibition of CCR5-mediated HIV-1 Infection by ccr5Δ32. *The Journal of Biological Chemistry* 1997; 272:30603-30606.
25. O'Brien TR, Winkler C, Dean M, et al. HIV-1 infection in a man homozygous for CCR5 delta 32. Lancet 1997; 349:1219.
26. Michael NL, Nelson JA, KewalRamani VN, et al. Exclusive and persistent use of the entry coreceptor CXCR4 by human immunodeficiency virus type 1 from a subject homozygous for CCR5 delta32. J Virol. 1998;72:6040-7.
27. de Roda Husman AM, Koot M, Cornelissen M, et al. Association between CCR5 genotype and the clinical course of HIV-1 infection. *Ann. Int. Med* 1997; 127:882-890.
28. Michael NL, Chang G, Louie LG, et al. The role of viral phenotype and CCR-5 gene defects in HIV-1 transmission and disease progression. Nat Med. 1997;3:338-40.
29. Cairns JS, D'Souza MP. Chemokines and HIV-1 second receptors: The therapeutic connection. *Nature Medicine* 1998; 4.
30. Smith MW, Dean M, Carrington M, et al. Contrasting genetic influence of *CCR2* and *CCR5* variants on HIV-1 infection and disease progression. *Science* 1997; 277:959-965.
31. Kostrikis LG, Huang Y, Moore JP, et al. A chemokine receptor CCR2 allele delays HIV-1 disease progression and is associated with a CCR5 promoter mutation. *Nature Med.* 1998; 4:350-353.
32. Mellado M, Rodriguez-Frade JM, Vila-Coro AJ, de Ana AM, Martinez AC. Chemokine control of HIV-1 infection. Nature 1999; 400:723-724.
33. Martin MP, Dean M, Smith MW, et al. Genetic acceleration of AIDS progression by a promoter variant of CCR5. Science 1998; 282:1907-1911.
34. Mummidi S, Ahuja SS, Gonzalez E, et al. Genealogy of the CCR5 locus and chemokine system gene variants associated with altered rates of HIV-1 disease progression. Nat Med 1998; 4:786-93.

6

Human Genetic Variability and Susceptibility to Infectious Diseases

Laurent Abel
INSERM U550, Necker Medical School, Paris, France

INTRODUCTION

The profound influence of the genetic makeup of the host on resistance to infections has been established in experiments on animals (1,2) in which disease phenotypes, environmental factors, and mating can be controlled. Furthermore, the recent development of gene knockout, mutant, and transgenic mice has advanced the genetic analysis of complex traits involved in susceptibility and resistance to infectious pathogens (2,3). One important result of these developments was the isolation of the *Lsh/Ity/Bcg* gene (on mouse chromosome 1) which controls innate susceptibility to several intracellular pathogens [reviewed in (2,4)]. This gene was subsequently identified and designated *Nramp1* (natural resistance associated macrophage protein 1) (5).

In humans, the role of genetic factors in infectious diseases has been suggested by several observations. One of the most important, and probably the earliest, was the very large variability in response observed among individuals who were exposed to the same infectious agent. Evidence of this variability includes: 1) a fraction of subjects exposed to certain agents never becomes infected; 2) among infected subjects, infection levels (e.g., HIV-1 RNA level) often vary greatly; 3) some infected subjects do not develop clinical evidence of disease; and 4) among symptomatic patients, clinical manifestations of disease (e.g., severity, time to onset, etc) may vary widely. Furthermore, this wide interpersonal variability often contrasts with intra-ethnic and intra-familial similarities. Familial clustering is found for most infectious diseases, raising the problem of distinguishing between environmental (i.e., shared exposures that increase the risk of infection) and genetic causes of familial aggregation. Twin studies, demonstrating higher disease concordance rates among monozygotic twins compared to dizygotic twins, have helped estimate the genetic contribution to susceptibility for many infectious diseases (detailed below in the malaria, tuberculosis, and leprosy sections). The specific methods of genetic epidemiology (6) can be used to further investigate this genetic contribution and to identify the main genes involved in the control of infectious disease related phenotypes.

GENETIC EPIDEMIOLOGY METHODS

Methods that combine epidemiological and genetic information are often used to initially identify genes that influence the expression of complex human traits, such as infectious disease related phenotypes (6-8). Epidemiological data include measured risk factors that could influence the trait under study (e.g., factors influencing exposure to the infectious agent, age). Genetic information includes the familial relationship between study subjects (e.g., collections of families) and the typing of genetic markers. Recent developments, such as the establishment of a genetic map of the human genome based on highly polymorphic markers (9) and the growing availability of single nucleotide polymorphisms (SNPs) located within candidate genes (10,11), have created fundamental tools for these genetic studies.

The ultimate goal of genetic epidemiology is to identify genes (and the polymorphisms of these genes) that significantly influence the phenotype under study, as well as possible interactions of these genes with environmental factors. To achieve this goal, numerous methods have been (and are being) developed. The respective advantages and disadvantages of these methods are described in the following paragraphs. These methods generally fall into two categories: linkage studies, which seek to locate a chromosomal region that segregates non-randomly with the phenotype of interest within families; and association studies, which test for a statistical association between a specific genetic polymorphism and a phenotype within a population (Figure 1) (8,12). There is no single optimal strategy to investigate genes involved in human infectious diseases. Consequently, the choice of a design for a particular study depends on several factors including the phenotype (nature, frequency, etc), the population, the capacity to measure environmental factors accurately, and the known genetic background information.

Linkage Studies

In the analysis of complex traits such as infectious diseases, linkage studies designed to locate chromosomal regions containing genes of interest may focus on a few candidate regions or use a genome-wide search. The whole genome approach ensures that all major loci involved in the control of a phenotype are identified and provides the opportunity to discover new major genes (and, consequently,

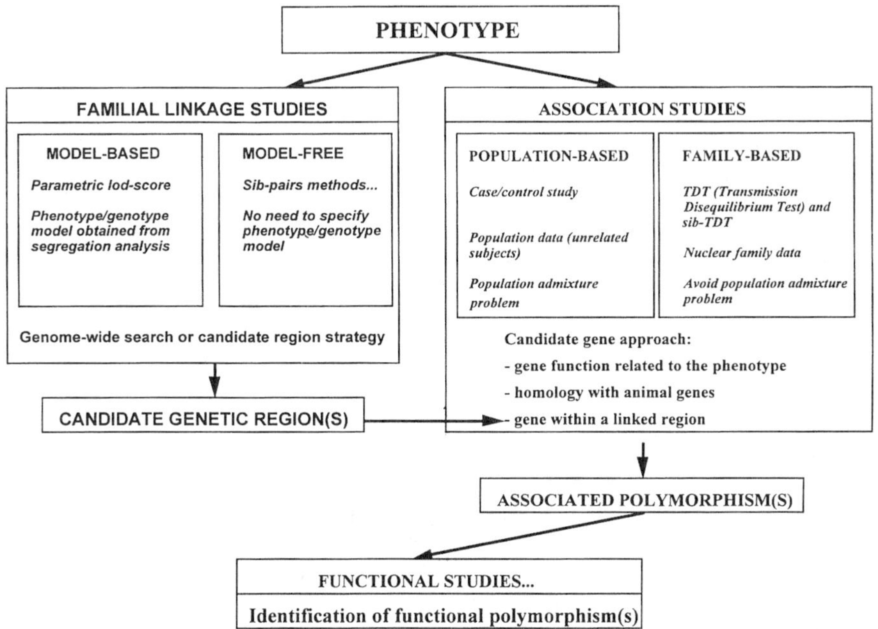

Figure 1 Summary of genetic epidemiology methods used to identify genes and genetic polymorphisms involved in human infectious diseases. Linkage studies locate a chromosomal region that segregates nonrandomly with the infectious disease related phenotype within families. Model-based linkage analysis requires a defined model, which is usually provided by segregation analysis. Model-free linkage approaches are used when little is known about this model. Successful linkage analyses identify a chromosomal region that may contain hundreds of genes. The role of polymorphisms of candidate genes located within a region can be tested in population-based or family-based association studies. Candidate genes may also be identified on the basis of their function or their homology with animal loci. Evidence for an association should be validated by functional studies which examine whether the detected polymorphism modifies gene expression or the gene product in a manner that can affect susceptibility to the disease.

pathophysiologic pathways) that were not previously suspected of contributing to a phenotype. Unlike the analysis of simple monogenic diseases, fine mapping of genes of interest for complex infectious phenotypes cannot be expected from linkage studies. When successful, linkage analyses generally identify regions of about 10-20 centiMorgans (a centiMorgan is a unit of genetic distance that corresponds to about 1,000,000 bases on the human genome) that may contain hundreds of genes. Linkage studies, which are performed on familial data, are classically divided into parametric and nonparametric approaches (8,13).

Parametric linkage methods

Parametric, or model-based, linkage analysis uses the classical lod (logarithm of the odds) score method as a statistical measure of the evidence for linkage (14). Parametric linkage methods require a defined model specifying the relationship between the phenotype and factors that may influence its expression, mainly a putative gene with two alleles (d, D) and other relevant factors. For the example of a clinical phenotype (affected/unaffected), this model should specify the frequency of the deleterious allele (D), the probability that an individual with given genotype (dd, Dd, or DD) and covariate characteristics (e.g., age and history of exposure to the infectious agent) will be affected.

The genetic information required for this phenotype/genotype model is generally provided by segregation analysis, which uses family data to determine the mode of inheritance of a given phenotype. The aim of segregation analysis is to discriminate between factors that may cause familial resemblance in an effort to test for the existence of a major gene that affects the phenotype. The term "major gene" does not mean that only one gene is involved in the expression of the phenotype, but that, among a set of involved genes, at least one gene has an effect important enough to be distinguished from the other genes. For a binary clinical phenotype (e.g., affected or not), this effect can be expressed in terms of relative risks (e.g., the ratio of the probability of being affected given a DD genotype to the probability of being affected given a dd genotype). For a quantitative phenotype (e.g. infection levels), this effect is measured by the proportion of the phenotypic variance explained by the major gene (the heritability due to the gene).

When there is evidence for a major gene, parametric linkage analysis allows one to confirm and locate this gene (denoted below as the phenotype locus). This method tests whether the phenotype locus co-segregates in families with genetic markers of known chromosomal location (13). Linkage with the phenotype locus can be tested marker by marker (two-point analysis) or by considering a set of linked markers (multi-point analysis). In a parametric linkage analysis, as in a segregation analysis, all inferences for individual genotypes at the phenotype locus are made from the individual phenotypes and the specified phenotype/genotype model. When this model is well defined, the lod-score approach is the most powerful linkage method. However, an incorrect phenotype/genotype model can lead to severe loss of power to detect linkage (and, therefore, false exclusion of the region containing the phenotype locus) and to an inaccurate estimation of the recombination fraction (i.e., the genetic distance) between the phenotype locus and the marker locus (15). Nevertheless, an incorrect phenotype/genotype model does not affect the robustness of the method (i.e., it does not lead to false conclusions in favor of linkage) as long as only one phenotype/genotype model is tested. The use of several phenotype/genotype models requires a correction for multiple testing and the same problem occurs when multiple markers are tested. Guidelines have been proposed to adapt lod score thresholds to the context of a genome-wide search (16). Another problem arises when marker data are missing for some family members. In this case, linkage analysis depends on estimates of marker allele frequencies. Inaccurate allele frequency data can affect both the power and the robustness of the method. The problems of multiple marker testing and errors in marker allele frequencies are also common to nonparametric methods.

Nonparametric linkage methods

Nonparametric, or model-free, linkage approaches (allele sharing methods such as sib-pair studies) allow one to locate the genetic factors influencing a phenotype without specifying the phenotype/genotype model. Therefore, these methods are strongly recommended when little is known about this model (i.e., when segregation analysis has not been performed or when a major gene model cannot be clearly inferred from segregation analysis). The general principle of model-free linkage analyses is to test whether or not relatives who have a certain phenotypic resemblance (e.g., affected relatives) share more marker alleles that are identical by descent (IBD) than expected under random segregation. IBD alleles are identical because they have been inherited from the same common ancestor.

The most commonly used nonparametric linkage analysis approach is the sib-pair method. Two sibs can share 0, 1, or 2 parental alleles IBD at any locus, and the respective proportions of this IBD sharing under random segregation are simply 0.25, 0.5, and 0.25. When the clinical phenotype under study can be classified as either affected or unaffected, the method tests whether affected sib-pairs share more parental alleles than would be expected randomly. A simple χ^2 test can be used to examine this allele sharing, particularly when all parental marker data are known. Maximum likelihood methods have also been developed to analyze affected sib-pair data [i.e., maximum likelihood score (17) and maximum likelihood binomial approach (18)], and these methods can lead to more powerful statistical tests. When the phenotype under study is quantitative, these tests examine whether sib-pairs having close phenotype values share more alleles IBD than sib-pairs that having more distant values. This approach is the basis of the classical method developed by Haseman and Elston (19), which regresses the squared difference of the sib-pair phenotypes on the expected proportion of alleles shared IBD by the sib-pair. Other recent methodological developments for model-free linkage studies are implemented in popular packages such as MAPMAKER/SIBS (20) and GENEHUNTER (21), but these advances will not be detailed here. Model-free methods share the same problems as parametric linkage analysis with respect to missing parental marker data and testing multiple markers. In particular, significance levels of statistical tests should be adapted to the number of comparisons that are being made and confirmatory studies are required to verify suggested linkages.

Association studies

Classical association studies are population-based case-control and cohort studies in which the frequency of a given allele is compared among unrelated affected (cases) and unaffected (controls) subjects (6,7). As an example, we will consider a situation in which there are two loci, denoted as G and M, each of which contains a single nucleotide polymorphism (SNP). G has two alleles, G_1 and G_2; G_1 is the functional polymorphism that increases the risk of disease (G_1 may be understood as the deleterious allele D described previously). M, which also has two alleles (M_1 and M_2), is the SNP that has been genotyped and which will be tested as a marker. Association studies examine the role of a particular allele of M, such as allele M_1 (in the case of a two allele marker, testing M_1 or M_2 would be equivalent). Allele M_1 is said to be associated with the phenotype under study if it is found at a significantly higher or lower frequency in cases compared to controls. This comparison is usually made with a simple 2x2 contingency table. The simplest explanation for the association between M_1 and the phenotype is that allele M_1 itself is the functional polymorphism G_1 itself (i.e., M and G are the same locus). A more likely explanation is that M_1 has no direct role in determining the phenotype, but is in linkage disequilibrium with allele G_1.

Linkage disequilibrium is the nonrandom association of alleles at linked loci. Two conditions must be fulfilled for M_1 and G_1 to be in linkage disequilibrium. First, there must be linkage between M and G (i.e., M and G lie close to one on the same chromosome, often within the same gene). Second, allele M_1 must be preferentially associated with allele G_1 (i.e., the frequency of the M_1-G_1 haplotype exceeds that which would be expected given the respective frequencies of M_1 and G_1). A classical explanation for linkage disequilibrium is that many people who bear the disease causing allele (G_1) inherited that allele from a single common ancestor who bore the M_1-G_1 haplotype. It should be noted that linkage alone (fulfillment of condition one), even very close linkage, does not lead to association, and that the absence of association does not exclude linkage. Therefore, in the candidate gene approach, association studies are most useful for considering markers that lie within a gene that has a known relationship with the phenotype or for considering markers that are in close linkage with such a gene.

Finally, an association between a marker allele and a phenotype may be an artifact due to population admixture. For example, if a case-control study is conducted in a population that is a mixture of two sub-populations, allele M_1 will be positively associated with the disease if one of the sub-populations has both a higher frequency of disease and a higher frequency of the M_1 allele.

To avoid the problem of population admixture, family-based association methods, such as the transmission disequilibrium test (TDT) (22) and the sib TDT (23), have been developed. The sampling unit in the standard TDT (22) is two parents with an affected child. Parental alleles that are not transmitted to affected children are considered control alleles. Specifically, the TDT method considers affected children who are born of parents who are heterozygous for allele M_1, (i.e., M_1M_2 parents) and tests whether or not these children have received M_1 with a probability of 0.5 (i.e., the expected value under random segregation). The TDT is a very efficient method when M_1 is the functional polymorphism G_1 itself (24). For this situation, Risch and Merikangas (24) demonstrated that the TDT was more powerful than the sib-pair method, even in the context of a theoretical genome-wide search involving 500,000 diallelic polymorphisms (5 polymorphisms per gene for a total of 100,000 genes). However, in the more common situation in which M_1 is not the same allele as G_1, the power of TDT (and that of other association study methods) is highly dependent on both the respective frequencies of M_1 and G_1, and the strength of the linkage disequilibrium between M_1 and G_1 (25,26). For these reasons, linkage methods will remain useful for identifying genes involved in infectious diseases at least until molecular resources become available for full screening of the human genome. Note also that association studies share the same problems as linkage studies with respect to multiple comparisons, and significance levels of tests must take into account the number of alleles that are examined.

HUMAN GENETICS OF INFECTIOUS DISEASES

The study of the genetics of human infectious diseases presents several advantages compared to the genetic study of other complex phenotypes and these studies also raise some other specific considerations. First, there is a known causative agent that is absolutely required for infection and the development of disease. Second, environmental factors that influence the risk of infection are generally known and can be considered in the analysis. Third, candidate genes may be chosen on the basis of the function of the gene and its known role in the response to the pathogen of interest, or by exploiting mouse-human chromosome homology and identified murine resistance loci. Fourth, several complementary traits may be examined for a given pathogen. These traits include clinical phenotypes, which may be binary (i.e., affected or unaffected) or which may measure the time to onset of disease (e.g., time from HIV infection to development of AIDS); biological measures of infection, which can be quantitative (e.g. infection intensities measured by fecal egg counts in schistosomiasis) or binary (HIV antibody seropositive/seronegative); and phenotypes that measure the immune response (antibody levels, cytokine levels, skin test response, etc). The panel of phenotypes available for a given infectious disease allows one to perform complementary studies in order to investigate the genetic control of the different steps of the pathogenic process leading to the disease itself (12). This section presents the main findings obtained in the study of human genes influencing susceptibility to parasitic, mycobacterial, and viral infections.

Parasitic Infections

With the exception of malaria, the role of host genes in susceptibility to human parasitic infections has not been readily accepted, probably because environmental factors (i.e., vectors and reservoirs) play an important role in transmission. It was also thought that the changing properties of parasites accounted for a large part of the heterogeneity observed between individuals in endemic areas. However, this view has evolved in recent years and solid evidence now indicates that intrinsic resistance to parasitic infections may vary widely between individuals. Host genetics may strongly influence the outcome of infection in major parasitic diseases such as schistosomiasis and leishmaniasis, as well as for malaria.

Malaria

Severe malaria clinical phenotype. Most genetic epidemiology studies of malaria have searched for genes involved in the severe clinical phenotype (e.g., cerebral malaria with coma or severe anemia due to *Plasmodium falciparum* infection). As this phenotype is relatively rare, familial studies are extremely difficult, and, instead, population-based association studies have been performed that compare the frequency of candidate gene polymorphisms among severe malaria cases and different types of control subjects (e.g., general population or mild malaria controls).

The existence of genetic polymorphisms that affect susceptibility to severe malaria has been suggested for more than 40 years on the basis of an increased frequency of alleles that encode mutant hemoglobin chains (e.g., sickle cell anemia) in areas that are endemic for malaria [reviewed in (27,28)]. A recent study also confirmed the protective effect of α^+-thalassemia in children living in Papua New Guinea, an area where α^+-thalassemia affects more than 90% of the population (29). A previous study in the same region showed, unexpectedly, that the incidence of malaria infections (mainly due to *P. vivax)* was increased in young children with α^+-thalassemia (30). This finding led the authors to propose that this enhanced number of infections could be due to a higher proportion of young erythrocytes in α^+-thalassemic children. Earlier infection might result in the induction of an earlier immunization against severe disease, an interpretation consistent with the subsequent findings of Allen et al. (29). Other genetic red cell variants, such as glucose-6-phosphate dehydrogenase (G6PD) deficiency, also are involved in the outcome of malaria. A recent case-control study showed that the *G6PD A-* polymorphism (the most common allele that causes G6PD deficiency in Africa) was associated with a 50% reduced risk of severe malaria for both female heterozygotes and male hemizygotes (31). Other studies have shown that erythrocytes of West Africans who are Duffy negative resist entry by *P. vivax* (32), and that Melanesian ovalocytosis with a band 3 mutation partially resist invasion by *P. vivax* and *P. falciparum* (33). However, despite the remarkable frequency of some inherited red cell polymorphisms in areas that are endemic for malaria (34), none of the polymorphisms confers absolute resistance to *P. falciparum*, which has been a major killer over the years. Thus, even though the genetic red cell variants have achieved high allele frequencies in many populations, the individual degree of protection afforded by them may be quite small (27).

Besides genetic red cell variants, the most highly studied polymorphisms for severe malaria are those located within the major histocompatibility complex (MHC). The most information about these polymorphisms comes from a case-control study in The Gambia that compared about 600 children with severe malaria (2/3 with cerebral malaria and 1/3 with severe anemia) to 1400 controls (35). An initial study reported a protective effect of *HLA-B53* (and to a lesser degree of *HLA-DRB1*1302* which is not in linkage disequilibrium with *HLA-B53*), which was found at a lower frequency among severe malaria cases (15.7%) than among different groups of controls (23-25%) (35). However, the immunological mechanism of this protection, which may relate to the activity of cytotoxic T cells against malaria liver-stage antigen epitopes (36), has been debated (37). Furthermore, the protective role of *HLA-B53* was not confirmed in a population from Kenya (38). These conflicting results may be explained by an interaction of HLA type and polymorphisms in the malaria parasite. This hypothesis is supported by a recent study showing that the distribution of variants of an antigenic epitope of *P. falciparum* that induces cytotoxic T cell response is influenced by the presence of *HLA-B35*, the most common class I antigen of the Gambian population (39).

Two other studies performed in the same population examined polymorphisms within the tumor necrosis factor alpha (*TNF*-α) promoter region. The *TNF*-α gene is a good candidate because high blood levels of TNF are observed in children with severe cerebral malaria (40). The first study analyzed the diallelic polymorphism $TNF_{-308G/-308A}$, located at position –308 base pairs relative to the transcription start site, and found an increased frequency of TNF_{-308A} homozygosity among patients with severe cerebral malaria (41). After some debate (42), it was shown that the rare TNF_{-308A} allele functions to allow higher levels of transcription of the *TNF*-α gene than the more common TNF_{-308G} allele (43). A second study investigated the role of two other SNPs within the *TNF*-α promoter, $TNF_{-238G/-238A}$, and $TNF_{-376G/-376A}$. The rare TNF_{-376A} allele augments the production of TNF by recruiting the transcription factor OCT-1 (44), but the functional role of TNF_{-238A} has not been established. It is important to note that there is complete linkage disequilibrium between TNF_{-238A} and TNF_{-376A}, (i.e., the TNF_{-376A} allele is always associated with TNF_{-238A} and the haplotype TNF_{-238G}- TNF_{-376A} does not exist). Multivariate analysis of these polymorphisms in the Gambian population showed that TNF_{-376A} was associated with an increased risk of cerebral malaria, whereas TNF_{-238A} had no effect and TNF_{-308A} (for homozygous subjects) had a borderline significant effect (44). The same analysis in a population from Kenya provided results that were more difficult to interpret. In that study, a protective effect of TNF_{-238A} appeared to be counterbalanced by the deleterious effect of TNF_{-376A}. Furthermore, the effect of TNF_{-308A} was not found in the Kenyan population. In conclusion, the roles of polymorphisms of the TNF-α promoter appear to be quite interesting and need to be refined by studies in other populations.

Associations between severe malaria and other genetic polymorphisms have also been reported. The most significant result was the association between a coding polymorphism in the gene for intercellular adhesion molecule 1 (ICAM-1), a molecule that influences the adherence of parasitised red cells to small vessel endothelium, and cerebral malaria in Kenya (45). In smaller samples, polymorphisms of the *nitric oxide synthase* gene, *NOS2*, (46,47) and the *mannose–binding lectin* gene, *MBL* (48) have been reported to be associated with severe malaria. All three of these results require replication.

Malaria biological phenotypes. A second group of genetic epidemiological studies of malaria have investigated factors involved in the control of quantitative phenotypes that measure either the intensity of infection or the immune response to the parasite. Considerable evidence suggests the role of genetic factors in the regulation of these biological phenotypes. As an example, an elegant study in Burkina Faso demonstrated clear interethnic differences in infection rates, malaria febrile episodes, and antibody response to a major *Plasmodium* surface protein. These differences were not explained by differences in malaria protective measures, socio-cultural factors, environmental exposures, or known genetic factors of resistance (49). Strong evidence for the role of genetic factors in the regulation of the immune response to plasmodial antigens also came from twin studies in which humoral and cellular responses were more concordant within monozygotic than dizygotic pairs (50). Furthermore, the comparison of dizygotic pairs showed that genes lying both within and outside of the MHC regulate these immune responses, with a greater contribution from the non-MHC genes (51).

Segregation analyses on malaria infection levels have been performed in villagers from Cameroon and Burkina Faso. Infection levels were assessed by multiple measurements of *P. falciparum* blood parasitemia and the data were adjusted for factors known to influence parasitemia, such as season, area of residence, and age of the subject. Whereas an initial study indicated that a recessive major gene controlled blood parasite levels (52), two subsequent reports found evidence for a more complex genetic mechanism (53,54). These discrepancies can be explained by factors related to the host, the parasite, and the vectorial transmission. However, all studies underlined the presence of sibling correlation and the dramatic effect of age, with children being much more heavily infected than adults. Therefore, two further linkage analyses were conducted among sib-pairs. The first analysis (55), performed in Cameroon, investigated a few candidate regions and produced evidence that suggested linkage with the 5q31-q33 region, an area previously shown to be linked to *Schistosoma mansoni* infection levels (56). The sample size of this study was too small to reach a definitive conclusion. The second sib-pair study, performed in a larger sample from Burkina Faso, confirmed the linkage of *P. falciparum* infection levels to chromosome 5q31-q33 (57). This region contains several candidate genes implicated in the regulation of the immune responses to *Plasmodium* species and in malaria pathogenesis, such as those coding for interleukin (IL)-4, IL-12, and interferon (IFN) regulatory factor. The direct role of polymorphisms located within these genes is under investigation.

Schistosomiasis

Infection levels - Schistosoma mansoni. Model-based approaches have been particularly successful in the search for susceptibility genes for human schistosomiasis. In a first step, segregation analysis in a Brazilian population showed that the intensity of infection by *S. mansoni* was controlled by a major gene (58). This gene, referred to as *SM1*, accounts for 66% of the infection intensity variance that is residual after other risk factor effects (water contact levels, age, gender) are considered. Under this major gene model, about 3% of the population are homozygous and predisposed to very high infection levels, 68% are homozygous and resistant, and 29% are heterozygous with an intermediate level of resistance. The second step of the study was to locate this gene by parametric linkage analysis using the model estimated from segregation analysis. A genome-wide search was carried out and *SM1* was mapped to human chromosome 5q31-q33 (56,59), a genetic region that contains a cluster of T helper (Th) 2-related cytokine genes such as IL-4, IL-5, and IL-9. More recently, a study performed in a Senegalese population confirmed the presence of a locus influencing *S. mansoni* infection levels on chromosome 5q31-q33 (60). Furthermore, this region has also been linked with loci related to IgE and eosinophilia production [i.e., a locus regulating IgE levels (61,62), a locus controlling bronchial hyper-responsiveness in asthma (63), and a locus involved in familia hypereosinophilia (64)].

Other data strongly support the hypothesis that differences in human susceptibility to schistosomiasis are influenced by polymorphisms in a gene controlling T-lymphocyte subset differentiation. Human resistance to schistosomiasis is regulated by lymphokines that are characteristic of Th2 subsets (65). Resistant *SM1* homozygotes mount a Th2 response against schistosomes, while susceptible *SM1* homozygotes exhibit a Th1 response (66). In addition, a segregation analysis in the Brazilian population mentioned above showed that IL-5 levels are also under the control of a major gene (67). This finding raises the possibility that this major gene plays a critical role in resistance, a view consistent with the known role of IL-5 in the defense against schistosome infections. It is also notable that a recent association study suggests that polymorphisms within the IL-4 locus may be involved in the regulation of Th1/Th2 differentiation in immune response to mycobacterial antigens (68). Association studies testing the role of polymorphisms within candidate genes in the 5q31-q33 region in human schistosomiasis are ongoing.

Severe hepatic fibrosis due to *Schistosoma mansoni*. Another trait of interest in schistosomiasis is hepatic periportal fibrosis, which occurs in 2-10% of subjects infected by *S. mansoni* in endemic regions such as Sudan. The reason why only a fraction of infected individuals develop severe disease is not known, and several observations suggest that inherited factors may play a role in the development of fibrosis (69). A segregation analysis in pedigrees from a Sudanese village (70) provided evidence for a codominant major gene (i.e., a gene for which disease frequency for heterozygous subjects differs from that for in homozygotes) that controls the development of severe hepatic fibrosis and portal hypertension. The frequency of allele D, which predisposes to advanced periportal fibrosis, was estimated to be 0.16. A 50% penetrance (i.e., disease frequency) was reached after 9, 14 and 19 years of residency in the area for DD males, DD females, and Dd heterozygous males, respectively. For other subjects, the penetrance remained lower than 0.02 after 20 years of exposure. Using this phenotype/genotype model, a parametric linkage analysis performed in four candidate regions (including the 5q31-q33 region) showed that this major locus mapped to chromosome 6q22-q23 and was closely linked to the *IFNGR1* gene encoding the ligand-binding chain for the receptor of the strongly anti-fibrogenic cytokine IFN-γ (70). Therefore, infection levels and advanced hepatic fibrosis in human schistosomiasis are controlled by distinct loci, and polymorphisms within the *IFNGR1* gene could determine severe hepatic disease due to *S. mansoni* infection. These results also suggest that the *IFNGR1* gene is a strong candidate for the control of fibrosis observed in other diseases.

Leishmaniasis

Susceptibility to leishmaniasis has been extensively studied in experimental models (71-73), and most of the identified mouse chromosomal regions carrying leishmanial susceptibility genes are homologous to corresponding regions in the human genome. Interestingly, one of these regions, which is located at the proximal end of mouse chromosome 11, is homologous to human region 5q21-q33 where *SM1* has been mapped. Other homologous human regions include 2q35 (candidate gene *NRAMP1*), 9p (candidate *Jak2 kinase*), 17q11.2-q12 (candidate gene *NOS2*), and the MHC (6p21) where the *TNF-α* gene is located (74).

In humans, classical epidemiological studies have shown familial aggregation of visceral (75,76) and mucocutaneous (77) leishmaniasis, as well as ethnic differences in both initial severity and progression of cutaneous lesions due to *Leishmania braziliensis* (78). The role of genetic factors in mucocutaneous leishmaniasis (MCL) was underlined by two recent segregation analyses. A study performed in a *L. peruviana* endemic area of Peru (79) showed that genetics played a role in controlling susceptibility to MCL and influencing the severity of the disease. This observation was confirmed in a study among families who were recently exposed to *L. braziliensis* because of migration into an endemic area in Bolivia (80). This second study provided evidence that a recessive major gene controls the onset of the primary cutaneous lesion of MCL, especially among young subjects. Therefore, host genetics may effect mechanisms involved in the development of protection from MCL during childhood. Familial linkage studies with the HLA region using parametric (81) or sib-pair (82) methods failed to show an HLA linked susceptibility locus for MCL. However, more interesting results with the MHC genes were found by association studies. The most consistent results for HLA genes were obtained with *HLA-DQ3*, which was found to be associated with *L. braziliensis* infections (81,83). Furthermore, a recent case-control study carried out in a *L. braziliensis* endemic area of Venezuela (84) has shown evidence for association between MCL and *TNF* genes. Homozygotes for an intron2/exon3 polymorphism in *TNF-β* gene had a relative risk (RR) of 7.5 for developing MCL. Homozygotes and heterozygotes for allele TNF_{-308A} of the *TNF-α* gene, which also predisposes to cerebral malaria, had a RR of 3.5. These associations with *TNF* gene polymorphisms are consistent with observations showing high circulating levels of TNF-α in patients with *L. braziliensis* infections (85) and suggest that susceptibility to MCL may be influenced by functional variants affecting TNF-α production.

Mycobacterial Infections

In humans, mycobacterial pathogenicity strongly depends on the species of the infecting mycobacterium. Tuberculosis and leprosy, the most common human mycobacterial diseases, are caused by *Mycobacterium tuberculosis*, and *M. leprae*, respectively. Numerous other mycobacterial species present in the environment, denoted as non-tuberculous mycobacteria (NTM), are generally less pathogenic, although they can cause a variety of infections under certain conditions. There is now clear evidence that the intrinsic virulence of a mycobacterial species is not the sole factor determining clinical severity and that the outcome of mycobacterial infection depends to a large extent on the genetic background of the infected subject. Many experimental studies have demonstrated the role of genetic factors in mycobacterial infections [reviewed in (1,2,4)]. As detailed below, genetic epidemiological studies have shown that human genes have an important role in the expression of leprosy and tuberculosis, although the molecular basis of this genetic control remains largely unknown. However, major advances have been made through the genetic dissection of disseminated infections caused by mycobacteria that are not usually virulent (i.e., NTM).

Leprosy

Leprosy, caused by *M. leprae*, is a chronic mycobacterial disease that affects an estimated 5-6 million persons worldwide (86). The expression of the disease results from the interactions between the bacillus and the immune system of the infected host (87). Whereas most infected individuals develop an effective immunity without disease, some develop disease manifestations along a wide spectrum that is correlated with the immunological response of the patient. At one pole of this spectrum, tuberculoid leprosy patients show well-developed specific cellular responses and low *M. leprae* antibody levels, while, at the other pole, lepromatous patients have poorly-developed specific cellular responses and high *M. leprae* antibody levels. In humans, numerous studies of familial aggregation, as well as twin studies and, more recently, segregation analyses have clearly shown that leprosy susceptibility has a significant genetic component [reviewed in (88)]. In particular, a segregation analysis performed in Desirade Island, French West Indies found evidence for the presence of a recessive major gene that controls susceptibility to leprosy *per se* [i.e., leprosy regardless of the clinically defined subtype (89)]. The frequency of the deleterious allele was estimated to be 0.3 (9% of subjects were homozygotes who were predisposed to leprosy]. By age 60, the penetrance (i.e., percentage of individuals who are phenotypically affected among persons with a given genotype) was about 0.6 for predisposed homozygotes, whereas it remained below 0.02 for other subjects.

Association studies of leprosy and HLA have provided other evidence for the role of genetic factors in diseases caused by *M. leprae*. In tuberculoid leprosy, the most consistent results were obtained for *HLA-DR2* [reviewed in (90,91)]. By using molecular typing of HLA, a recent study (92) refined these results to show a positive association between tuberculoid leprosy and two specific *DR2* alleles (*DRB1*1501* and *DRB1*1502*). Lepromatous leprosy also was associated with *HLA-DR3* in several studies [reviewed in (90,91)]. Sib-pair linkage analyses have shown a nonrandom segregation of parental HLA haplotypes both among sets of tuberculoid leprosy children and among lepromatous leprosy siblings [reviewed in (88,90,93)]. However, the random segregation of HLA haplotypes among all leprosy patients and among healthy siblings in multicase leprosy families argues against a role for HLA in susceptibility to leprosy *per se*.

The identification of the human gene *NRAMP1* (94), homologue of the mouse gene *NRAMP1*, has provided an excellent candidate gene for the study of susceptibility to leprosy *per se*. In mice, a point mutation in the *Nramp1* gene that results in a single nonconservative amino acid substitution is causally associated with susceptibility to several intracellular pathogens including *M. lepraemurium*, bacille Calmette-Guerin (BCG), and *L. donovani* (95-97). Functional studies showed that the *Nramp1* gene plays an important role early in the macrophage activation pathway and has many pleiotropic effects on macrophage function [reviewed in (98)]. In humans, a recent sib-pair study in Vietnam showed significant linkage between leprosy *per se* and *NRAMP1* haplotypes that consisted of six intragenic variants of *NRAMP1* and four polymorphic flanking markers (99). This finding yields the first evidence that *NRAMP1* could be a leprosy susceptibility locus. This study, combined with the segregation analysis performed in the same population (88), suggested a genetic heterogeneity according to the ethnic origin of the families (Vietnamese or Chinese). Genetic heterogeneity may explain, at least in part, the results of two previous reports that failed to detect linkage between leprosy and distal chromosome 2q where *NRAMP1* is located (100,101). In the same Vietnamese study, the *NRAMP1* region was also found to be linked with the *in vivo* Mitsuda reaction measuring the delayed immune response against intradermally injected lepromin (102). This latter result supports the view of Blackwell et al that *NRAMP1* can be involved in the development of immune responses to mycobacterial antigens with a putative role in the regulation of the Th1/Th2 differentiation (103). Increasing evidence indicates that tuberculoid leprosy (generally displaying positive Mitsuda reactions) is associated with a predominantly Th1 response, while a more Th2-type response is observed in lepromatous leprosy (104,105).

A recent leprosy association study in India indicates that *Vitamin D Receptor* (*VDR*) genotype may also influence this Th1/Th2 balance (106). In this study, the two alleles of a polymorphism at codon 352 of the *VDR* gene denoted as T and t (t being the less frequent) were found to be positively associated with lepromatous and tuberculoid leprosy, respectively. This finding suggests that TT homozygotes may tend to produce a Th2-type immune response and that tt homozygotes produce a Th1-type response. These results, together with the previously described observations in parasitic diseases, highlight the considerable interest in identifying the genetic factors regulating the Th1/Th2 balance in response to foreign antigens.

Tuberculosis

Tuberculosis, a chronic mycobacterial disease due to *M. tuberculosis*, affects about one third of the world's population and causes an estimated 3 million deaths each year (107). As with leprosy, the disease likely results from complex interactions between *M. tuberculosis*, environmental factors, and host genes. Among the vast number of infected persons, only 10 million people actually develop the disease each year. In humans, the role of genetic factors in tuberculosis was first suggested on the basis of strong ethnic differences, in particular a higher prevalence of the disease among blacks than among whites (108). Twin studies confirmed the importance of host genes by showing differences in concordance rates between monozygotic (~60%) and dizygotic (~20%) twins [reviewed in (75)]. Compared to leprosy, very few familial studies have been performed for tuberculosis. A segregation analysis that was performed recently in Brazil (109) found evidence for a complex genetic model involving oligogenic inheritance. A weak linkage was observed with the *NRAMP1* region in this study, but, so far, no definitive results of ongoing genome-wide linkage studies (38) have been reported.

Numerous association studies have been performed between tuberculosis and HLA alleles - the most consistent results have been obtained for class II alleles [reviewed in (38), (110)]. A recent study in The Gambia found that four *NRAMP1* variants predisposed subjects to tuberculosis. Subjects who were heterozygous for the two variants located in intron 4 (INT4) and the 3' untranslated region (3'UTR) of the gene had a particularly high risk of disease (111). In the same population, tuberculosis patients were less likely to be homozygous for allele t of the *VDR* polymorphism (described above in the leprosy section) (112). Finally, a recent study found that polymorphisms located within the genes for the IL-1 receptor antagonist and IL-1β may influence tuberculosis expression (113).

Disseminated infections with weakly pathogenic mycobacteria

Idiopathic disseminated infections with weakly pathogenic mycobacterias, such as NTM and the attenuated strain of *M. bovis* used for vaccination (BCG), are very rare and severe conditions. Familial forms of this condition, along with the high rates of parental consanguinity among affected children, strongly suggest the involvement of a recessive genetic disorder [reviewed in (114)]. Using a linkage study based on homozygosity mapping (115) in affected children from two consanguineous families, two groups located a genetic defect on chromosome region 6q22-q23, and identified mutations in the *IFNGR1* gene that encodes the IFN-γ-receptor ligand-binding chain (IFN-γR1) (116,117). In the first family, four Maltese children infected with NTM were homozygous for a nonsense mutation (116), and in the second, one child with disseminated BCG infection was homozygous for a frameshift deletion (117). Several *in vitro* experiments established the causative relationship between the presence of two mutated *IFNGR1* alleles and the impaired response to IFN-γ by the cells of these patients [reviewed in (114)]. Another child was found to be a compound heterozygote for two null *IFNGR1* mutations (118), and additional patients with complete IFN-γR1 deficiency were reported (119). Subsequently, a missense homozygous mutation causing partial, as opposed to complete, IFN-γR1 deficiency was identified in a child with tuberculoid BCG infection (120). This finding suggested a correlation between *IFNGR1* genotype and cellular, histopathological and clinical phenotypes (121). More recently, a hotspot (i.e., sequence with an abnormally high frequency of mutations) for small deletions in *IFNGR1* that confer dominant susceptibility to NTM and BCG was reported in 12 independent families (122). Homozygous mutations causing these disseminated infections have also been found in three other genes involved in IFN-γ mediated immunity. These mutations are: a null mutation in the *IFNGR2* gene, which encodes the IFN-γ receptor signalling chain (IFN-γR2) (123); a large deletion in the *IL12B* gene, which encodes the p40 subunit of IL-12 (a potent IFN-γ-inducing heterodimeric cytokine secreted by phagocytes and dendritic cells) (124); and several mutations in the *IL12RB1* gene, which encodes the β1 subunit of the IL-12 receptor (IL-12Rβ1) that is expressed on NK and T cells (125,126).

These genetically distinct, but immunologically related, disorders highlight the importance of IFN-γ mediated immunity in the control of mycobacteria infection (127). The severity of the phenotype depends on the type of genetic defect. Complete IFN-γR1 and IFN-γR2 deficiencies predispose to overwhelming infection with impaired granuloma formation in early childhood. Partial IFN-γR1 deficiency, and complete IL-12 p40 and IL-12Rβ1 deficiencies predispose to curable infection with mature granulomas at various ages. These findings provide new candidate genes for the investigation of susceptibility to tuberculosis and leprosy. An appealing hypothesis is that less severe variants of these genes may predispose to more common mycobacterial diseases. It is important to note that the elucidation of these genetic disorders has major therapeutic implications (114). IFN-γ therapy appears to be the treatment of choice for patients with IL-12 p40 or IL-12Rβ1 deficiencies, but is not likely to be effective in children with complete IFN-γR1 and IFN-γR2 deficiencies (for whom bone marrow transplantation is probably the treatment of choice).

Viral Infections

The most important recent results with regard to genetic susceptibility and resistance to human viral infections were found in HIV-1 infection. Two main phenotypes were studied, the predisposition to infection itself (i.e., HIV-1 seronegative or seropositive) and the clinical phenotype (e.g., time to AIDS onset for HIV-1 infected patients). These findings are detailed in chapter 7 of this book and will not be described here. The present section reviews recent results obtained for another retrovirus, the human T cell leukemia/lymphoma virus type I (HTLV-I), as well as for hepatitis viruses.

HTLV-I

HTLV-I causes a lymphoproliferative malignancy called adult T-cell leukemia/lymphoma (ATLL), as well as a chronic myelopathy called tropical spastic paraparesis/HTLV-I associated myelopathy (TSP/HAM) (128). Three modes of transmission are recognized for HTLV-I: mother-to-child (through breast-feeding), sexual, and intravenous. Several arguments strongly suggest that host genetic factors are involved in susceptibility to HTLV-I infection, as well as in the development of HTLV-I associated diseases. Familial aggregation of HTLV-I seropositive individuals in endemic areas such as Japan, the Caribbean and South America (128-132) raises the problem of distinguishing familial exposure factors from genetic factors. Furthermore, mother-to-child transmission of HTLV-I occurs in only 15% to 20% of children born who are born of infected mothers, despite similar exposure to HTLV-I infection in infected and uninfected children (129,133). Recently a segregation analysis was performed using familial data from two villages in French Guiana where HTLV-I infection seroprevalence is ~10%. The investigators found evidence for a dominant major gene that predisposes to HTLV-I infection (133a). Under a phenotype/genotype model that considered expected familial correlation due to the transmission routes of the virus, as well as other risk factors for infection (e.g., age and gender), about 1.5% of the population was predicted to be highly predisposed to HTLV-I infection. Under this model, almost all HTLV-I infections among children <15 years born of seropositive mothers were attributable to genetic makeup, whereas most new infections among adults were not. As ATLL is highly associated with infection through breast-feeding (134,135) and exhibits familial aggregation (136,137), investigation of the possible role of this gene in the development of ATLL will be of major interest. Linkage studies are ongoing to identify this gene.

Familial aggregation is also exhibited for the HTLV-I-associated pathologies ATLL (136,137) and TSP/HAM (138,139). Several association studies have shown that persons who develop ATLL or TSP/HAM have a different HLA distribution than healthy carriers of HTLV-I in Japanese (140,141) and Black populations (142). Jeffery et al recently showed that the class I allele *HLA-A*02* strongly protected against TSP/HAM in Japanese subjects, whereas *HLA-DRB1*0101* increased the risk of TSP/HAM in the absence of *HLA-A*02* (143). Among healthy HTLV-I carriers, those with the *HLA-A*02+* allele had a lower proviral load than those with the *HLA-A*02-* allele. Overall, the results of Jeffery et al. suggest that MHC class I-restricted cytotoxic T lymphocytes can reduce the proviral load of HTLV-I and, consequently, the risk of TSP/HAM.

Hepatitis virus

Several association studies have examined the role of host genetics in infection with hepatitis B (HBV) virus or hepatitis C (HCV) virus. The most consistent results have been observed between HBV persistence and HLA class II alleles. The *HLA-DRB1*1302* allele was shown to be associated with protection from chronic HBV infection in Gambian (144) and Caucasian (145) populations. This protective role was not found in a recent study conducted in a smaller sample of adult African American subjects (146) that instead reported an association of HBV persistence with alleles *DQA1*0501* and *DQB1*0301*. Furthermore, this latter study, as well as a previous one performed in Gambia (147), showed that HBV persistence was associated with HLA class II homozygosity. This heterozygote advantage, which has also been observed for HLA class I alleles in delaying progression towards AIDS (148), may be explained by a greater number of HLA-viral antigen combinations (149). Associations between chronic HBV infection and several other genetic variants have been reported, such as a mutation of the *mannose-binding protein* gene (150), the $TNF_{-238G/-238A}$ polymorphism of the TNF-α promoter (151), and the t/T polymorphism at codon 352 of the *VDR* gene (112).

The influence of HLA class II alleles in chronic HCV infection has also been investigated in numerous studies [reviewed in (38,152)]. Two independent studies performed in Caucasian populations (152,153) found remarkably concordant results for the role of *DRB1*11* and *DQB1*0301* alleles, which were highly associated with clearance of circulating HCV. As these two alleles are in strong linkage disequilibrium, their respective influence (or the role of another linked polymorphism) remains to be determined more precisely.

CONCLUSION

The essential tools for identifying genes that influence human infectious diseases have been developed recently. These tools include genetic epidemiology methods, a dense human genetic map, and a growing number of candidate genes identified on the basis of their function or location (through linkage results or homology with mouse resistance loci). Progress in the genetic dissection of infectious diseases will also come from the complementary analysis of different phenotypes (clinical, intensity of infection, immunological) for the same infectious agent. At this point, there is strong evidence that genetic factors play a major role in most infectious diseases, but the molecular basis of genetic susceptibility and resistance remains largely unknown, except for some rare Mendelian disorders such as disseminated mycobacterial infections. It is likely that several distinct genes and several functional polymorphisms within the same gene influence the outcome for many infectious agents. This situation raises methodological problems due to interaction and linkage disequilibrium between intragenic variants, as observed for the *TNF-α* gene in cerebral malaria (44) and the *CCR5-CCR2* complex in AIDS (154). This tremendous challenge will require new analytical strategies. We cannot yet fully appreciate how genetic information will modify our approach to the prevention and treatment of infectious diseases. However, the identification of susceptibility/resistance genes in malaria, schistosomiasis, mycobacterial, and HIV infections has already opened new avenues for understanding pathogenic mechanisms, screening genetically predisposed subjects, designing vaccines, and developing novel drugs.

REFERENCES

1. D Wakelin, JM Blackwell. Genetics of resistance to bacterial and parasitic infection. London: Taylor & Francis, 1988.
2. R McLeod, E Buschman, LD Arbuckle, E Skamene. Immunogenetics in the analysis of resistance to intracellular pathogens. Curr Opin Immunol 7: 539-552, 1995.
3. JH Nadeau, LD Arbuckle, E Skamene. Genetic dissection of inflammatory responses. J Inflamm 45: 27-48, 1995.
4. JM Blackwell, CH Barton, JK White, TI Roach, MA Shaw, SH Whitehead, BA Mock, S Searle, H Williams, AM Baker. Genetic regulation of leishmanial and mycobacterial infections: the Lsh/Ity/Bcg gene story continues. Immunol Lett 43: 99-107, 1994.
5. SM Vidal, D Malo, K Vogan, E Skamene, P Gros. Natural resistance to infection with intracellular parasites: isolation of a candidate for Bcg. Cell 73: 469-485, 1993.
6. MJ Khoury, TH Beaty, BH Cohen. Fundamentals of genetic epidemiology. New York: Oxford University Press, 1993.
7. ES Lander, NJ Schork. Genetic dissection of complex traits. Science 265: 2037-2048, 1994.
8. L Abel, AJ Dessein. Genetic epidemiology of infectious diseases in humans: design of population-based studies. Emerg Infect Dis 4: 593-603, 1998.
9. C Dib, S Faure, C Fizames, D Samson, N Drouot, A Vignal, P Millasseau, S Marc, J Hazan, E Seboun, M Lathrop, G Gyapay, J Morissette, J Weissenbach. A comprehensive genetic map of the human genome based on 5,264 microsatellites. Nature 380: 152-154, 1996.
10. DG Wang, JB Fan, CJ Siao, A Berno, P Young, R Sapolsky, G Ghandour, N Perkins, E Winchester, J Spencer, L Kruglyak, L Stein, L Hsie, T Topaloglou, E Hubbell, E Robinson, M Mittmann, MS Morris, N Shen, D Kilburn, J Rioux, C Nusbaum, S Rozen, TJ Hudson, ES Lander, et al. Large-scale identification, mapping, and genotyping of single- nucleotide polymorphisms in the human genome. Science 280: 1077-1082, 1998.
11. L Kruglyak. Prospects for whole-genome linkage disequilibrium mapping of common disease genes. Nat Genet 22: 139-144, 1999.
12. L Abel, AJ Dessein. The impact of host genetics on susceptibility to human infectious diseases. Curr Opin Immunol 9: 509-516, 1997.
13. J Ott. Analysis of human genetic linkage. Baltimore: Johns Hopkins University Press, 1991.
14. NE Morton. Sequential tests for the detection of linkage. Am J Hum Genet 7: 277-318, 1955.
15. F Clerget-Darpoux, C Bonaiti-Pellie, J Hochez. Effects of misspecifying genetic parameters in lod score analysis. Biometrics 42: 393-399, 1986.

16. E Lander, L Kruglyak. Genetic dissection of complex traits: guidelines for interpreting and reporting linkage results. Nat Genet 11: 241-247, 1995.
17. N Risch. Linkage strategies for genetically complex traits. III. The effect of marker polymorphism on analysis of affected relative pairs. Am J Hum Genet 46: 242-253, 1990.
18. L Abel, B Muller-Myhsok. Robustness and power of the maximum-likelihood-binomial and maximum- likelihood-score methods, in multipoint linkage analysis of affected- sibship data. Am J Hum Genet 63: 638-647, 1998.
19. JK Haseman, RC Elston. The investigation of linkage between a quantitative trait and a marker locus. Behav Genet 2: 3-19, 1972.
20. L Kruglyak, ES Lander. Complete multipoint sib-pair analysis of qualitative and quantitative traits. Am J Hum Genet 57: 439-454, 1995.
21. L Kruglyak, MJ Daly, MP Reeve-Daly, ES Lander. Parametric and nonparametric linkage analysis: a unified multipoint approach. Am J Hum Genet 58: 1347-1363, 1996.
22. RS Spielman, RE McGinnis, WJ Ewens. Transmission test for linkage disequilibrium: the insulin gene region and insulin-dependent diabetes mellitus (IDDM). Am J Hum Genet 52: 506-516, 1993.
23. RS Spielman, WJ Ewens. A sibship test for linkage in the presence of association: the sib transmission/disequilibrium test. Am J Hum Genet 62: 450-458, 1998.
24. N Risch, K Merikangas. The future of genetic studies of complex human diseases. Science 273: 1516-1517, 1996.
25. B Muller-Myhsok, L Abel. Genetic analysis of complex diseases. Science 275: 1328-1329, 1997.
26. L Abel, B Muller-Myhsok. Maximum-likelihood expression of the transmission/disequilibrium test and power considerations. Am J Hum Genet 63: 664-667, 1998.
27. DJ Weatherall. Common genetic disorders of the red cell and the 'malaria hypothesis'. Ann Trop Med Parasitol 81: 539-548, 1987.
28. RL Nagel, EF Roth, Jr. Malaria and red cell genetic defects. Blood 74: 1213-1221, 1989.
29. SJ Allen, A O'Donnell, ND Alexander, MP Alpers, TEA Peto, JB Clegg, DJ Weatherall. alpha+-Thalassemia protects children against disease caused by other infections as well as malaria. Proc Natl Acad Sci USA 94: 14736-14741, 1997.
30. TN Williams, K Maitland, S Bennett, M Ganczakowski, TE Peto, CI Newbold, DK Bowden, DJ Weatherall, JB Clegg. High incidence of malaria in alpha-thalassaemic children. Nature 383: 522-525, 1996.
31. C Ruwende, SC Khoo, RW Snow, SN Yates, D Kwiatkowski, S Gupta, P Warn, CE Allsopp, SC Gilbert, N Peschu, et al. Natural selection of hemi- and heterozygotes for G6PD deficiency in Africa by resistance to severe malaria. Nature 376: 246-249, 1995.
32. LH Miller, SJ Mason, DF Clyde, MH McGinniss. The resistance factor to *Plasmodium vivax* in blacks. The Duffy-blood- group genotype, FyFy. N Engl J Med 295: 302-304, 1976.
33. P Jarolim, J Palek, D Amato, K Hassan, P Sapak, GT Nurse, HL Rubin, S Zhai, KE Sahr, SC Liu. Deletion in erythrocyte band 3 gene in malaria-resistant Southeast Asian ovalocytosis. Proc Natl Acad Sci USA 88: 11022-11026, 1991.
34. LH Miller. Impact of malaria on genetic polymorphism and genetic diseases in Africans and African Americans. Proc Natl Acad Sci USA 91: 2415-2419, 1994.

35. AV Hill, CE Allsopp, D Kwiatkowski, NM Anstey, P Twumasi, PA Rowe, S Bennett, D Brewster, AJ McMichael, BM Greenwood. Common west African HLA antigens are associated with protection from severe malaria. Nature 352: 595-600, 1991.
36. AV Hill, J Elvin, AC Willis, M Aidoo, CE Allsopp, FM Gotch, XM Gao, M Takiguchi, BM Greenwood, AR Townsend, et al. Molecular analysis of the association of HLA-B53 and resistance to severe malaria. Nature 360: 434-439, 1992.
37. A Dieye, C Rogier, JF Trape, JL Sarthou, D P. HLA class I-associated resistance to severe malaria: a parasitological re-assessment. Parasitol today 13: 48-49, 1997.
38. AV Hill. The immunogenetics of human infectious diseases. Annu Rev Immunol 16: 593-617, 1998.
39. SC Gilbert, M Plebanski, S Gupta, J Morris, M Cox, M Aidoo, D Kwiatkowski, BM Greenwood, HC Whittle, AV Hill. Association of malaria parasite population structure, HLA, and immunological antagonism. Science 279: 1173-1177, 1998.
40. D Kwiatkowski, AV Hill, I Sambou, P Twumasi, J Castracane, KR Manogue, A Cerami, DR Brewster, BM Greenwood. TNF concentration in fatal cerebral, non-fatal cerebral, and uncomplicated *Plasmodium falciparum* malaria. Lancet 336: 1201-1204, 1990.
41. W McGuire, AV Hill, CE Allsopp, BM Greenwood, D Kwiatkowski. Variation in the TNF-alpha promoter region associated with susceptibility to cerebral malaria. Nature 371: 508-510, 1994.
42. AE Goldfeld, EY Tsai. TNF-alpha and genetic susceptibility to parasitic disease. Exp Parasitol 84: 300-303, 1996.
43. AG Wilson, JA Symons, TL McDowell, HO McDevitt, GW Duff. Effects of a polymorphism in the human tumor necrosis factor alpha promoter on transcriptional activation. Proc Natl Acad Sci USA 94: 3195-3199, 1997.
44. JC Knight, I Udalova, AV Hill, BM Greenwood, N Peshu, K Marsh, D Kwiatkowski. A polymorphism that affects OCT-1 binding to the TNF promoter region is associated with severe malaria. Nat Genet 22: 145-150, 1999.
45. D Fernandez-Reyes, AG Craig, SA Kyes, N Peshu, RW Snow, AR Berendt, K Marsh, CI Newbold. A high frequency African coding polymorphism in the N-terminal domain of ICAM-1 predisposing to cerebral malaria in Kenya. Hum Mol Genet 6: 1357-1360, 1997.
46. D Burgner, W Xu, K Rockett, M Gravenor, IG Charles, AV Hill, D Kwiatkowski. Inducible nitric oxide synthase polymorphism and fatal cerebral malaria. Lancet 352: 1193-1194, 1998.
47. JF Kun, B Mordmuller, B Lell, LG Lehman, D Luckner, PG Kremsner. Polymorphism in promoter region of inducible nitric oxide synthase gene and protection against malaria. Lancet 351: 265-266, 1998.
48. AJ Luty, JF Kun, PG Kremsner. Mannose-binding lectin plasma levels and gene polymorphisms in *Plasmodium falciparum* malaria. J Infect Dis 178: 1221-1224, 1998.
49. D Modiano, V Petrarca, BS Sirima, I Nebie, D Diallo, F Esposito, M Coluzzi. Different response to *Plasmodium falciparum* malaria in west African sympatric ethnic groups. Proc Natl Acad Sci USA 93: 13206-13211, 1996.
50. K Sjoberg, JP Lepers, L Raharimalala, A Larsson, O Olerup, NT Marbiah, M Troye-Blomberg, P Perlmann. Genetic regulation of human anti-malarial antibodies in twins. Proc Natl Acad Sci USA 89: 2101-2104, 1992.

51. A Jepson, W Banya, F Sisay-Joof, M Hassan-King, C Nunes, S Bennett, H Whittle. Quantification of the relative contribution of major histocompatibility complex (MHC) and non-MHC genes to human immune responses to foreign antigens. Infect Immun 65: 872-876, 1997.
52. L Abel, M Cot, L Mulder, P Carnevale, J Feingold. Segregation analysis detects a major gene controlling blood infection levels in human malaria. Am J Hum Genet 50: 1308-1317, 1992.
53. A Garcia, M Cot, JP Chippaux, S Ranque, J Feingold, F Demenais, L Abel. Genetic control of blood infection levels in human malaria: evidence for a complex genetic model. Am J Trop Med Hyg 58: 480-488, 1998.
54. P Rihet, L Abel, Y Traore, T Traore-Leroux, C Aucan, F Fumoux. Human malaria: segregation analysis of blood infection levels in a suburban area and a rural area in Burkina Faso. Genet Epidemiol 15: 435-450, 1998.
55. A Garcia, S Marquet, B Bucheton, D Hillaire, M Cot, N Fievet, AJ Dessein, L Abel. Linkage analysis of blood *Plasmodium falciparum* levels: interest of the 5q31-q33 chromosome region. Am J Trop Med Hyg 58: 705-709, 1998.
56. S Marquet, L Abel, D Hillaire, H Dessein, J Kalil, J Feingold, J Weissenbach, AJ Dessein. Genetic localization of a locus controlling the intensity of infection by *Schistosoma mansoni* on chromosome 5q31-q33. Nat Genet 14: 181-184, 1996.
57. P Rihet, Y Traore, L Abel, C Aucan, T Traore-Leroux, F Fumoux. Malaria in humans: *Plasmodium falciparum* blood infection levels are linked to chromosome 5q31-q33. Am J Hum Genet 63: 498-505, 1998.
58. L Abel, F Demenais, A Prata, AE Souza, A Dessein. Evidence for the segregation of a major gene in human susceptibility/resistance to infection by *Schistosoma mansoni*. Am J Hum Genet 48: 959-970, 1991.
59. S Marquet, L Abel, D Hillaire, A Dessein. Full results of the genome-wide scan which localises a locus controlling the intensity of infection by *Schistosoma mansoni* on chromosome 5q31-q33. Eur J Hum Genet 7: 88-97, 1999.
60. B Muller-Myhsok, FF Stelma, F Guisse-Sow, B Muntau, T Thye, GD Burchard, B Gryseels, RD Horstmann. Further evidence suggesting the presence of a locus, on human chromosome 5q31-q33, influencing the intensity of infection with *Schistosoma mansoni*. Am J Hum Genet 61: 452-454, 1997.
61. DG Marsh, JD Neely, DR Breazeale, B Ghosh, LR Freidhoff, E Ehrlich-Kautzky, C Schou, G Krishnaswamy, TH Beaty. Linkage analysis of IL4 and other chromosome 5q31.1 markers and total serum immunoglobulin E concentrations. Science 264: 1152-1156, 1994.
62. DA Meyers, DS Postma, CI Panhuysen, J Xu, PJ Amelung, RC Levitt, ER Bleecker. Evidence for a locus regulating total serum IgE levels mapping to chromosome 5. Genomics 23: 464-470, 1994.
63. DS Postma, ER Bleecker, PJ Amelung, KJ Holroyd, J Xu, CI Panhuysen, DA Meyers, RC Levitt. Genetic susceptibility to asthma--bronchial hyperresponsiveness coinherited with a major gene for atopy. N Engl J Med 333: 894-900, 1995.
64. JD Rioux, VA Stone, MJ Daly, M Cargill, T Green, H Nguyen, T Nutman, PA Zimmerman, MA Tucker, T Hudson, AM Goldstein, E Lander, AY Lin. Familial eosinophilia maps to the cytokine gene cluster on human chromosomal region 5q31-q33. Am J Hum Genet 63: 1086-1094, 1998.
65. P Couissinier-Paris, AJ Dessein. Schistosoma-specific helper T cell clones from subjects resistant to infection by *Schistosoma mansoni* are Th0/2. Eur J Immunol 25: 2295-2302, 1995.

66. V Rodrigues Jr, K Piper, P Couissinier-Paris, O Bacelar, H Dessein, AJ Dessein. Genetic control of schistosome infections by the SM1 locus of the 5q31- q33 region is linked to differentiation of type 2 helper T lymphocytes. Infect Immun 67: 4689-4692, 1999.
67. V Rodrigues Jr, L Abel, K Piper, AJ Dessein. Segregation analysis indicates a major gene in the control of interleukine-5 production in humans infected with *Schistosoma mansoni*. Am J Hum Genet 59: 453-461, 1996.
68. JM Blackwell, GF Black, CS Peacock, EN Miller, D Sibthorpe, D Gnananandha, JJ Shaw, F Silveira, Z Lins-Lainson, F Ramos, A Collins, MA Shaw. Immunogenetics of leishmanial and mycobacterial infections: the Belem Family Study. Philos Trans R Soc Lond B Biol Sci 352: 1331-1345, 1997.
69. Q Mohamed-Ali, NE Elwali, AA Abdelhameed, A Mergani, S Rahoud, KE Elagib, OK Saeed, L Abel, MM Magzoub, AJ Dessein. Susceptibility to Periportal (Symmers) Fibrosis in Human Schistosoma mansoni Infections: Evidence That Intensity and Duration of Infection, Gender, and Inherited Factors Are Critical in Disease Progression. J Infect Dis 180: 1298-1306, 1999.
70. AJ Dessein, D Hillaire, NE Elwali, S Marquet, Q Mohamed-Ali, A Mirghani, S Henri, AA Abdelhameed, OK Saeed, MM Magzoub, L Abel. Severe hepatic fibrosis in Schistosoma mansoni infection is controlled by a major locus that is closely linked to the interferon-gamma receptor gene. Am J Hum Genet 65: 709-721, 1999.
71. JM Blackwell. Genetic susceptibility to leishmanial infections: studies in mice and man. Parasitology 112: S67-74, 1996.
72. AM Beebe, S Mauze, NJ Schork, RL Coffman. Serial backcross mapping of multiple loci associated with resistance to *Leishmania major* in mice. Immunity 6: 551-557, 1997.
73. LJ Roberts, TM Baldwin, JM Curtis, E Handman, SJ Foote. Resistance to *Leishmania major* is linked to the H2 region on chromosome 17 and to chromosome 9. J Exp Med 185: 1705-1710, 1997.
74. JM Blackwell. Genetics of host resistance and susceptibility to intramacrophage pathogens: a study of multicase families of tuberculosis, leprosy and leishmaniasis in north-eastern Brazil. Int J Parasitol 28: 21-28, 1998.
75. PE Fine. Immunogenetics of susceptibility to leprosy, tuberculosis, and leishmaniasis. An epidemiological perspective. Int J Lepr Other Mycobact Dis 49: 437-454, 1981.
76. PH Cabello, AM Lima, ES Azevedo, H Krieger. Familial aggregation of *Leishmania chagasi* infection in northeastern Brazil. Am J Trop Med Hyg 52: 364-365, 1995.
77. TC Jones, WD Johnson, Jr., AC Barretto, E Lago, R Badaro, B Cerf, SG Reed, EM Netto, MS Tada, TF Franca, et al. Epidemiology of American cutaneous leishmaniasis due to *Leishmania braziliensis braziliensis*. J Infect Dis 156: 73-83, 1987.
78. BC Walton, L Valverde. Racial differences in espundia. Ann Trop Med Parasitol 73: 23-29, 1979.
79. MA Shaw, CR Davies, EA Llanos-Cuentas, A Collins. Human genetic susceptibility and infection with *Leishmania peruviana*. Am J Hum Genet 57: 1159-1168, 1995.
80. A Alcais, L Abel, C David, ME Torrez, P Flandre, JP Dedet. Evidence for a major gene controlling susceptibility to tegumentary leishmaniasis in a recently exposed Bolivian population. Am J Hum Genet 61: 968-979, 1997.
81. ML Lara, Z Layrisse, JV Scorza, E Garcia, Z Stoikow, J Granados, W Bias. Immunogenetics of human American cutaneous leishmaniasis. Study of HLA haplotypes in 24 families from Venezuela. Hum Immunol 30: 129-135, 1991.

82. D Barbier, F Demenais, JF Lefait, B David, M Blanc, J Hors, N Feingold. Susceptibility to human cutaneous leishmaniasis and HLA, Gm, Km markers. Tissue Antigens 30: 63-67, 1987.
83. ML Petzl-Erler, MP Belich, F Queiroz-Telles. Association of mucosal leishmaniasis with HLA. Hum Immunol 32: 254-260, 1991.
84. M Cabrera, MA Shaw, C Sharples, H Williams, M Castes, J Convit, JM Blackwell. Polymorphism in tumor necrosis factor genes associated with mucocutaneous leishmaniasis. J Exp Med 182: 1259-1264, 1995.
85. M Castes, D Trujillo, ME Rojas, CT Fernandez, L Araya, M Cabrera, J Blackwell, J Convit. Serum levels of tumor necrosis factor in patients with American cutaneous leishmaniasis. Biol Res 26: 223-238, 1993.
86. SK Noordeen, L Lopez Bravo, TK Sundaresan. Estimated number of leprosy cases in the world. Bull World Health Organ 70: 7-10, 1992.
87. P Sansonetti, PH Lagrange. The immunology of leprosy: speculations on the leprosy spectrum. Rev Infect Dis 3: 422-469, 1981.
88. L Abel, DL Vu, J Oberti, VT Nguyen, VC Van, M Guilloud-Bataille, E Schurr, PH Lagrange. Complex segregation analysis of leprosy in southern Vietnam. Genet Epidemiol 12: 63-82, 1995.
89. L Abel, F Demenais. Detection of major genes for susceptibility to leprosy and its subtypes in a Caribbean island: Desirade island. Am J Hum Genet 42: 256-266, 1988.
90. W van Eden, RRP de Vries. HLA and leprosy: a reevaluation. Lepr Rev 55: 89-104, 1984.
91. TH Ottenhoff, RR de Vries. HLA class II immune response and suppression genes in leprosy. Int J Lepr Other Mycobact Dis 55: 521-534, 1987.
92. L Zerva, B Cizman, NK Mehra, SK Alahari, R Murali, CM Zmijewski, M Kamoun, DS Monos. Arginine at positions 13 or 70-71 in pocket 4 of HLA-DRB1 alleles is associated with susceptibility to tuberculoid leprosy. J Exp Med 183: 829-836, 1996.
93. W van Eden, NM Gonzalez, RR de Vries, J Convit, JJ van Rood. HLA-linked control of predisposition to lepromatous leprosy. J Infect Dis 151: 9-14, 1985.
94. M Cellier, G Govoni, S Vidal, T Kwan, N Groulx, J Liu, F Sanchez, E Skamene, E Schurr, P Gros. Human natural resistance-associated macrophage protein: cDNA cloning, chromosomal mapping, genomic organization, and tissue-specific expression. J Exp Med 180: 1741-1752, 1994.
95. D Malo, K Vogan, S Vidal, J Hu, M Cellier, E Schurr, A Fuks, N Bumstead, K Morgan, P Gros. Haplotype mapping and sequence analysis of the mouse Nramp gene predict susceptibility to infection with intracellular parasites. Genomics 23: 51-61, 1994.
96. SM Vidal, E Pinner, P Lepage, S Gauthier, P Gros. Natural resistance to intracellular infections: Nramp1 encodes a membrane phosphoglycoprotein absent in macrophages from susceptible (Nramp1 D169) mouse strains. J Immunol 157: 3559-3568, 1996.
97. G Govoni, S Vidal, S Gauthier, E Skamene, D Malo, P Gros. The Bcg/Ity/Lsh locus: genetic transfer of resistance to infections in C57BL/6J mice transgenic for the Nramp1 Gly169 allele. Infect Immun 64: 2923-2929, 1996.
98. JM Blackwell, S Searle. Genetic regulation of macrophage activation: understanding the function of Nramp1 (=Ity/Lsh/Bcg). Immunol Lett 65: 73-80, 1999.
99. L Abel, FO Sanchez, J Oberti, NV Thuc, LV Hoa, VD Lap, E Skamene, PH Lagrange, E Schurr. Susceptibility to leprosy is linked to the human NRAMP1 gene. J Infect Dis 177: 133-145, 1998.

100. MA Shaw, S Atkinson, H Dockrell, R Hussain, Z Lins-Lainson, J Shaw, F Ramos, F Silveira, SQ Mehdi, F Kaukab, et al. An RFLP map for 2q33-q37 from multicase mycobacterial and leishmanial disease families: no evidence for an Lsh/Ity/Bcg gene homologue influencing susceptibility to leprosy. Ann Hum Genet 57: 251-271, 1993.
101. G Levee, J Liu, B Gicquel, S Chanteau, E Schurr. Genetic control of susceptibility to leprosy in French Polynesia; no evidence for linkage with markers on telomeric human chromosome 2. Int J Lepr Other Mycobact Dis 62: 499-511, 1994.
102. A Alcaïs, F Sanchez, NV Thuc, VD Lap, J Oberti, PH Lagrange, E Schurr, L Abel. Granulomatous reaction to intradermal injection of lepromin (Mitsuda reaction) is linked to the human NRAMP1 gene in Vietnamese leprosy sibships. J Infect Dis 181:302-308, 2000.
103. JM Blackwell, GF Black, C Sharples, SS Soo, CS Peacock, N Miller. Roles of Nramp1, HLA, and a gene(s) in allelic association with IL-4, in determining T helper subset differentiation. Microbes Infect 1: 95-102, 1999.
104. M Yamamura, K Uyemura, RJ Deans, K Weinberg, TH Rea, BR Bloom, RL Modlin. Defining protective responses to pathogens: cytokine profiles in leprosy lesions. Science 254: 277-279, 1991.
105. N Misra, A Murtaza, B Walker, NP Narayan, RS Misra, V Ramesh, S Singh, MJ Colston, I Nath. Cytokine profile of circulating T cells of leprosy patients reflects both indiscriminate and polarized T-helper subsets: T-helper phenotype is stable and uninfluenced by related antigens of *Mycobacterium leprae*. Immunology 86: 97-103, 1995.
106. S Roy, A Frodsham, B Saha, SK Hazra, CG Mascie-Taylor, AV Hill. Association of vitamin D receptor genotype with leprosy type. J Infect Dis 179: 187-191, 1999.
107. PJ Dolin, MC Raviglione, A Kochi. Global tuberculosis incidence and mortality during 1990-2000. Bull World Health Organ 72: 213-220, 1994.
108. WW Stead, JW Senner, WT Reddick, JP Lofgren. Racial differences in susceptibility to infection by *Mycobacterium tuberculosis*. N Engl J Med 322: 422-427, 1990.
109. MA Shaw, A Collins, CS Peacock, EN Miller, GF Black, D Sibthorpe, Z Lins-Lainson, JJ Shaw, F Ramos, F Silveira, JM Blackwell. Evidence that genetic susceptibility to *Mycobacterium tuberculosis* in a Brazilian population is under oligogenic control: linkage study of the candidate genes NRAMP1 and TNFA. Tuber Lung Dis 78: 35-45, 1997.
110. AE Goldfeld, JC Delgado, S Thim, MV Bozon, AM Uglialoro, D Turbay, C Cohen, EJ Yunis. Association of an HLA-DQ allele with clinical tuberculosis. Jama 279: 226-228, 1998.
111. R Bellamy, C Ruwende, T Corrah, KP McAdam, HC Whittle, AV Hill. Variations in the NRAMP1 gene and susceptibility to tuberculosis in West Africans. N Engl J Med 338: 640-644, 1998.
112. R Bellamy, C Ruwende, T Corrah, KP McAdam, M Thursz, HC Whittle, AV Hill. Tuberculosis and chronic hepatitis B virus infection in Africans and variation in the vitamin D receptor gene. J Infect Dis 179: 721-724, 1999.
113. RJ Wilkinson, P Patel, M Llewelyn, CS Hirsch, G Pasvol, G Snounou, RN Davidson, Z Toossi. Influence of polymorphism in the genes for the interleukin (IL)-1 receptor antagonist and IL-1beta on tuberculosis. J Exp Med 189: 1863-1874, 1999.
114. F Altare, E Jouanguy, S Lamhamedi, R Doffinger, A Fischer, JL Casanova. Mendelian susceptibility to mycobacterial infection in man. Curr Opin Immunol 10: 413-417, 1998.

117. E Jouanguy, F Altare, S Lamhamedi, P Revy, JF Emile, M Newport, M Levin, S Blanche, E Seboun, A Fischer, JL Casanova. Interferon-gamma-receptor deficiency in an infant with fatal bacille Calmette-Guerin infection. N Engl J Med 335: 1956-1961, 1996.
118. F Altare, E Jouanguy, S Lamhamedi-Cherradi, MC Fondaneche, C Fizame, F Ribierre, G Merlin, Z Dembic, R Schreiber, B Lisowska-Grospierre, A Fischer, E Seboun, JL Casanova. A causative relationship between mutant IFNgR1 alleles and impaired cellular response to IFNgamma in a compound heterozygous child. Am J Hum Genet 62: 723-726, 1998.
119. SM Holland, SE Dorman, A Kwon, IF Pitha-Rowe, DM Frucht, SM Gerstberger, GJ Noel, P Vesterhus, MR Brown, TA Fleisher. Abnormal regulation of interferon-gamma, interleukin-12, and tumor necrosis factor-alpha in human interferon-gamma receptor 1 deficiency. J Infect Dis 178: 1095-1104, 1998.
120. E Jouanguy, S Lamhamedi-Cherradi, F Altare, MC Fondaneche, D Tuerlinckx, S Blanche, JF Emile, JL Gaillard, R Schreiber, M Levin, A Fischer, C Hivroz, JL Casanova. Partial interferon-gamma receptor 1 deficiency in a child with tuberculoid bacillus Calmette-Guerin infection and a sibling with clinical tuberculosis. J Clin Invest 100: 2658-2664, 1997.
121. S Lamhamedi, E Jouanguy, F Altare, J Roesler, JL Casanova. Interferon-gamma receptor deficiency: relationship between genotype, environment, and phenotype. Int J Mol Med 1: 415-418, 1998.
122. E Jouanguy, S Lamhamedi-Cherradi, D Lammas, SE Dorman, MC Fondaneche, S Dupuis, R Doffinger, F Altare, J Girdlestone, JF Emile, H Ducoulombier, D Edgar, J Clarke, VA Oxelius, M Brai, V Novelli, K Heyne, A Fischer, SM Holland, DS Kumararatne, RD Schreiber, JL Casanova. A human IFNGR1 small deletion hotspot associated with dominant susceptibility to mycobacterial infection. Nat Genet 21: 370-378, 1999.
123. SE Dorman, SM Holland. Mutation in the signal-transducing chain of the interferon-gamma receptor and susceptibility to mycobacterial infection. J Clin Invest 101: 2364-2369, 1998.
124. F Altare, D Lammas, P Revy, E Jouanguy, R Doffinger, S Lamhamedi, P Drysdale, D Scheel-Toellner, J Girdlestone, P Darbyshire, M Wadhwa, H Dockrell, M Salmon, A Fischer, A Durandy, JL Casanova, DS Kumararatne. Inherited interleukin 12 deficiency in a child with bacille Calmette-Guerin and *Salmonella enteritidis* disseminated infection. J Clin Invest 102: 2035-2040, 1998.
125. F Altare, A Durandy, D Lammas, JF Emile, S Lamhamedi, F Le Deist, P Drysdale, E Jouanguy, R Doffinger, F Bernaudin, O Jeppsson, JA Gollob, E Meinl, AW Segal, A Fischer, D Kumararatne, JL Casanova. Impairment of mycobacterial immunity in human interleukin-12 receptor deficiency. Science 280: 1432-1435, 1998.
126. R de Jong, F Altare, IA Haagen, DG Elferink, T Boer, PJ van Breda Vriesman, PJ Kabel, JM Draaisma, JT van Dissel, FP Kroon, JL Casanova, TH Ottenhoff. Severe mycobacterial and Salmonella infections in interleukin-12 receptor-deficient patients. Science 280: 1435-1438, 1998.
127. E Jouanguy, R Doffinger, S Dupuis, A Pallier, F Altare, JL Casanova. IL-12 and IFN-gamma in host defense against mycobacteria and salmonella in mice and men. Curr Opin Immunol 11: 346-351, 1999.
128. N Mueller, W Blattner. Retroviruses-Human T cell Lymphotropic Virus. In: AS Evans and RA Kaslow, eds. Viral infections of humans : epidemiology and control. New York: Plenum Medical Book Co., 1997, pp 785-814.

127. E Jouanguy, R Doffinger, S Dupuis, A Pallier, F Altare, JL Casanova. IL-12 and IFN-gamma in host defense against mycobacteria and salmonella in mice and men. Curr Opin Immunol 11: 346-351, 1999.
128. N Mueller, W Blattner. Retroviruses-Human T cell Lymphotropic Virus. In: AS Evans and RA Kaslow, eds. Viral infections of humans : epidemiology and control. New York: Plenum Medical Book Co., 1997, pp 785-814.
129. K Tajima, S Tominaga, T Suchi, T Kawagoe, H Komoda, Y Hinuma, T Oda, K Fujita. Epidemiological analysis of the distribution of antibody to adult T- cell leukemia-virus-associated antigen: possible horizontal transmission of adult T-cell leukemia virus. Gann 73: 893-901, 1982.
130. W Kajiyama, S Kashiwagi, H Ikematsu, J Hayashi, H Nomura, K Okochi. Intrafamilial transmission of adult T cell leukemia virus. J Infect Dis 154: 851-857, 1986.
131. JM Trujillo, M Concha, A Munoz, G Bergonzoli, C Mora, I Borrero, CJ Gibbs, Jr., C Arango. Seroprevalence and cofactors of HTLV-I infection in Tumaco, Colombia. AIDS Res Hum Retroviruses 8: 651-657, 1992.
132. GJ Miller, LL Lewis, SM Colman, JA Cooper, G Lloyd, N Scollen, N Jones, RS Tedder, MF Greaves. Clustering of human T lymphotropic virus type I seropositive in Montserrat, West Indies: evidence for an environmental factor in transmission of the virus. J Infect Dis 170: 44-50, 1994.
133. S Hino, H Sugiyama, H Doi, T Ishimaru, T Yamabe, Y Tsuji, T Miyamoto. Breaking the cycle of HTLV-I transmission via carrier mothers' milk. Lancet 2: 158-159, 1987.
133a. Plancoulaine S, Gessain A, Joubert M, Tortevoye P, Jeanne I, Talarmin A, de The G, Abel L. Detection of a major gene predisposing to human T lymphotropic virus type I infection in children among an endemic population of African origin. J Infect Dis. 182:405-412, 2000.
134. EL Murphy, B Hanchard, JP Figueroa, WN Gibbs, WS Lofters, M Campbell, JJ Goedert, WA Blattner. Modelling the risk of adult T-cell leukemia/lymphoma in persons infected with human T-lymphotropic virus type I. Int J Cancer 43: 250-253, 1989.
135. C Bartholomew, N Jack, J Edwards, W Charles, D Corbin, FR Cleghorn, WA Blattner. HTLV-I serostatus of mothers of patients with adult T-cell leukemia and HTLV-I-associated myelopathy/tropical spastic paraparesis. J Hum Virol 1: 302-305, 1998.
136. S Momita, S Ikeda, T Amagasaki, H Soda, Y Yamada, S Kamihira, M Tomonaga, K Kinoshita, M Ichimaru. Survey of anti-human T-cell leukemia virus type I antibody in family members of patients with adult T-cell leukemia. Jpn J Cancer Res 81: 884-889, 1990.
137. M Ichimaru, K Kinoshita, S Kamihira, S Ikeda, Y Yamada, J Suzuyama, S Momita, T Amagasaki. Familial disposition of adult T-cell leukemia and lymphoma. Hematol Oncol 4: 21-29, 1986.
138. K Kayembe, P Goubau, J Desmyter, R Vlietinck, H Carton. A cluster of HTLV-1 associated tropical spastic paraparesis in Equateur (Zaire): ethnic and familial distribution. J Neurol Neurosurg Psychiatry 53: 4-10, 1990.
139. HF Liu, AM Vandamme, K Kazadi, H Carton, J Desmyter, P Goubau. Familial transmission and minimal sequence variability of human T- lymphotropic virus type I (HTLV-I) in Zaire. AIDS Res Hum Retroviruses 10: 1135-1142, 1994.
140. K Usuku, S Sonoda, M Osame, S Yashiki, K Takahashi, M Matsumoto, T Sawada, K Tsuji, M Tara, A Igata. HLA haplotype-linked high immune responsiveness against

HTLV-I in HTLV- I-associated myelopathy: comparison with adult T-cell leukemia/lymphoma. Ann Neurol 23: S143-150, 1988.
141. S Sonoda, T Fujiyoshi, S Yashiki. Immunogenetics of HTLV-I/II and associated diseases. J Acquir Immune Defic Syndr Hum Retrovirol 13: S119-123, 1996.
142. A Manns, B Hanchard, OS Morgan, R Wilks, B Cranston, JM Nam, M Blank, M Kuwayama, S Yashiki, T Fujiyoshi, W Blattner, S Sonoda. Human leukocyte antigen class II alleles associated with human T-cell lymphotropic virus type I infection and adult T-cell leukemia/lymphoma in a Black population. J Natl Cancer Inst 90: 617-622, 1998.
143. KJ Jeffery, K Usuku, SE Hall, W Matsumoto, GP Taylor, J Procter, M Bunce, GS Ogg, KI Welsh, JN Weber, AL Lloyd, MA Nowak, M Nagai, D Kodama, S Izumo, M Osame, CR Bangham. HLA alleles determine human T-lymphotropic virus-I (HTLV-I) proviral load and the risk of HTLV-I-associated myelopathy. Proc Natl Acad Sci USA 96: 3848-3853, 1999.
144. MR Thursz, D Kwiatkowski, CE Allsopp, BM Greenwood, HC Thomas, AV Hill. Association between an MHC class II allele and clearance of hepatitis B virus in the Gambia. N Engl J Med 332: 1065-1069, 1995.
145. Hohler, G Gerken, A Notghi, R Lubjuhn, H Taheri, U Protzer, HF Lohr, PM Schneider, KH Meyer zum Buschenfelde, C Rittner. HLA-DRB1*1301 and *1302 protect against chronic hepatitis B. J Hepatol 26: 503-507, 1997.
146. CL Thio, M Carrington, D Marti, SJ O'Brien, D Vlahov, KE Nelson, J Astemborski, DL Thomas. Class II HLA alleles and hepatitis B virus persistence in African Americans. J Infect Dis 179: 1004-1006, 1999.
147. MR Thursz, HC Thomas, BM Greenwood, AV Hill. Heterozygote advantage for HLA class-II type in hepatitis B virus infection. Nat Genet 17: 11-12, 1997.
148. M Carrington, GW Nelson, MP Martin, T Kissner, D Vlahov, JJ Goedert, R Kaslow, S Buchbinder, K Hoots, SJ O'Brien. HLA and HIV-1: heterozygote advantage and B*35-Cw*04 disadvantage. Science 283: 1748-1752, 1999.
149. PC Doherty, RM Zinkernagel. Enhanced immunological surveillance in mice heterozygous at the H-2 gene complex. Nature 256: 50-52, 1975.
150. HC Thomas, GR Foster, M Sumiya, D McIntosh, DL Jack, MW Turner, JA Summerfield. Mutation of gene of mannose-binding protein associated with chronic hepatitis B viral infection. Lancet 348: 1417-1419, 1996.
151. T Hohler, A Kruger, G Gerken, PM Schneider, KH Meyer zum Buschenefelde, C Rittner. A tumor necrosis factor-alpha (TNF-alpha) promoter polymorphism is associated with chronic hepatitis B infection. Clin Exp Immunol 111: 579-582, 1998.
152. EJ Minton, D Smillie, KR Neal, WL Irving, JC Underwood, V James, and Members of the Trent Hepatitis C Virus Study Group. Association between MHC class II alleles and clearance of circulating hepatitis C virus. J Infect Dis 178: 39-44, 1998.
153. L Alric, M Fort, J Izopet, JP Vinel, JP Charlet, J Selves, J Puel, JP Pascal, M Duffaut, M Abbal. Genes of the major histocompatibility complex class II influence the outcome of hepatitis C virus infection. Gastroenterology 113: 1675-1681, 1997.
154. MP Martin, M Dean, MW Smith, C Winkler, B Gerrard, NL Michael, B Lee, RW Doms, J Margolick, S Buchbinder, JJ Goedert, TR O'Brien, MW Hilgartner, D Vlahov, SJ O'Brien, M Carrington. Genetic acceleration of AIDS progression by a promoter variant of CCR5. Science 282: 1907-1911, 1998.

7

The Role of Human Genetics in HIV-1 Infection

Maureen P. Martin and Mary Carrington
National Cancer Institute, Frederick, Maryland

INTRODUCTION

Over the last two decades HIV-1 has spread worldwide and has now surpassed malaria as the leading cause of adult infectious disease mortality (1). Studies of large cohorts of HIV-1 infected individuals have shown that the clinical course and outcome of HIV-1 infection are highly variable among individuals. Most individuals infected with HIV develop AIDS within ten years, but about 1-5% of individuals who become infected remain relatively healthy for 15 years or more (long-term nonprogressors), while others progress to AIDS within the first 2 to 3 years after infection (rapid progressors) (2-7). A small number of individuals are resistant to infection (8-10), and there is evidence that some individuals who become infected apparently eliminate the virus and are subsequently protected (11). The factors that influence disease progression are not entirely known, but probably include both viral and host factors. Host genetic variability has been a fundamental component in determining the fate of individuals exposed to several highly pathogenic microorganisms. Mutations in the *β-globin* and *duffy antigen receptor for chemokines* (*DARC*) genes have undergone positive selection in regions of Africa endemic for malaria because of their extreme protective effects against *P. falciparum* and *P. vivax*, respectively (12,13). More recently, a mutation in the chemokine receptor gene *CCR5* has been shown to provide strong protection from infection with HIV-1 (8-10), but the frequency of the genotype rendering this effect is quite low and other factors must account for the majority of protected individuals. Unlike the clear mechanisms by which genotypes of *β-globin*, *DARC*, and *CCR5,* protection against most infectious diseases is likely to involve an exceedingly complex array of host genetic effects that are complicated further by pathogen diversity.

In recent years, a growing body of evidence has accumulated pointing to the influence of host genes on HIV-1 infection and progression to AIDS These genes fall into two major groups: 1) genes that encode chemokine receptors which mediate HIV-1 cellular entry and 2) genes that regulate the immune response, particularly those encoded in the human major histocompatibility complex (MHC). Although some of these genetic effects are pronounced, most are weak and detectable only in large cohorts that are well-defined with regard to clinical parameters. These findings fulfill predictions of the complex genetic interactions between host and pathogen. This chapter will address the current evidence substantiating the influence of host genes on HIV-1 infection and disease progression.

BACKGROUND

Chemokine Receptors as HIV-1 Co-receptors

HIV-1 entry into target cells is mediated by binding of the viral envelope glycoprotein to CD4 on the target cell membrane (14,15), but CD4 expression is not sufficient for HIV-1 infection of target cells. Different HIV-1 isolates show distinct tropism for various CD4+ target cells, preferentially infecting either T cell lines or macrophages depending on usage of distinct chemokine receptors as coreceptors for infection (16-27). R5 (also referred to as M-tropic) isolates of HIV-1 primarily utilize CCR5 found on macrophages and primary CD4+ T cells, while X4 (T-tropic) isolates utilize CXCR4 found on CD4+ T cell lines and primary CD4+ T cells. The R5 isolates are the most commonly transmitted strains and are present throughout the entire course of the infection. X4 strains are rarely involved in the initial infection, but rather emerge in about 50% of infected individuals around the time that AIDS develops (23-27).

Although the vast majority of primary isolates of HIV-1 utilize either CCR5 or CXCR4 as co-receptors, and to a lesser extent CCR2 (19) and CCR3 (17), some isolates of HIV-1 are able to use other chemokine receptors in viral entry assays. These include STRL33 (28-30), GPR15 (28,29), GPR1 (29), CCR8 (31,32), and US28 (33), the last of which is encoded by cytomegalovirus. Primary HIV-2 isolates also utilize CCR5 predominantly, but have been found to utilize multiple coreceptors in vitro (34). Although only rare isolates of HIV-1 use CCR2 as a coreceptor for infection, primary isolates of SIV found in red-capped macaques efficiently use this receptor to gain entry into cells (35). CCR3 has also been shown to function as a co-receptor for some primary strains of HIV-1 (17,19) as well as HIV-2 (34). CCR3 may play a role in HIV-1 infection of microglial cells in the central nervous system (36,37), raising the possibility that use of CCR3 may correlate with neuropathogenesis of AIDS.

Just as high serum levels of MIP-1α, MIP-1β and RANTES have been shown to be associated with resistance to HIV-1 infection, these CCR5 ligands inhibit HIV-1 infection of peripheral blood mononuclear cells (PBMCs) *in vitro* by blocking viral fusion and entry (38,39). Recently, RANTES was shown to mediate cytotoxic activity of HIV-specific CD8+ T cells by binding to CCR3 (40). The cytolytic activity of CD8+ T cells is mediated by two mechanisms (41): the release of perforin which kills target cells by forming pores in their plasma membranes; and the expression of Fas ligand (FasL) which on interaction with Fas-bearing targets, induces apoptosis of these cells. Following binding of RANTES or eotaxin (the selective ligand for CCR3) to CCR3 FasL expression is upregulated on effector T cells (42). These cells are then able to induce apoptosis of virally infected cells expressing Fas, through the Fas/FasL pathway.

Cellular Immune Response to HIV-1

After becoming infected with HIV-1, individuals become acutely viremic and develop HIV-specific cytotoxic T lymphocytes (CTLs). CTLs control the viremia and infected individuals then enter a period of clinical latency that is highly variable in length (43,44). When the virus has sufficiently weakened the host immune system by destruction of the host's CD4+ T cells, the individual becomes symptomatic with the development of opportunistic infections and an increase in viral load (45).

T cell receptors on the surface of CTLs recognize viral peptides assembled in the groove of MHC class I proteins on the surface of the infected cell (46). *In vitro* studies have also demonstrated that CTLs can dramatically inhibit HIV replication (47). HIV-specific CTLs are present in high risk individuals who remain uninfected despite repeated exposures to HIV, as well as in transiently infected individuals, suggesting that these individuals have mounted a protective CTL response. A prospective study of HIV-1-exposed sex workers in Nairobi revealed that individuals who remained HIV-1 negative developed a strong CTL response to HIV-1 (11,48,49). These individuals also had HIV-1-specific IgA in genital secretions, which is absent in individuals who become seropositive (50). Several of the HIV-1-resistant women in this study were related, suggesting the possibility of protective genetic factors. Additional data indicating the importance of CTL responses in controlling HIV-1 infection was shown by depletion of CD8+ cells with an anti-CD8+ antibody *in vivo* in macaques (51,52). Under this regimen, dramatic increases in viral load occurred and recovery of CD8+ cell numbers was accompanied by a coincident decline in viral load. Anti-HIV CTLs also secrete soluble substances such as chemokines (53) and CD8+ T lymphocyte antiviral factor (CAF) (54) that can potently inhibit infection. While anti-HIV CTL responses may prolong an asymptomatic phase of HIV infection, they fail to prevent development of AIDS in most infected individuals. Viral proteins such as nef, which have been reported to down-regulate MHC class I HLA-A and –B expression (but not HLA-C) on infected cells, may play a role in evading an effective

CTL response (55,56). HIV-1 tat has also been shown to inhibit NK cell cytolytic function via the intracellular signaling pathways in these cells (57).

GENETIC EFFECTS CONTROLLING HIV-1 INFECTION AND DISEASE PROGRESSION

CCR5-Δ32

The *CCR5* gene has been mapped to the short arm of chromosome 3 within a chemokine receptor gene cluster that includes *CCR1, CCR2, CCR3, CCR4, CCR6, CCR8,* and *CX3CR1* (58-60). The *CCR5* gene became an obvious disease gene candidate for HIV-1 infection upon the discovery of CCR5 as a co-receptor for HIV-1 and screening the coding region of the gene was easily performed since it contains a single open reading frame (exon 4) of only 1,055 base pairs. A common, severe mutation characterized by a 32 base pair deletion, *CCR5-Δ32*, was rapidly identified (8-10). The deletion begins in the region encoding the third extracellular domain of CCR5, and results in a frame shift and premature stop codon in the fifth transmembrane domain. The truncated protein product is not expressed on the cell surface (9), explaining the nearly complete protection against HIV-1 infection (see Table 1), despite repeated exposures, in individuals homozygous for the mutant allele (8-10,61,62). Accordingly, peripheral blood lymphocytes (PBLs) from individuals homozygous for *CCR5-Δ32* are resistant to infection with R5 (but not X4) strains of HIV-1 *in vitro* (9,10,63,64). The normal CCR5 function appears to be dispensable, perhaps because of the redundancy of the chemokine receptor system, since individuals who are homozygous for the *CCR5-Δ32* are generally unremarkable (see Chapter 10).

Rare cases of HIV-1 infection in *CCR5-Δ32/Δ32* homozygotes have been reported (65-70) in spite of the strong protection afforded by this genotype, suggesting that rare isolates of HIV-1 may use other chemokine receptors to initiate infection. X4 isolates were identified in serum from one of these patients relatively soon after seroconversion (71), suggesting the potential for X4 isolates to initiate viral infection under some conditions. Despite an early decline in CD4+ T cell numbers, this subject did not show rapid progression to disease symptoms (71), as is usually the case with the switch to the X4 viral phenotype.

Table 1 *CCR5-Δ32* genotype distribution. Data updated from those reported in Ref. 8.

	+/+ (%)	+/*Δ32* (%)	*Δ32/Δ32* (%)
HIV-	793 (80)	174 (17)	29 (3)
HIV+	1988 (82)	440 (18)	2 (0.08)

OR=0.03, p<0.0001

Individuals who are heterozygous for the normal (+) and *CCR5-Δ32* alleles (*+/Δ32*) are not protected from infection, but they show slower progression to AIDS (by 2-4 years on average) after HIV-1 seroconversion, and there is an increased frequency of this genotype among long-term non-progressors (8,61,62,72). The average amount of cell surface expression of CCR5 is lower on PBMCs from *+/Δ32* individuals than on cells from individuals homozygous for the normal *CCR5* allele (73). Rather than simply a gene dosage effect, formation of CCR5-Δ32/CCR5 heterocomplexes causes normal CCR5 to be retained in the endoplasmic reticulum,resulting in reduced cell surface expression of the normal molecule (74). Accordingly, *CCR5-Δ32* heterozygotes demonstrate impaired R5 HIV-1 replication *in vitro*, and reduced virus load *in vivo* (62,72,75).

The *+/Δ32* genotype is also associated with protection against AIDS-related non-Hodgkin's B cell lymphoma (76,77). B cells express CCR5 on their cell surfaces and the CCR5 ligand RANTES, which is increased in HIV-1 infected individuals, is mitogenic for B cells (77). A reduced response to mitogenic stimulation by RANTES in *CCR5-Δ32* heterozygotes could provide a basis for the lower frequency of lymphoma in *+/Δ32* individuals. A somewhat reduced frequency of *CCR5-Δ32* among patients with AIDS dementia complex has also been reported (78), suggesting that *CCR5-Δ32* heterozygosity may protect against the development of this condition. Finally, *CCR5-Δ32* may be associated with an improved response to antiretroviral therapy (79) and reduced risk of toxoplasmosis (80). Thus, the effects of *CCR5-Δ32* are quite broad, and it is clear that this mutation has the most significant impact on disease progression of any genetic factor identified to date.

Additional *CCR5* Polymorphisms

The *CCR5-Δ32* mutation is estimated to have occurred ~700-2000 years ago (81,82) and since then it has increased to an allele frequency of 15% in some regions of Northern Europe (81,83). This rapid increase in frequency over a relatively short period of time suggests that *CCR5-Δ32* has been subject to positive selection. Recently, Lalani et al. (84) reported evidence that poxviruses can use several chemokine receptors to infect leukocytes and suggested the possibility that mutant alleles of *CCR5* may have been selected by providing resistance to variola (smallpox) virus. In addition to *CCR5-Δ32*, other mutations that result in severe functional alterations may be subject to selective pressures. Twenty-one additional polymorphisms of the *CCR5* coding region (Figure 1,Table 2) have been described (85-87), two of which cause premature termination of translation (C101X, and 299 FS). Among the 22 total *CCR5* variants identified thus far, 18 (82%) are protein altering (non-synonymous) and only four are synonymous variants. This high predominance of codon-altering variants is consistent with an adaptive accumulation of function-altering alleles (88). Seven of the mutations occurred at positions that are highly conserved throughout the β-chemokine

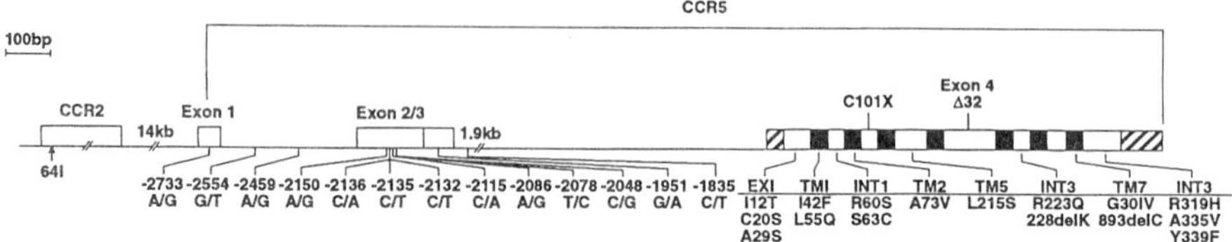

Figure 1. Map illustrating the *CCR2* and *CCR5* genes and the variations identified in them. The numbering system used designates the first nucleotide of the translation start site of *CCR5* as position 1, and the nucleotide immediately upstream of this as position −1. (From Ref. 87)

Table 2. Genetic variants of the *CCR5* gene

Variant	Nucleic acid substitution	Reference
I12T	A25C	86
C20S	T58A	86
A29S	G85T	86
I42F	A24T	86
L55Q	T164A	85,86
R60S	G180T	86
S63C	A187T	87
A73V	C218T	86
S75S	T215C	86
C101X	T303A	86
Δ32 (185)	D32	
L215S	C664T	85
R223Q	G668A	85,86
228delK	680del3	86
299FS	893delC	85
V300V	C900A	86
G301V	G902T	86
R319H	G956A	87
P332P	C996T	85
A335V	C1004T	85,86
Y339F	A1016T	85,86

receptor family, and three of these are also conserved in the α-chemokine receptor CXCR4, as well. The variants were observed throughout the entire molecule, including the transmembrane, intracellular, and extracellular domains, with a slight concentration near the N-terminus.

The *CCR5* variants are relatively uncommon, with allele frequencies of 4% or less (apart from *CCR5-Δ32*). Thus, the epidemiological consequences on HIV-1 infection or progression to AIDS cannot be evaluated. While no individual sampled was homozygous for any of the *CCR5* variants (apart from *CCR5-Δ32*), six of the codon-altering variants have been identified in individuals carrying *CCR5-Δ32* on the other haplotype (86,87). Therefore, only the product of the variant allele is expressed on their cell surfaces. Individuals expressing three of these variants (C20S, I42F, C101X) were HIV negative despite the high likelihood of multiple exposures to the virus, while individuals expressing the other three variants (I12T, A73V, L55Q) were HIV-1 seropositive. Recently, a second individual with the genotype encoding for C101X plus CCR5-Δ32 who was at high risk of HIV-1 infection was identified (89). The C101X mutation causes premature termination of translation, resulting in a truncated non-functional protein product. PBLs from this individual were resistant to infection with primary isolates of R5 HIV-1 virus strains, but were susceptible to infection with X4 isolates, as is the case for *CCR5-Δ32* homozygotes.

Functional analyses to test the effect of six of the naturally occurring variants in the amino terminal third of the CCR5 molecule (I12T, C20S, A29S, I42F, L55Q, A73V) on chemokine binding and HIV-1 infection in vitro have been performed (90). Binding of the normal CCR5 ligands, Rantes and MIP-1β, to variants in the first extracellular domain (I12T, C20S, A29S) was completely abrogated or severely reduced. Two variants, I12T and C20S, were also unable to function as co-receptors for R5 HIV-1 isolates suggesting that these variants radically alter the normal conformation of the CCR5 molecule. Conversely, the transmembrane variants (I42F, L55Q, and A73V), located in a region of the molecule that is not thought to interact directly with ligands, demonstrated a 4-8-fold enhanced affinity for RANTES. Further, these transmembrane variants did not exhibit the typical attenuation of chemotactic response in the presence of high concentrations of RANTES, perhaps resulting from their strong affinity for the chemokine ligands. These variants also supported HIV-1 infection. Thus, several of the naturally occurring variants alter the function of CCR5, further supporting the contention that this molecule is dispensable.

CCR5 Promoter Polymorphisms

CCR5 is expressed on activated and memory T cells, monocytes/macrophages, microglia (91-94) and, to a lesser extent, B cells (77). Although heterozygotes for *CCR5-Δ32* express less CCR5 on their cell surfaces than those with two normal alleles, the level of CCR5 expression among individuals with the *CCR5-+/+* genotype is quite variable (73). PBLs from individuals with the *CCR5-+/Δ32* genotype, which generally express relatively low levels of cell surface CCR5, are not as easily infected with R5 isolates *in vitro* as are cells from individuals who have the *CCR5-+/+* genotype (9). Therefore, it is reasonable to expect that the level of cell surface CCR5 expression correlates with infectability by R5 HIV-1 strains. This hypothesis has led to a search for polymorphisms in the *CCR5* promoter region that may alter transcription levels of this gene.

The *CCR5* promoter region has been characterized by several groups (95-99), and it appears that transcription is initiated from two distinct promoters, one of which lies upstream of exon 1 (P_U), and another that lies downstream within the region that includes intron 1, exon 2, and part of exon 3 (P_D) (97) (Figure 1). The downstream promoter is the stronger of the two when tested in a variety of cells, including monocytic and lymphocytic cell lines, and CD4+ T cells (97). Sequence motifs similar to consensus sequences for a variety of transcription factors have been identified in the P_D promoter region (98). Polymorphisms in cis-regulatory sequences can affect the strength of the promoter by altering the affinity of regulatory proteins for these elements. Such polymorphisms could account for some of the heterogeneity in both CCR5 expression and the rate of HIV disease progression that has been observed among individuals.

Another stimulus for testing the possibility that promoter region variation accounts for altered expression of CCR5 was that a variant in the *CCR2* gene (*CCR2-64I*), which maps only ~14 Kb from *CCR5,* has been shown to be associated with delayed progression to AIDS (100,101). Because CCR2 is used only by rare isolates of HIV-1 to gain entry into cells and because the *CCR2* and *CCR5* genes are in very close proximity, *CCR2-64I* could simply be marking a variant in the *CCR5* gene, perhaps a promoter variant, through linkage disequilibrium. At least 12 single nucleotide polymorphims have been identified thus far (97,99,101-104) that distinguish ten promoter region alleles (*CCR5P1- CCR5P10*), four of which are common (*CCR5P1-CCR5P4*) in Caucasians (102). The variants, *CCR5-Δ32* and *CCR2-64I* (see a description of *CCR2-64I* below) appear to have arisen independently on a haplotype containing the most common promoter allele, *CCR5P1* (102). Survival analyses were performed on data from individuals partitioned by the following genotypes: (i) those homozygous for the haplotype *CCR2+-CCR5P1-CCR5+* (where "+" indicates the normal allele of that gene); (ii) those with haplotypes containing at least one copy of the protective alleles *CCR5-Δ32* or *CCR2-64I*; and (iii) those with any other haplotypic combination (102). Individuals homozygous for the *CCR2+-CCR5P1-CCR5+* haplotype showed an accelerated rate of progression to AIDS compared to the other two groups. This effect was most marked in the first four to six years after infection, which is consistent with CCR5 being the primary HIV-1 co-receptor in the early years after infection. Genotypes containing the protective alleles (group ii) had appreciably delayed onset of AIDS, while individuals with other haplotypic combinations (group iii) developed AIDS at an intermediate rate. Similar results were observed in another study for a common variant (*A/G*) at position *–2459* (relative to the translation start site, ref. 87), where homozygosity for *–2459A* was associated with rapid progression to AIDS (104). This finding relates to the results of the previously mentioned study in that the variant *-2459A* is a component only of the haplotype characterized by *CCR5P1*, and the *-2459G* variant is found on haplotypes characterized by *CCR5P2-P4*.

Quantitative analysis of CCR5 on PBMCs from healthy volunteers with *CCR5P1/P1, P1/P4,* and *P4/P4* genotypes (all lacking the protective alleles *CCR5-Δ32* and *CCR2-64I*), revealed no significant differences in expression of CCR5, efficiency of promoting a luciferase reporter construct, nor infectivity by R5 or R5/X4 strains of HIV-1 (102). However, McDermott et al. (104) observed a modest decrease in promoter activity in a luciferase vector using the *CCR5* promoter characterized by *–2459G*. More recently, gel-shift assays have been used to determine whether the variants at each of five positions (*-2554G/T, -2459A/G, -2135C/T, -2086A/G* and *-1835C/T*) differ in their ability to bind nuclear factors in T cell extracts (105). A clear difference in binding of one or more nuclear factors to oligonucleotides containing *–2554T* (found on the *P4* allele) as compared with *–2554G* (found on the *P1* allele) was observed. Further studies to identify subtle effects of variation in the *CCR5* promoter region on *CCR5* transcription are underway to explain the epidemiological effects observed on AIDS progression.

CCR2 Polymorphisms

The importance of CCR5 and CXCR4 in HIV-1 pathogenesis has resulted in a search for polymorphisms in other chemokine receptor genes that may also play a role in HIV-1 disease progression. Screening of the entire *CCR2* gene for variants revealed a *G→A* transition at DNA position 190 (counting from the *ATG* start site), that causes a conservative change from valine to isoleucine at amino acid position 64 (*CCR2-64I*) in the first transmembrane domain of the molecule (100). CCR5 also has an isoleucine at position 64 and shares sequence identity to the first transmembrane domain of CCR2 at all other positions, as well. The *CCR2-64I* allele is relatively common, with frequencies of 10% in Caucasians, 15% in African Americans, 17% in Hispanics, and 25% in Asians (100). Several studies have shown that individuals bearing this allele progress to AIDS two to four years later than individuals who are homozygous for the normal allele, and this protection is independent of that conferred by *CCR5-Δ32* since these variants are never found on the same haplotype (100,101). Consistent with delayed progression, seroconverters with the *CCR2-64I* allele have significantly lower viral load 9-12 months after seroconversion (101). However, a study of 395 men whose seroconversion dates were unknown (seroprevalents) did not confirm this association (62), perhaps due to chance or the lack of information on the dates of seroconversion. Although a potential mechanism for *CCR2-64I* in protection against AIDS has not been identified, an association between the *+/64I* genotype and slightly reduced levels of CXCR4 on PBMCs from healthy volunteers has been noted (106). In addition, *in vitro* studies suggested possible formation of heterodimers between

CXCR4 and CCR2-64I, but not wild type CCR2, which could affect HIV-1 binding to PBMCs (107).

Several observations have led to speculation that *CCR2-64I* is simply marking (through linkage disequilibrium) a true disease associated variant that is located in the *CCR5* gene (101). First, CCR2 is used as a co-receptor by only rare isolates of HIV-1 (18,19,108).Second, the *CCR2-64I* variant does not markedly affect co-receptor expression, chemokine ligand binding, or HIV-1 co-receptor activity (106).Third, *CCR2* and *CCR5* are in very close physical proximity. One candidate allele is the variant *–1835C→T* located in intron 2 of *CCR5*, which was found to be in 100% linkage disequilibrium with *CCR2-64I* (101). However, there are no data indicating a functional role for this polymorphism in the control of *CCR5* expression.

CXCR4 **Polymorphisms**

Analysis of the *CXCR4* gene has indicated that this gene is highly conserved. A screen of the entire transcription unit of the gene in 232 individuals revealed only the single rare synonymous polymorphism *C→T* at position 3952 (I261I)(109). A survey of the *CXCR4* coding sequence in 11 HIV-1 positive long-term nonprogressors identified one synonymous variant (*A→G*; K204K) and one nonsynonymous (amino acid changing) variant (*T→C*; F278S) (110). The F278S variant was tested in an HIV envelope fusion assay, but no significant differences were observed between the variant and the normal control. CXCR4 and its only ligand, SDF-1, demonstrate exclusive binding. Knockout mutations of either gene are lethal in mice (111-113), suggesting that both are critical to normal physiology. Thus, there is likely to be strong selective pressure to avoid variation in this gene that would alter its function.

SDF-1

As the chemokine ligand for CXCR4, SDF-1 specifically blocks the use of CXCR4 by X4 isolates (22,114). The *SDF-1* gene produces two isoforms, designated SDF-1α and SDF-1β, by alternative splicing of the mRNA (115). A polymorphism in the 3' untranslated region of *SDF-1*, which results in a *G→A* transition at position 801 from the *ATG* start codon, has been identified (116). This polymorphism, designated *SDF-1 3'A*, is found in all racial groups tested, with allele frequencies of 0.211 in Caucasians, 0.160 in Hispanics, 0.057 in African Americans, and 0.257 in Asians (116). The *SDF-1 3'A* variant is located in a conserved segment of the 3'UTR of the *SDF-1β* transcript (115) (69% homology between human and mouse), and it could potentially serve as a target for cis-acting factors which influence production or transport of the product (117-120). In one study, HIV-1 infected individuals homozygous for this polymorphism were shown to exhibit delayed progression to AIDS (116). Its association with delayed progression to AIDS was suggested to occur by up-regulating the quantity of SDF-1 protein available to bind CXCR4, thereby blocking X4 viruses from infecting T cells. Delayed progression to AIDS associated with *SDF1-3'A* homozygosity was also observed in the French GRIV cohort, although not significantly (121). However, no functional data supporting a role for *SDF1-3'A* has been forthcoming, and additional epidemiologic studies have not supported the original observations. Three subsequent studies have reported the opposite effect of an acceleration in disease progression with the *SDF1-3'A/3'A* genotype (103,122,123). Although statistical power issues may explain some of the differences among studies, (since only about 5% of Caucasian individuals are homozygous for the variant), the effect of *SDF1 3'A* on progression to AIDS is not clear at present.

RANTES

The CCR5 chemokine ligand RANTES (regulated on activation normal T cell expressed and secreted), potently suppresses R5 HIV-1 infection of cells by blocking CCR5 (38,124). PBLs from different individuals show wide variations in their ability to secrete RANTES and MIP-1β (125,126), and there is an inverse correlation between levels of chemokine secreted and rate of disease progression. Similarly, CD4+ lymphocytes from exposed uninfected individuals secrete higher levels of RANTES than those from HIV-1 infected individuals (125,127). Thus, differences in levels of secretion of RANTES have led to a search for polymorphisms in the promoter region of the gene. Two variants were identified amongst 272 HIV-1 infected and 193 uninfected Japanese individuals characterized by a *C→G* substitution at position –28, and a *G→A* substitution at position –403 (128). Three haplotypes of the *RANTES* promoter could account for all genotypes observed: *-403G/-28C* (haplotype I); *-403A/-28C* (haplotype II); and *–403A/-28G* (haplotype III). Haplotype III was associated with significantly slower rates of CD4+ lymphocyte depletion relative to the other haplotypes ($p = 0.008$) and the effect was dominant. Although no significant difference in serum RANTES levels among the three haplotypes was detected, stimulation of CD4+ lymphocytes with PHA *in vitro* induced significantly more RANTES secretion in individuals with haplotype III relative to those without this haplotype. Also, haplotype III had slightly higher promoter activity in a luciferase reporter assay. While the effect of *–28G* needs to be confirmed in larger cohorts, these results support the importance of chemokines in delaying progression to AIDS and the potential clinical use of chemokines as anti-viral factors.

HLA AND HIV-1

The human major histocompatibility complex (MHC) on the short arm of chromosome 6 contains the polymorphic *HLA* class I and class II loci which encode products that are fundamental to the immune response (129,130). HLA molecules present antigenic peptides to T cells, thereby initiating an immune response resulting in clearance of the foreign material. The extraordinary polymorphism of

HLA genes is believed to be maintained through selective forces such as infectious disease morbidity (131,132). Examples of *HLA* influence on the host immune response to human pathogens include malaria and hepatitis B (133-135).

The hypothesis of overdominant selection (heterozygote advantage) proposes that individuals heterozygous at HLA loci are able to present a greater variety of antigenic peptides than are homozygotes, resulting in a more productive immune response to a large array of pathogens (136,137). A definitive study of the effects of HLA class I homozygosity on infectious diseases requires particularly large numbers of subjects because of the highly polymorphic nature of these loci and the relatively even distribution of their alleles (131,132). The largest epidemiological study addressing the validity of overdominant selection at the *HLA* class I loci entailed an analysis of 498 HIV-1 positive individuals whose seroconversion date was known within a 6 month period (138). The basic hypothesis tested was that heterozygosity at *HLA* class I loci confers relative resistance to AIDS progression because an individual who is homozygous at *HLA-A, HLA-B*, and *HLA-C* presents a limited repertoire of antigenic epitopes relative to an individual who is heterozygous at these loci. A highly significant association between *HLA* class I homozygosity (at one or more loci) and rapid progression to AIDS was observed in both Caucasians and African Americans (Figure 2A). All three class I loci contributed independently to the association and the effect was most pronounced in individuals who were homozygous at two or three loci. The most parsimonious explanation for this data is that heterozygotes are able to present a broader range of HIV-1 peptides, thereby prolonging the time it takes for an escape mutant to arise. Similar results for homozygosity at *HLA-A* and *HLA-B* were observed in 140 Dutch homosexual men and 202 Rwandan heterosexual women infected with HIV-1 (139). There was a stronger association with homozygosity at the *HLA-B* locus in the Amsterdam cohort, and at the *HLA-A* locus in the Rwandan cohort, consistent with previous evidence that *HLA-A* and *HLA-B* genes are subject to varying degrees of gene flow and natural selection in human populations (140). Oddly, there was no effect seen for homozygosity at the *HLA-C* locus in either of these two cohorts.

More than 50 reports examining a role for *HLA* alleles or haplotypes (for HLA nomenclature see ref. 141) in AIDS pathogenesis have been published (reviewed in ref. 142) and two extended haplotypes have been consistently associated with accelerated progression to AIDS: *HLA-A1-Cw7-B8-DR3-DQ2*, and *HLA-A11-Cw4-B35-DR1-DQ1* (142-144). Recently, a strong effect of *B*35-Cw*04* on rapid disease progression was observed in a large study of 330 Caucasian and 144 African American seroconverters (138), leaving little doubt as to the inadequacy of this haplotype in controlling HIV-1 disease relative to other haplotypes. The *B*35-Cw*04* haplotype has a co-dominant effect in that homozygotes for this haplotype progress more rapidly than heterozygotes and heterozygotes progress more rapidly than individuals without *B*35-Cw*04* (Figure 2B).

Viral epitopes for both B*3501 and Cw*04 have been identified (145-148), but no viral epitopes have been reported for the other B35 alleles (149). Given the

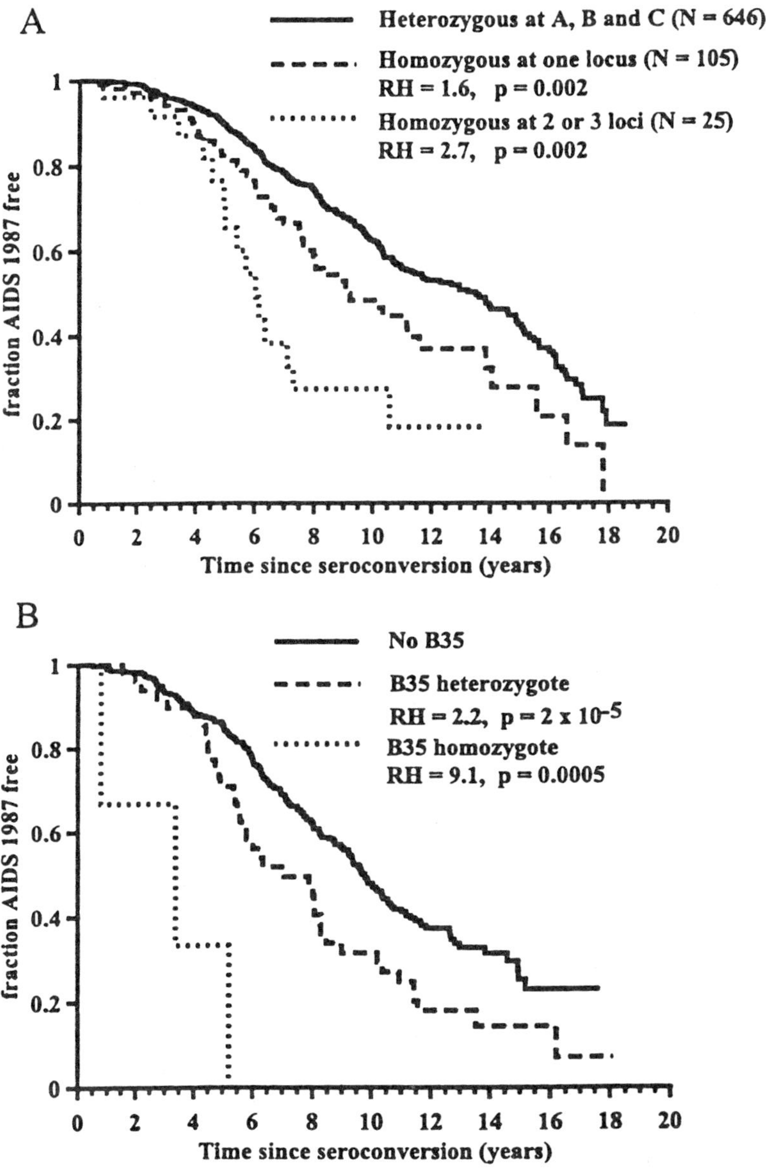

Figure 2 (A) Kaplan Meier survival curves illustrating association between homozygosity at one or more HLA class I loci and progression to AIDS (1987 definition). (B) Kaplan Meier survival curves showing the influence of HLA-B*35 on progression to AIDS (1987 definition) (from ref. 138).

association of the *B*35-Cw*04* alleles with progression to AIDS, it will be interesting to determine whether these alleles are inferior in some way in inducing a productive CTL response.

Decreased natural killer cell activity was suggested as a potential mechanism to explain the rapid progression to AIDS in individuals with *B*35-Cw*04* (150), instigated by previously reported data that *HLA* homozygosity and the *B35-Cw04* haplotype are associated with reduction in NK cell number and activity (151). Unlike CTL cytotoxity that occurs via recognition of antigenic epitope in the context of MHC class I, NK cells kill targets that lack class I expression (152,153). The HIV-1-encoded *nef* gene product has been shown to downregulate HLA-A and HLA-B expression, perhaps rendering some protection of infected cells from CTL-mediated killing (55). HLA-C molecules, the ligands for a variety of NK cell receptors, are not downregulated by nef, which may protect the infected cell from NK cell mediated killing (55,56). Thus, functional analysis of NK cell activity in HIV-1 disease along with genetic analysis of the complex of genes encoding NK cell receptors warrant further investigation.

Many other associations between *HLA* haplotype and the rate of HIV disease progression have been reported, but most of these findings have been difficult to confirm in multiple cohorts (154-158). This situation is probably due to a combination of small patient sample size, limitations in patient clinical descriptions, use of low resolution *HLA* typing methods (i.e., serologic typing), and failure to correct for multiple comparisons.

OTHER GENES INVOLVED IN IMMUNE REGULATION

Tumor Necrosis Factor

Tumor necrosis factor-α (TNF-α) is a potent proinflammatory cytokine that has been implicated in the pathogenesis of autoimmune and infectious diseases (159,160). The *TNF-α* gene lies in the class III region of the human *MHC* approximately 250 kb centromeric of the *HLA-B* locus. In view of its biological effects and the location of the gene near the *HLA* class I and class II loci, it has been speculated that polymorphisms within this gene might contribute to some of the associations seen between *HLA* and disease (161). Indeed, haplotypes containing *HLA-DR3* and *HLA-DR4* are associated with higher levels of TNF-α (162,163), while *HLA-DR2* haplotypes are associated with low production (162,164), suggesting the possibility of a functional polymorphism within the regulatory region of the gene that may contribute to disease phenotype. Polymorphisms in the *TNF-α* promoter at positions -376, -308, -238, and –163 have been identified (165-167), all of which are characterized by *G→ A* transitions. The *-308A* variant is part of the most common Caucasian *HLA* haplotype *HLA-A1-B8-DR3-DQ2*, which is associated with high TNF-α production (165,168). Associations between the *-308A* allele and susceptibility to cerebral malaria (169), lepromatous leprosy (170), and mucocutaneous leishmaniasis (171) have been observed, perhaps as a consequence of high TNF-α production.

Both TNF-α and lymphotoxin (TNF-β) are potent inducers of HIV replication and expression *in vitro* through activation of the transcription factor NF-κB (172,173). TNF-α and TNF-β may induce apoptosis of HIV-infected and uninfected lymphocytes, thereby accelerating CD4 depletion and disease progression (174,175). Increased levels of TNF-α have also been reported in patients with AIDS (176). The four *G* to *A* transition polymorphisms in the promoter region of the *TNF-α* gene have been examined in a Dutch HIV-1 seropositive cohort and none of the polymorphisms were significantly associated with disease progression in this study (176). A more recent study of homosexual men from CDC- and NIH-sponsored cohorts suggested a weak association of homozygosity for *-308A* (also referred to as *TNF2*) with long-term nonprogression, but no effect on susceptibility to infection was observed (177). The numbers of individuals studied in both reports were small, so the studies were not powerful enough to draw any solid conclusions. A recent report (178) also demonstrated a strong association between the *TNF c2* microsatellite allele, which lies within the first intron of the lymphotoxin gene (179), and slower rate of progression to AIDS.

Mannose-Binding Lectin

Mannose-binding lectin (MBL) is a member of the collectin family of proteins and is an important constituent of the innate immune system (180-182). MBL activates complement (183) and acts in the first line of defense against various bacterial, viral, and parasitic infections, before the establishment of adaptive immune protection by B and T cells (180). Low serum levels of MBL are associated with opsonization defects and impaired phagocytosis (184-186). The *MBL* gene is located on chromosome 10q (187,188), and polymorphisms in the first exon have been shown to be important in determining the level of circulating MBL (189,190). Single amino acid variants associated with lower MBL serum concentrations include G→D at codon 54 (allele B) (191), G→E at codon 57 (allele C) (189), and R→C at codon 52 (allele D) (190). Polymorphisms in the promoter region of the *MBL* gene have also been shown to affect serum concentration of MBL (192).

Early studies by Ezekowitz et al. demonstrated that MBL was able to inhibit HIV infection *in vitro* (193). Genetic analysis of *MBL* variants in an HIV-1 Danish homosexual cohort showed an association between homozygosity for any combination of the variant alleles (*B*, *C*, and *D*) and increased susceptibility to HIV-1 infection (194). These variant alleles were also associated with a significantly shorter survival time after AIDS diagnosis. Similar findings have been reported in a Finnish HIV-1 cohort where there was significant enrichment of homozygotes for the variant alleles in the HIV patient group compared to normal controls (195). However, analysis of an Amsterdam HIV-1 cohort suggested a weak association of the variant alleles with slower progression to AIDS, and no association with survival time after AIDS diagnosis (196). Sample sizes were relatively small once again, perhaps accounting for the discrepancies in the studies.

SUMMARY

Despite apparent inconsistencies between some genetic studies, it is clear that host genetic effects on HIV-1 disease are exceedingly complex and likely to involve multiple loci. The discovery of the *CCR5-Δ32* allele in particular has been instrumental in our understanding of how human genetic factors influence outcome in HIV-1 infection, and provides good evidence that genetic analysis is indeed a strong tool for understanding the heterogeneous characteristics of infectious diseases. The strong associations of certain *HLA* haplotypes with disease progression support the theory that the genes involved in the host immune response play a central role in containing HIV-1 infection. It is clear, however, that there is no simple inheritance pattern. Rather, the observed phenotype may be the result of

Table 3 Genes that affect HIV-1 infection and AIDS progression.

Gene	Genotype	Effect	Reference
CCR5	*Δ32/Δ32*	Prevent infection	8-10
CCR5	*+/Δ32*	Delay AIDS	8,61,62,72
CCR5	*+/Δ32*	↓Risk of lymphoma	76,77
CCR5	*+/Δ32*	↑Response to therapy	79
CCR5	*A303/Δ32*	Prevent infection	89
CCR5P	*P1/P1*	Accelerate AIDS	102,104
CCR2	*+/64I*	Delay AIDS	100,101
SDF1	*3'A/3'A*	?Delay AIDS	116,121
RANTES	*+/-403A/-28G*	Delay AIDS	128
HLA	*HLA- A,-B,-C* homozygosity	Accelerate AIDS	138,139
HLA	*B*35*	Accelerate AIDS	138
HLA	*Cw*04*	Accelerate AIDS	138
HLA	*A1-B8-DR3*	Accelerate AIDS	142
TNF-α	*-308A/-308A*	?Delay AIDS	177
TNF-β	*TNF c2*	Delay AIDS	178
MBL	Homozygosity for variant alleles	?Accelerate AIDS	194,195

multiple genes working independently or synergistically. In addition, the role of viral factors in determining disease outcome is becoming more apparent. The HIV-1 *nef* gene, for example, protects infected cells from anti-HIV CTL recognition by down-regulating MHC class I expression. HIV also undergoes a high rate of mutation increasing the likelihood that the virus will evade the host immune system. This clearly reinforces the notion that in order to adequately control this devastating infection, the mechanisms involved in the interaction of the virus with the host immune system must be understood.

Apart from the genes discussed here (summarized in Table 3), there are likely to be other genes affecting AIDS outcome that will be discovered in the near future. As a result of the progress made so far, we now have a better understanding of the mechanisms underlying HIV-1 disease pathogenesis. This information has far-reaching implications for the development of novel therapies and vaccines against HIV-1.

ACKNOWLEDGMENTS

The content of this publication does not necessarily reflect the views or policies of the Department of Health and Human Services, nor does mention of trade names, commercial products, or organizations imply endorsement by the U.S. government.

This project has been funded in whole or in part with Federal funds from the National Cancer Institute, National Institutes of Health, under Contract No. NO1-CO-56000. The publisher or recipient acknowledges right of the U.S. Government to retain a nonexclusive, royalty-free license in and to any copyright covering the article.

REFERENCES

1. Michael NL. Host genetic influences on HIV-1 pathogenesis. Curr Opin Immunol 1999; 11:466-474.
2. Phair JP. Keynote address: variations in the natural history of HIV infection. AIDS Res Hum Retroviruses 1994; 10:883-885.
3. Pantaleo G, Menzo S, Vaccarezza M, Graziosi C, Cohen OJ, Demarest JF, Montefiori D, Orenstein JM, Fox C, Schrager LK, Margolick JB, Buchbinder S, Giorgi JV, Fauci AS. Studies in subjects with long-term nonprogressive human immunodeficiency virus infection. N Engl J Med 1995; 332:209-216.
4. Schrager LK, Young JM, Fowler MG, Mathieson BJ, Vermund SH. Long-term survivors of HIV infection. Acquir Immune Defic Syndr 1994; 8:S95-S108.
5. Klein MR, Miedema F. Long-term survivors of HIV-1 infection. Trends Microbiol 1995; 3:386-391.
6. Sheppard HW, Lang W, Ascher MS, Vittinghoff E, Winkelstein W. The characterization of non-progressors: long-term HIV-1 infection with stable CD4+ T-cell levels. AIDS 1993; 7:1159-1166.

7. Phair J, Jacobson L, Detels R, Rinaldo C, Saah A, Schrager L, Munoz A. Acquired immune deficiency syndrome occurring within 5 years of infection with human immunodeficiency virus type-1: the Multicenter AIDS Cohort Study. J Acquir Immune Defic Syndr 1992; 5:490-496.
8. Dean M, Carrington M, Winkler C, Huttley GA, Smith MW, Allikmets R, Goedert JJ, Buchbinder SP, Vittinghoff E, Gomperts E, Donfield S, Vlahov D, Kaslow R, Saah A, Rinaldo C, Detels R, Hemophilia Growth and Development Study, Multicenter AIDS Cohort Study, Multicenter Hemophilia Cohort Study, San Francisco City Cohort, ALIVE Study, O'Brien SJ. Genetic restriction of HIV-1 infection and progression to AIDS by a deletion allele of the CKR5 structural gene. Science 1996; 273:1856-1862.
9. Liu R, Paxton WA, Choe S, Ceradini D, Martin SR, Horuk R, MacDonald ME, Stuhlmann H, Koup RA, Landau NR. Homozygous defect in HIV-1 coreceptor accounts for resistance of some multiply-exposed individuals to HIV-1 infection. Cell 1996; 86:367-377.
10. Samson M, Frédérick L, Doranz B, Rucker J, Liesnard C, Farber C-M, Saragosti S, Lapouméroulie C, Cognaux J, Forceille C, Muyldermans G, Verhofstede C, Burtonboy G, Georges M, Imai T, Rana S, Yi Y, Smyth RJ, Collman RG, Doms RW, Vassart G, and Parmentier M. Resistance to HIV-1 infection in caucasian individuals bearing mutant alleles of the CCR-5 chemokine receptor gene. Nature 1996; 382:722-725.
11. Fowke K, Nagelkerke N, Kimani J, Simonsen JN, Anzala AO, Bwayo JJ, MacDonald KS, Ngugi EN, Plummer FA. Resistance to HIV-1 infection amongst persistently seronegative prostitutes in Nairobi, Kenya. Lancet 1996; 348:1347-1351.
12. Pasvol G, Weatherall DJ, Wilson RJ. Cellular mechanism for the protective effect of haemoglobin S against P. falciparum malaria. Nature 1978; 274:701-703.
13. Miller LH, Mason SJ, Clyde DF, McGinniss MH. The resistance factor to Plasmodium vivax in blacks. The Duffy-blood-group genotype, FyFy. N Engl J Med 1976; 295:302-304.
14. Dalgleish AG, Beverley PC, Clapham PR, Crawford DH, Greaves MF, Weiss RA. The CD4 (T4) antigen is an essential component of the receptor for the AIDS retrovirus. Nature 1984; 312:763-767.
15. Klatzmann D, Champagne E, Chamaret S, Gruest J, Guetard D, Hercend T, Gluckman JC, Montagnier L. T-lymphocyte T4 molecule behaves as the receptor for human retrovirus LAV. Nature 1984; 312:767-768.
16. Alkhatib G, Combadiere C, Broder CC, Feng Y, Kennedy PE, Murphy PM, Berger EA. CC CKR5: a RANTES, MIP-1α, MIP-1β receptor as a fusion cofactor for macrophage-tropic HIV-1. Science 1996; 272:1955-1958.
17. Choe H, Farzan M, Sun Y, Sullivan N, Rollins B, Ponath PD, Wu L, Mackay CR, LaRosa G, Newman W, Gerard N, Gerard C, Sodroski J. The beta-chemokine receptors CCR3 and CCR5 facilitate infection by primary HIV-1 isolates. Cell 1996; 85:1135-1148.
18. Deng H, Liu R, Ellmeier W, Choe S, Unutmaz D, Burkhart M, Di Marzio P, Marmon S, Sutton RE, Hill CM, Davis CB, Peiper SC, Schall TJ, Littman DR, Landau NR. Identification of a major co-receptor for primary isolates of HIV-1. Nature 1996; 381:661-666.
19. Doranz BJ, Rucker J, Yi Y, Smyth RJ, Samson M, Peiper SC, Parmentier M, Collman RG, Doms RW. A dual-tropic primary HIV-1 isolate that uses fusin and the beta-chemokine receptors CKR-5, CKR-3, and CKR-2b as fusion cofactors. Cell 1996; 85:1149-1158.

20. Dragic T, Litwin V, Allaway GP, Martin SR, Huang Y, Nagashima KA, Cayanan C, Maddon PJ, Koup RA, Moore JP, Paxton WA. HIV-1 entry into CD4+ cells is mediated by the chemokine receptor CC-CKR-5. Nature 1996; 381:667-673.
21. Berson JF, Long D, Doranz GJ, Rucker J, Jirik FR, Doms RW. A seven-transmembrane domain receptor involved in fusion and entry of T-cell-tropic human immunodeficiency virus type 1 strains. J Virol 1996; 70:6288-6295.
22. Feng Y, Broder CC, Kennedy PE, Berger EA. HIV-1 entry cofactor: functional cDNA cloning of a seven-transmembrane, G protein-coupled receptor. Science 1996; 272:872-877.
23. Moore JP, Trkola A, Dragic T. Co-receptors for HIV-1 entry. Curr Opin Immunol 1997; 9:551-562.
24. Berger EA. HIV entry and tropism: the chemokine receptor connection. AIDS 1997; 11:S3-S16.
25. Berger EA, Doms RA, Fenyo EM, Korber BTM, Littman DR, Moore JP, Sattentau QJ, Schuitemaker H, Sodroski J, Weiss RA. A new classification for HIV-1. Nature 1998; 391:240.
26. Zhu T, Mo H, Wang N, Nam DS, Cao Y, Koup RA, Ho DD. Genotypic and phenotypic characterization of HIV-1 patients with primary infection. Science 1993; 261:1179-1181.
27. Richman DD, Bozzette SA. The impact of the synctium-inducing phenotype of human immunodeficiency virus on disease progression. J Infect Dis 1996; 169:968-974.
28. Deng H, Unutmaz D, Kewal-Ramani VN, Littman DR. Expression cloning of new receptors used by simian and human immunodeficiency viruses. Nature 1997; 388:296-300.
29. Edinger AL, Hoffman TL, Sharron M, Lee B, O'Dowd B, Doms RW. Use of GPR1, GPR15, and STRL33 as coreceptors by diverse human immunodeficiency virus type 1 and simian immunodeficiency virus envelope proteins. Virology 1998; 249:367-378.
30. Loetscher M, Amara A, Oberlin E, Brass N, Legler D, Loetscher P, D'Apuzzo M, Meese E, Rousset D, Virelizier JL, Baggiolini M, Arenzana-Seisdedos F, Moser B. TYMSTR, a putative chemokine receptor selectively expressed in activated T cells, exhibits HIV-1 coreceptor function. Curr Biol 1997; 7:652-660.
31. Rucker J, Edinger AL, Sharron M, Samson M, Lee B, Berson JF, Yi Y, Margulies B, Collman RG, Doranz BJ, Parmentier M, Doms RW. Utilization of chemokine receptors, orphan receptors, and herpesvirus-encoded receptors by diverse human and simian immunodeficiency viruses. J Virol 1997;71:8999-9007.
32. Horuk R, Hesselgesser J, Zhou Y, Faulds D, Halks-Miller M, Harvey S, Taub D, Samson M, Parmentier M, Rucker J, Doranz BJ, Doms RW. The CC chemokine I-309 inhibits CCR8-dependent infection by diverse HIV-1 strains. J Biol Chem 1998; 273:386-391.
33. Pleskoff O, Treboute C, Alizon M. The cytomegalovirus-encoded chemokine receptor US28 can enhance cell-cell fusion mediated by different viral proteins. J Virol 1998; 72:6389-6397.
34. Bron R, Klasse PJ, Wilkinson D, Clapham PR, Pelchen-Matthews A, Power C, Wells TN, Kim J, Peiper SC, Hoxie JA, Marsh M. Promiscuous use of CC and CXC chemokine receptors in cell-to-cell fusion mediated by a human immunodeficiency virus type 2 envelope protein. J Virol 1997; 71:8405-8415.
35. Chen Z, Kwon D, Jin Z, Monard S, Telfer P, Jones MS, Lu CY, Aguilar RF, Ho DD, Marx PA. Natural infection of a homozygous delta24 CCR5 red-capped mangabey with an R2b-tropic simian immunodeficiency virus. J Exp Med 1998; 188:2057-2065.

36. He J, Chen Y, Farzan M, Choe H, Ohagen A, Gartner S, Busciglio J, Yang X, Hofmann W, Newman W, Mackay CR, Sodroski J, Gabuzda D. CCR3 and CCR5 are coreceptors for HIV-1 infection of microglia. Nature 1997; 385:645-649.
37. Albright AV, Shieh JT, Itoh T, Lee B, Pleasure D, O'Connor MJ, Doms RW, Gonzalez-Scarano F. Microglia express CCR5, CXCR4, and CCR3, but of these, CCR5 is the principal coreceptor for human immunodeficiency virus type 1 dementia isolates. J Virol 1999; 73:205-213.
38. Paxton WA, Martin SR, Tse D, O'Brien TR, Skurnick J, VanDevanter NL, Padian N, Braun JF, Kotler DP, WolinskySM, Koup RA. Relative resistance to HIV-1 infection of CD4 lymphocytes from persons who remain uninfected despite multiple high-risk sexual exposure. Nat Med 1996; 2:412-417.
39. Cocchi F, DeVico AL, Garzino-Demo A, Arya SK, Gallo RC, Lusso P. Identification of RANTES, MIP-1 alpha, and MIP-1 beta as the major HIV-suppressive factors produced by CD8+ T cells. Science 1995; 270:1811-1815.
40. Hadida F, Vieillard V, Autran B, Clark-Lewis I, Baggiolini M, Debre P. HIV-specific T cell cytotoxicity mediated by RANTES via the chemokine receptor CCR3. J Exp Med 1998;188:609-614.
41. Kagi D, Vignaux F, Ledermann B, Burki K, Depraetere V,Nagata S, Hengartner H, Golstein P. Fas and perforin pathways as major mechanisms of T cell-mediated cytotoxicity. Science 1994; 265:528-530.
42. Hadida F, Vieillard V, Mollet L, Clark-Lewis I, Baggiolini M, Debre P. Cutting edge: RANTES regulates Fas ligand expression and killing by HIV-specific CD8 cytotoxic T cells. J Immunol 1999; 163:1105-1109.
43. Borrow P, Lewicki H, Hahn BH, Shaw GM, Oldstone MB. Virus-specific CD8+ cytotoxic T-lymphocyte activity associated with control of viremia in primary human immunodeficiency virus type 1 infection. J Virol 1994; 68:6103-6110.
44. Koup RA, Safrit JT, Cao Y, Andrews CA, McLeod G, Borkowsky W, Farthing C, Ho DD. Temporal association of cellular immune responses with the initial control of viremia in primary human immunodeficiency virus type 1 syndrome. J Virol 1994; 68:4650-4655.
45. Feinberg MB, McLean AR. AIDS: decline and fall of immune surveillance? Curr Biol 1997; 7:R136-R140.
46. Yang OO, Kalams SA, Rosenzweig M, Trocha A, Jones N, Koziel M, Walker BD, Johnson RP. Efficient lysis of human immunodeficiency virus type 1-infected cells by cytotoxic T lymphocytes. J Virol 1996; 70:5799-5806.
47. Yang OO, Kalams SA, Trocha A, Cao H, Luster A, Johnson RP, Walker BD. Suppression of human immunodeficiency virus type 1 replication by CD8+ cells: evidence for HLA class I-restricted triggering of cytolytic and noncytolytic mechanisms. J Virol 1997; 71:3120-3128.
48. Rowland-Jones SL, Dong T, Fowke KR, Kimani J, Krausa P, Newell H, Blanchard T, Arlyoshi K, Oyugi J, Ngugi E, Bwayo J, MacDonald KS, McMichael AJ. Cytotoxic T cell responses to multiple conserved HIV epitopes in HIV-resistant prostitutes in Nairobi. J Clin Invest 1998; 102:1758-1765.
49. Kaul R, Plummer FA, Kimani J, Dong T, Kiama P, Rostron T, Njagi E, MacDonald KS, Bwayo JJ, McMichael AJ, Rowland-Jones SL. HIV-1-specific mucosal CD8+ lymphocyte responses in the cervix of HIV-1-resistant prostitutes in Nairobi. J Immunol 2000; 164:1602-1611.

50. Kaul R, Trabattoni D, Bwayo JJ, Arienti D, Zagliani A, Mwangi FM, Kariuki C, Ngugi EN, MacDonald KS, Ball TB, Clerici M, Plummer FA. HIV-1-specific mucosal IgA in a cohort of HIV-1-resistant Kenyan sex workers. AIDS 1999; 13:23-29.
51. Schmitz JE, Kuroda MJ, Santra S, Sasseville VG, Simon MA, Lifton MA, Racz P, Tenner-Racz K, Dalesandro M, Scallon BJ, Ghrayeb J, Forman MA, Montefiori DC, Rieber EP, Letvin NL, Reimann KA. Control of viremia in simian immunodeficiency virus infection by CD8+ lymphocytes. Science 1999; 283:857-860.
52. Jin X, Bauer DE, Tuttleton SE, Lewin S, Gettie A, Blanchard J, Irwin CE, Safrit JT, Mittler J, Weinberger L, Kostrikis LG, Zhang L, Perelson AS, Ho DD. Dramatic rise in plasma viremia after CD8(+) T cell depletion in simian immunodeficiency virus-infected macaques. J Exp Med 1999; 189:991-998.
53. Wagner L, Yang OO, Garcia-Zepeda EA, Ge Y, Kalams SA, Walker BD, Pasternack MS, Luster AD. Beta-chemokines are released from HIV-1-specific cytolytic T-cell granules complexed to proteoglycans. Nature 1998; 391:908-11.
54. Levy JA, Mackewicz CE, Barker E. Controlling HIV pathogenesis: the role of the noncytotoxic anti-HIV response of CD8+ T cells. Immunol Today 1996; 17:217-224.
55. Collins KL, Chen BK, Kalams SA, Walker BD, Baltimore D. HIV-1 Nef protein protects infected primary cells against killing by cytotoxic T lymphocytes. Nature 1998; 391:397-401.
56. Kerkau T, Schmitt-Landgraf R, Schimpl A, Wecker E. Downregulation of HLA class I antigens in HIV-1-infected cells. AIDS Res Hum Retroviruses 1989; 5:613-620.
57. Zocchi MR, Rubartelli A, Morgavi P, Poggi A. HIV-1 Tat inhibits human natural killer cell function by blocking L-type calcium channels. J Immunol 1998; 161:2938-2943.
58. Samson M, Soularue P, Vassart G, Parmentier M. The genes encoding the human CC-chemokine receptors CC-CKR1 to CC-CKR5 (CMKBR1-CMKBR5) are clustered in the p21.3-p24 region of chromosome 3. Genomics 1996; 36:522-526.
59. Combadiere C, Ahuja SK, Murphy PM. Cloning, chromosomal localization, and RNA expression of a human beta chemokine receptor-like gene. DNA Cell Biol 1995; 14:673-680.
60. Samson M, Stordeur P, Labbe O, Soularue P, Vassart G, Parmentier M. Molecular cloning and chromosomal mapping of a novel human gene, ChemR1, expressed in T lymphocytes and polymorphonuclear cells and encoding a putative chemokine receptor. Eur J Immunol 1996; 26:3021-3028.
61. Zimmerman PA, Buckler-White A, Alkhatib G, Spalding T, Kubofcik J, Combadiere C, Weissman D, Cohen O, Rubbert A, Lam G, Vaccarezza M, Kennedy PE, Kumaraswami V, Giorgi JV, Detels R, Hunter J, Chopek M, Berger EA, Fauci AS, Nutman TB, Murphy PM. Inherited resistance to HIV-1 conferred by an inactivating mutation in CC chemokine receptor 5: studies in populations with contrasting clinical phenotypes, defined racial background, and quantified risk. Mol Med 1997; 3:23-36.
62. Michael NL, Louie LG, Rohrbaugh AL, Schultz KA, Dayhoff DE, Wang CE, Sheppard HW. The role of CCR5 and CCR2 polymorphisms in HIV-1 transmission and disease progression. Nat Med 1997; 3:1160-1162.
63. Rana S, Besson G, Cook DG, Rucker J, Smyth RJ, Yi Y, Turner JD, Guo HH, Du JG, Peiper SC, Lavi E, Samson M, Libert F, Liesnard C, Vassart G, Doms RW, Parmentier M, Collman RG. Role of CCR5 in infection of primary macrophages and lymphocytes by macrophage-tropic strains of human immunodeficiency virus: resistance to patient-derived and prototype isolates resulting from the delta ccr5 mutation. J Virol 1997; 71:3219-3227.

64. Connor RI, Paxton WA, Sheridan KE, Koup RA. Macrophages and CD4+ T lymphocytes from two multiply exposed, uninfected individuals resist infection with primary non-syncytium-inducing isolates of human immunodeficiency virus type 1. J Virol 1996; 70:8758-8764.
65. Biti R, Ffrench R, Young J, Bennetts B, Stewart G, Liang T. HIV-1 infection in an individual homozygous for the CCR5 deletion allele. Nat Med 1997; 3:252-253.
66. O'Brien TR, Winkler C, Dean M, Nelson JA, Carrington M, Michael NL, White GC II. HIV-1 infection in a man homozygous for CCR5 delta 32. Lancet 1997; 349:1219.
67. Theodorou I, Meyer L, Magierowska M, Katlama C, Rouzioux C. HIV-1 infection in an individual homozygous for CCR5 delta 32. Seroco Study Group. Lancet 1997; 349:1219-1220.
68. Heiken H, Becker S, Bastisch I, Schmidt RE. HIV-1 infection in a heterosexual man homozygous for CCR-5 delta32. AIDS 1999; 13:529-530.
69. Kuipers H, Workman C, Dyer W, Geczy A, Sullivan J, Oelrichs R. An HIV-1-infected individual homozygous for the CCR-5 delta32 allele and the SDF-1 3'A allele. AIDS 1999; 13:433-434.
70. Balotta C, Bagnarelli P, Violin M, Ridolfo AL, Zhou D, Berlusconi A, Corvasce S, Corbellino M, Clementi M, Clerici M, Moroni M, Galli M. Homozygous delta 32 deletion of the CCR-5 chemokine receptor gene in an HIV-1-infected patient. AIDS 1997; 11:F67-F71.
71. Michael NL, Nelson JA, KewalRamani VN, Chang G, O'Brien SJ, Mascola JR, Volsky B, Louder M, White GC 2nd, Littman DR, Swanstrom R, O'Brien TR. Exclusive and persistent use of the entry coreceptor CXCR4 by human immunodeficiency virus type 1 from a subject homozygous for CCR5 delta32. J Virol 1998; 72:6040-6047.
72. de Roda Husman AM, Koot M, Cornelissen M, Keet IP, Brouwer M, Broersen SM, Bakker M, Roos MT, Prins M, de Wolf F, Coutinho RA, Miedema F, Goudsmit J, Schuitemaker H. Association between CCR5 genotype and the clinical course of HIV-1 infection. Ann Intern Med 1997; 127:882-890.
73. Wu L, Paxton WA, Kassam N, Ruffing N, Rottman JB, Sullivan N, Choe H, Sodroski J, Newman W, Koup RA, Mackay CR. CCR5 levels and expression pattern correlate with infectability by macrophage-tropic HIV-1, in vitro. J Exp Med 1997; 185:1681-1691.
74. Benkirane M, Jin DY, Chun RF, Koup RA, Jeang KT. Mechanism of transdominant inhibition of CCR5-mediated HIV-1 infection by ccr5delta32. J Biol Chem 1997; 272:30603-30606.
75. Bratt G, Leandersson AC, Albert J, Sandstrom E, Wahren B. MT-2 tropism and CCR-5 genotype strongly influence disease progression in HIV-1-infected individuals. AIDS 1998; 12:729-736.
76. Rabkin CS, Yang Q, Goedert JJ, Nguyen G, Mitsuya H, Sei S. Chemokine and chemokine receptor gene variants and risk of non-Hodgkin's lymphoma in human immunodeficiency virus-1-infected individuals. Blood 1999; 93:1838-1842.
77. Dean M, Jacobson LP, McFarlane G, Margolick JB, Jenkins FJ, Howard OM, Dong HF, Goedert JJ, Buchbinder S, Gomperts E, Vlahov D, Oppenheim JJ, O'Brien SJ, Carrington M. Reduced risk of AIDS lymphoma in individuals heterozygous for the CCR5-delta32 mutation. Cancer Res 1999; 59:3561-3564.
78. van Rij RP, Portegies P, Hallaby T, Lange JM, Visser J, Husman AM, van 't Wout AB, Schuitemaker H. Reduced prevalence of the CCR5 delta32 heterozygous genotype in human immunodeficiency virus-infected individuals with AIDS dementia complex. J Infect Dis 1999; 180:854-857.

79. Valdez H, Purvis SF, Lederman MM, Fillingame M, Zimmerman PA. Association of the CCR5delta32 mutation with improved response to antiretroviral therapy. JAMA 1999; 282:734.
80. Meyer L, Magierowska M, Hubert JB, Mayaux MJ, Misrahi M, Le Chenadec J, Debre P, Rouzioux C, Delfraissy JF, Theodorou I. CCR5 delta32 deletion and reduced risk of toxoplasmosis in persons infected with human immunodeficiency virus type 1. The SEROCO-HEMOCO-SEROGEST Study Groups. J Infect Dis 1999; 180:920-924.
81. Stephens JC, Reich DE, Goldstein DB, Shin HD, Smith MW, Carrington M, Winkler C, Huttley GA, Allikmets R, Schriml L, Gerrard B, Malasky M, Ramos MD, Morlot S, Tzetis M, Oddoux C, di Giovine FS, Nasioulas G, Chandler D, Aseev M, Hanson M, Kalaydjieva L, Glavac D, Gasparini P, Dean M, et al. Dating the origin of the CCR5-Delta32 AIDS-resistance allele by the coalescence of haplotypes. Am J Hum Genet 1998; 62:1507-1515.
82. Libert F, Cochaux P, Beckman G, Samson M, Aksenova M, Cao A, Czeizel A, Claustres M, de la Rua C, Ferrari M, Ferrec C, Glover G, Grinde B, Guran S, Kucinskas V, Lavinha J, Mercier B, Ogur G, Peltonen L, Rosatelli C, Schwartz M, Spitsyn V, Timar L, Beckman L, Vassart G, et al. The ΔCCR5 mutation conferring protection against HIV-1 in Caucasian populations has a single and recent origin in Northeastern Europe. Hum Mol Genet 1998; 7:399-406.
83. Martinson JJ, Chapman NH, Rees DC, Liu YT, Clegg JB. Global distribution of the CCR5 gene 32-basepair deletion. Nat Genet 1997; 16:100-103.
84. Lalani AS, Masters J, Zeng W, Barrett J, Pannu R, Everett H, Arendt CW, McFadden G. Use of chemokine receptors by poxviruses. Science 1999; 286:1968-1971.
85. Ansari-Lari MA, Liu XM, Metzker ML, Rut AR, Gibbs RA. The extent of genetic variation in the CCR5 gene. Nat Genet 1997; 16:221-222.
86. Carrington M, Kissner T, Gerrard B, Ivanov S, O'Brien SJ, Dean M. Novel alleles of the chemokine-receptor gene CCR5. Am J Hum Genet 1997; 61:1261-1267.
87. Carrington M, Dean M, Martin MP, O'Brien SJ. Genetics of HIV-1 infection: chemokine receptor CCR5 polymorphism and its consequences. Hum Mol Genet 1999; 8:1939-1945.
88. Li WH. Molecular Evolution. Sunderland, MA: Sinauer Association, 1997.
89. Quillent C, Oberlin E, Braun J, Rousset D, Gonzalez-Canali G, Metais P, Montagnier L, Virelizier JL, Arenzana-Seisdedos F, Beretta A. HIV-1-resistance phenotype conferred by combination of two separate inherited mutations of CCR5 gene. Lancet 1998; 351:14-18.
90. Howard OM, Shirakawa AK, Turpin JA, Maynard A, Tobin GJ, Carrington M, Oppenheim JJ, Dean M. Naturally occurring CCR5 extracellular and transmembrane domain variants affect HIV-1 Co-receptor and ligand binding function. J Biol Chem 1999; 274:16228-16234.
91. He J, Chen Y, Farzan M, Choe H, Ohagen A, Gartner S, Busciglio J, Yang X, Hofmann W, Newman W, Mackay CR, Sodroski J, Gabuzda D. CCR3 and CCR5 are co-receptors for HIV-1 infection of microglia. Nature 1997; 385:645-649.
92. Wu L, Gerard NP, Wyatt R, Choe H, Parolin C, Ruffing N, Borsetti A, Cardoso AA, Desjardin E, Newman W, Gerard C, Sodroski J. CD4-induced interaction of primary HIV-1 gp120 glycoproteins with the chemokine receptor CCR-5. Nature 1996; 384:179-183.
93. Wu L, LaRosa G, Kassam N, Gordon CJ, Heath H, Ruffing N, Chen H, Humblias J, Samson M, Parmentier M, Moore JP, Mackay CR. Interaction of chemokine receptor

CCR5 with its ligands: multiple domains for HIV-1 gp120 binding and a single domain for chemokine binding. J Exp Med 1997; 186:1373-1381.
94. Bleul CC, Wu L, Hoxie JA, Springer TA, Mackay CR. The HIV coreceptors CXCR4 and CCR5 are differentially expressed and regulated on human T lymphocytes. Proc Natl Acad Sci U S A 1997; 94:1925-1930.
95. Moriuchi H, Moriuchi M, Fauci AS. Cloning and analysis of the promoter region of CCR5, a coreceptor for HIV-1 entry. J Immunol 1997; 159:5441-5449.
96. Guignard F, Combadiere C, Tiffany HL, Murphy PM. Gene organization and promoter function for CC chemokine receptor 5 (CCR5). J Immunol 1998; 160:985-992.
97. Mummidi S, Ahuja SS, McDaniel BL, Ahuja SK. The human CC chemokine receptor 5 (CCR5) gene. Multiple transcripts with 5'-end heterogeneity, dual promoter usage, and evidence for polymorphisms within the regulatory regions and noncoding exons. J Biol Chem 1997; 272:30662-30671.
98. Liu R, Zhao X, Gurney TA, Landau NR. Functional analysis of the proximal CCR5 promoter. AIDS Res Hum Retroviruses 1998; 14:1509-1519.
99. Gonzalez E, Bamshad M, Sato N, Mummidi S, Dhanda R, Catano G, Cabrera S, McBride M, Cao XH, Merrill G, O'Connell P, Bowden DW, Freedman BI, Anderson SA, Walter EA, Evans JS, Stephan KT, Clark RA, Tyagi S, Ahuja SS, Dolan MJ, Ahuja SK. Race-specific HIV-1 disease-modifying effects associated with CCR5 haplotypes. Proc Natl Acad Sci U S A 1999; 96:12004-12009.
100. Smith MW, Dean M, Carrington M, Winkler C, Huttley GA, Lomb DA, Goedert JJ, O'Brien TR, Jacobson LP, Kaslow R, Buchbinder S, Vittinghoff E, Vlahov D, Hoots K, Hilgartner MW, O'Brien SJ. Contrasting genetic influence of CCR2 and CCR5 variants on HIV-1 infection and disease progression. Hemophilia Growth and Development Study (HGDS), Multicenter AIDS Cohort Study (MACS), Multicenter Hemophilia Cohort Study (MHCS), San Francisco City Cohort (SFCC), ALIVE Study. Science 1997; 277:959-965.
101. Kostrikis LG, Huang Y, Moore JP, Wolinsky SM, Zhang L, Guo Y, Deutsch L, Phair J, Neumann AU, Ho DD. A chemokine receptor CCR2 allele delays HIV-1 disease progression and is associated with a CCR5 promoter mutation. Nat Med 1998; 4:350-353.
102. Martin MP, Dean M, Smith MW, Winkler C, Gerrard B, Michael NL, Lee B, Doms RW, Margolick J, Buchbinder S, Goedert JJ, O'Brien TR, Hilgartner MW, Vlahov D, O'Brien SJ, Carrington M. Genetic acceleration of AIDS progression by a promoter variant of CCR5. Science 1998; 282:1907-1911.
103. Mummidi S, Ahuja SS, Gonzalez E, Anderson SA, Santiago EN, Stephan KT, Craig FE, O'Connell P, Tryon V, Clark RA, Dolan MJ, Ahuja SK. Genealogy of the CCR5 locus and chemokine system gene variants associated with altered rates of HIV-1 disease progression. Nat Med 1998; 4:786-793.
104. McDermott DH, Zimmerman PA, Guignard F, Kleeberger CA, Leitman SF, Murphy PM. CCR5 promoter polymorphism and HIV-1 disease progression. Multicenter AIDS Cohort Study (MACS). Lancet 1998; 352:866-870.
105. Bream JH, Young HA, Rice N, Martin MP, Smith MW, Carrington M, O'Brien SJ. CCR5 promoter alleles and specific DNA binding factors. Science 1999; 284:223a.
106. Lee B, Doranz BJ, Rana S, Yi Y, Mellado M, Frade JM, Martinez-A C, O'Brien SJ, Dean M, Collman RG, Doms RW. Influence of the CCR2-V64I polymorphism on human immunodeficiency virus type 1 coreceptor activity and on chemokine receptor function of CCR2b, CCR3, CCR5, and CXCR4. J Virol 1998; 72:7450-7458.

107. Mellado M, Rodriguez-Frade JM, Vila-Coro AJ, de Ana AM, Martinez-A C. Chemokine control of HIV-1 infection. Nature 1999; 400:723-724.
108. Frade JMR, Llorente M, Mellado M, Alcami J, Gutierrez-Ramos JC, Zaballos A, Real G, Martinez-A C. The amino-terminal domain of the CCR2 chemokine receptor acts as coreceptor for HIV-1 infection. J Clin Invest 1997; 100:497-502.
109. Martin MP, Carrington M, Dean M, O'Brien SJ, Sheppard HW, Wegner SA, Michael NL. CXCR4 polymorphisms and HIV-1 pathogenesis. J Acquir Immune Defic Syndr Hum Retrovirol 1998; 19:430.
110. Cohen OJ, Paolucci S, Bende SM, Daucher M, Moriuchi H, Moriuchi M, Cicala C, Davey RT Jr, Baird B, Fauci AS. CXCR4 and CCR5 genetic polymorphisms in long-term nonprogressive human immunodeficiency virus infection: lack of association with mutations other than CCR5-Delta32. J Virol 1998; 72:6215-6217.
111. Zou YR, Kottmann AH, Kuroda M, Taniuchi I, Littman DR. Function of the chemokine receptor CXCR4 in haematopoiesis and in cerebellar development. Nature 1998; 393:595-599.
112. Nagasawa T, Hirota S, Tachibana K, Takakura N, Nishikawa S, Kitamura Y, Yoshida N, Kikutani H, Kishimoto T. Defects of B-cell lymphopoiesis and bone-marrow myelopoiesis in mice lacking the CXC chemokine PBSF/SDF-1. Nature 1996; 382:635-638.
113. Ma Q, Jones D, Borghesani PR, Segal RA, Nagasawa T, Kishimoto T, Bronson RT, Springer TA. Impaired B-lymphopoiesis, myelopoiesis, and derailed cerebellar neuron migration in CXCR4- and SDF-1-deficient mice. Proc Natl Acad Sci U S A 1998; 95:9448-9453.
114. Bleul CC, Farzan M, Choe H, Parolin C, Clark-Lewis I, Sodroski J, Springer TA. The lymphocyte chemoattractant SDF-1 is a ligand for LESTR/fusin and blocks HIV-1 entry. Nature 1996; 382:829-833.
115. Shirozu M, Nakano T, Inazawa J, Tashiro K, Tada H, Shinohara T, Honjo T. Structure and chromosomal localization of the human stromal cell-derived factor 1 (SDF1) gene. Genomics 1995; 28:495-500.
116. Winkler C, Modi W, Smith MW, Nelson GW, Wu X, Carrington M, Dean M, Honjo T, Tashiro K, Yabe D, Buchbinder S, Vittinghoff E, Goedert JJ, O'Brien TR, Jacobson LP, Detels R, Donfield S, Willoughby A, Gomperts E, Vlahov D, Phair J, O'Brien SJ. Genetic restriction of AIDS pathogenesis by an SDF-1 chemokine gene variant. ALIVE Study, Hemophilia Growth and Development Study (HGDS), Multicenter AIDS Cohort Study (MACS), Multicenter Hemophilia Cohort Study (MHCS), San Francisco City Cohort. Science 1998; 279:389-393.
117. Tashiro K, Tada H, Heilker R, Shirozu M, Nakano T, Honjo T. Signal sequence trap: a cloning strategy for secreted proteins and type I membrane proteins. Science 1993; 261:600-603.
118. Ross J. Control of messenger RNA stability in higher eukaryotes. Trends Genet 1996; 12:171-175.
119. Tsai KC, Cansino VV, Kohn DT, Neve RL, Perrone-Bizzozero NI. Post-transcriptional regulation of the GAP-43 gene by specific sequences in the 3' untranslated region of the mRNA. J Neurosci 1997; 17:1950-1958.
120. McGowan KM, Police S, Winslow JB, Pekala PH. Tumor necrosis factor-alpha regulation of glucose transporter (GLUT1) mRNA turnover. Contribution of the 3'-untranslated region of the GLUT1 message. J Biol Chem 1997; 272:1331-1337.
121. Hendel H, Henon N, Lebuanec H, Lachgar A, Poncelet H, Caillat-Zucman S, Winkler CA, Smith MW, Kenefic L, O'Brien S, Lu W, Andrieu JM, Zagury D, Schachter F,

Rappaport J, Zagury JF. Distinctive effects of CCR5, CCR2, and SDF1 genetic polymorphisms in AIDS progression. J Acquir Immune Defic Syndr Hum Retrovirol 1998; 19:381-386.
122. van Rij RP, Broersen S, Goudsmit J, Coutinho RA, Schuitemaker H. The role of a stromal cell-derived factor-1 chemokine gene variant in the clinical course of HIV-1 infection. AIDS 1998; 12:F85-F90.
123. Brambilla A, Rizzardi GP, Veglia F, Sheppard HW, Lazzarin A, Poli G, Pantaleo G, Michael N, Vicenzi E. The SDF1-3'A genotype associates with accelerated time to death from AIDS diagnosis. Role of CD4+ T cell counts. 7th Conference on Retroviruses and Opportunistic Infections, Foundation for Retrovirology and Human Health, San Francisco, CA, Jan 29-Feb2, 2000.
124. Arenzana-Seisdedos F, Virelizier JL, Rousset D, Clark-Lewis I, Loetscher P, Moser B, Baggiolini M. HIV blocked by chemokine antagonist. Nature 1996; 383:400.
125. Paxton WA, Liu R, Kang S, Wu L, Gingeras TR, Landau NR, Mackay CR, Koup RA. Reduced HIV-1 infectability of CD4+ lymphocytes from exposed-uninfected individuals: association with low expression of CCR5 and high production of beta-chemokines. Virology 1998; 244:66-73.
126. Xiao L, Rudolph DL, Owen SM, Spira TJ, Lal RB. Adaptation to promiscuous usage of CC and CXC-chemokine coreceptors in vivo correlates with HIV-1 disease progression. AIDS 1998; 12:F137-F143.
127. Saha K, Bentsman G, Chess L, Volsky DJ. Endogenous production of beta-chemokines by CD4+, but not CD8+, T-cell clones correlates with the clinical state of human immunodeficiency virus type 1 (HIV-1)-infected individuals and may be responsible for blocking infection with non-syncytium-inducing HIV-1 in vitro. J Virol 1998; 72:876-881.
128. Liu H, Chao D, Nakayama EE, Taguchi H, Goto M, Xin X, Takamatsu JK, Saito H, Ishikawa Y, Akaza T, Juji T, Takebe Y, Ohishi T, Fukutake K, Maruyama Y, Yashiki S, Sonoda S, Nakamura T, Nagai Y, Iwamoto A, Shioda T. Polymorphism in RANTES chemokine promoter affects HIV-1 disease progression. Proc Natl Acad Sci U S A 1999; 96:4581-4585.
129. Dupont E, ed. Immunobiology of HLA. New York: Springer Verlag, 1995.
130. Klein J, ed. Natural History of the Major Histocompatibility Complex. New York: Wiley, 1986.
131. Parham P, Ohta T. Population biology of antigen presentation by MHC class I molecules. Science 1996; 272:67-74.
132. Hughes AL, Yeager M. Natural selection at major histocompatibility complex loci of vertebrates. Annu Rev Genet 1998; 32:415-435.
133. Gilbert SC, Plebanski M, Gupta S, Morris J, Cox M, Aidoo M, Kwiatkowski D, Greenwood BM, Whittle HC, Hill AV. Association of malaria parasite population structure, HLA, and immunological antagonism. Science 1998; 279:1173-1177.
134. Thursz MR, Kwiatkowski D, Allsopp CE, Greenwood BM, Thomas HC, Hill AV. Association between an MHC class II allele and clearance of hepatitis B virus in the Gambia. N Engl J Med 1995; 332:1065-1069.
135. Hill AV, Allsopp CE, Kwiatkowski D, Anstey NM, Twumasi P, Rowe PA, Bennett S, Brewster D, McMichael AJ, Greenwood BM. Common west African HLA antigens are associated with protection from severe malaria. Nature 1991; 352:595-600.
136. Doherty PC, Zinkernagel RM. Enhanced immunological surveillance in mice heterozygous at the H-2 gene complex. Nature 1975; 256:50-52.
137. Zinkernagel RM. Immunology taught by viruses. Science 1996; 271:173-178.

138. Carrington M, Nelson GW, Martin MP, Kissner T, Vlahov D, Goedert JJ, Kaslow R, Buchbinder S, Hoots K, O'Brien SJ. HLA and HIV-1: heterozygote advantage and B*35-Cw*04 disadvantage. Science 1999; 283:1748-1752.
139. Tang J, Costello C, Keet IP, Rivers C, Leblanc S, Karita E, Allen S, Kaslow RA. HLA class I homozygosity accelerates disease progression in human immunodeficiency virus type 1 infection. AIDS Res Hum Retroviruses 1999; 15:317-324.
140. Potts WK, Slev PR. Pathogen-based models favoring MHC genetic diversity. Immunol Rev 1995; 143:181-197.
141. Bodmer JG, Marsh SGE, Albert ED, Bodmer WF, Bontrop RE, Dupont B, Erlich HA, Hansen JA, Mach B, Mayr WR, Parham P, Petersdorf EW, Sasazuki T, Schreuder GM, Strominger JL, Svejgaard A, Terasaki PI. Nomenclature for factors of the HLA system, 1998. Hum Immunol 1999; 60:361-395.
142. Just JJ. Genetic predisposition to HIV-1 infection and acquired immune deficiency virus syndrome: a review of the literature examining associations with HLA. Hum Immunol 1995; 44:156-169.
143. Haynes BF, Pantaleo G, Fauci AS. Toward an understanding of the correlates of protective immunity to HIV infection. Science 1996; 271:324-328.
144. Rowland-Jones S, Tan R, McMichael A. Role of cellular immunity in protection against HIV infection. Adv Immunol 1997; 65:277-346.
145. Tomiyama H, Miwa K, Shiga H, Moore YI, Oka S, Iwamoto A, Kaneko Y, Takiguchi M. Evidence of presentation of multiple HIV-1 cytotoxic T lymphocyte epitopes by HLA-B*3501 molecules that are associated with the accelerated progression of AIDS. J Immunol 1997; 158:5026-5034.
146. Rowland-Jones S, Sutton J, Ariyoshi K, Dong T, Gotch F, McAdam S, Whitby D, Sabally S, Gallimore A, Corrah T, et al. HIV-specific cytotoxic T-cells in HIV-exposed but uninfected Gambian women. Nat Med 1995; 1:59-64.
147. Shiga H, Shioda T, Tomiyama H, Takamiya Y, Oka S, Kimura S, Yamaguchi Y, Gojoubori T, Rammensee HG, Miwa K, Takiguchi M. Identification of multiple HIV-1 cytotoxic T-cell epitopes presented by human leukocyte antigen B35 molecules. AIDS 1996; 10:1075-1083.
148. Johnson RP, Trocha A, Buchanan TM, Walker BD. Recognition of a highly conserved region of human immunodeficiency virus type 1 gp120 by an HLA-Cw4-restricted cytotoxic T-lymphocyte clone. J Virol 1993; 67:438-445.
149. Los Alamos HIV molecular immunology database. HTTP://hiv-web.lanl.gov/immunology.
150. Bruunsgaard H, Pedersen C, Skinhoj P, Pedersen BK. Clinical progression of HIV infection: role of NK cells. Scand J Immunol 1997; 46:91-95.
151. Dubey DP, Alper CA, Mirza NM, Awdeh Z, Yunis EJ. Polymorphic Hh genes in the HLA-B(C) region control natural killer cell frequency and activity. J Exp Med 1994; 179:1193-1203.
152. Trinchieri G. Biology of natural killer cells. Adv Immunol 1989; 47:187-376.
153. Ljunggren HG, Karre K. In search of the 'missing self': MHC molecules and NK cell recognition. Immunol Today 1990; 11:237-244.
154. Kaslow RA, Carrington M, Apple R, Park L, Munoz A, Saah AJ, Goedert JJ, Winkler C, O'Brien SJ, Rinaldo C, Detels R, Blattner W, Phair J, Erlich H, Mann DL. Influence of combinations of human major histocompatibility complex genes on the course of HIV-1 infection. Nat Med 1996; 2:405-411.
155. Keet IP, Tang J, Klein MR, LeBlanc S, Enger C, Rivers C, Apple RJ, Mann D, Goedert JJ, Miedema F, Kaslow RA. Consistent associations of HLA class I and II

and transporter gene products with progression of human immunodeficiency virus type 1 infection in homosexual men. J Infect Dis 1999; 180:299-309.
156. Hendel H, Caillat-Zucman S, Lebuanec H, Carrington M, O'Brien S, Andrieu JM, Schachter F, Zagury D, Rappaport J, Winkler C, Nelson GW, Zagury JF. New class I and II HLA alleles strongly associated with opposite patterns of progression to AIDS. J Immunol 1999; 162:6942-6946.
157. Costello C, Tang J, Rivers C, Karita E, Meizen-Derr J, Allen S, Kaslow RA. HLA-B*5703 independently associated with slower HIV-1 disease progression in Rwandan women. AIDS 1999; 13:1990-1991.
158. Rohowsky-Kochan C, Skurnick J, Molinaro D, Louria D. HLA antigens associated with susceptibility/resistance to HIV-1 infection. Hum Immunol 1998; 59:802-815.
159. Vassalli P. The pathophysiology of tumor necrosis factors. Annu Rev Immunol 1992; 10:411-452.
160. Brennan FM, Feldmann M. Cytokines in autoimmunity. Curr Opin Immunol 1996; 8:872-877.
161. Jacob CO. Tumor necrosis factor alpha in autoimmunity: pretty girl or old witch? Immunol Today 1992; 13:122-125.
162. Jacob CO, Fronek Z, Lewis GD, Koo M, Hansen JA, McDevitt HO. Heritable major histocompatibility complex class II-associated differences in production of tumor necrosis factor alpha: relevance to genetic predisposition to systemic lupus erythematosus. Proc Natl Acad Sci U S A 1990; 87:1233-1237.
163. Abraham LJ, French MA, Dawkins RL. Polymorphic MHC ancestral haplotypes affect the activity of tumour necrosis factor-alpha. Clin Exp Immunol 1993; 92:14-18.
164. Bendtzen K, Morling N, Fomsgaard A, Svenson M, Jakobsen B, Odum N, Svejgaard A. Association between HLA-DR2 and production of tumour necrosis factor alpha and interleukin 1 by mononuclear cells activated by lipopolysaccharide. Scand J Immunol 1988; 28:599-606.
165. Wilson AG, de Vries N, Pociot F, di Giovine FS, van der Putte LB, Duff GW. An allelic polymorphism within the human tumor necrosis factor alpha promoter region is strongly associated with HLA A1, B8, and DR3 alleles. J Exp Med 1993; 177:557-560.
166. Hamann A, Mantzoros C, Vidal-Puig A, Flier JS. Genetic variability in the TNF-alpha promoter is not associated with type II diabetes mellitus (NIDDM). Biochem Biophys Res Commun 1995; 211:833-839.
167. D'Alfonso S, Richiardi PM. A polymorphic variation in a putative regulation box of the TNFA promoter region. Immunogenetics 1994; 39:150-154.
168. Brinkman BM, Giphart MJ, Verhoef A, Kaijzel EL, Naipal AM, Daha MR, Breedveld FC, Verweij CL. Tumor necrosis factor alpha-308 gene variants in relation to major histocompatibility complex alleles and Felty's syndrome. Hum Immunol 1994; 41:259-266.
169. McGuire W, Hill AV, Allsopp CE, Greenwood BM, Kwiatkowski D. Variation in the TNF-alpha promoter region associated with susceptibility to cerebral malaria. Nature 1994; 371:508-510.
170. Roy S, McGuire W, Mascie-Taylor CG, Saha B, Hazra SK, Hill AV, Kwiatkowski D. Tumor necrosis factor promoter polymorphism and susceptibility to lepromatous leprosy. J Infect Dis 1997; 176:530-532.
171. Cabrera M, Shaw MA, Sharples C, Williams H, Castes M, Convit J, Blackwell JM. Polymorphism in tumor necrosis factor genes associated with mucocutaneous leishmaniasis. J Exp Med 1995; 182:1259-1264.

172. Duh EJ, Maury WJ, Folks TM, Fauci AS, Rabson AB. Tumor necrosis factor alpha activates human immunodeficiency virus type 1 through induction of nuclear factor binding to the NF-kappa B sites in the long terminal repeat. Proc Natl Acad Sci U S A 1989; 86:5974-5978.
173. Matsuyama T, Kobayashi N, Yamamoto N. Cytokines and HIV infection: is AIDS a tumor necrosis factor disease? AIDS 1991; 5:1405-1417.
174. Levy JA. HIV pathogenesis and long-term survival. AIDS 1993; 7:1401-1410.
175. Aukrust P, Liabakk NB, Muller F, Lien E, Espevik T, Froland SS. Serum levels of tumor necrosis factor-alpha (TNF alpha) and soluble TNF receptors in human immunodeficiency virus type 1 infection--correlations to clinical, immunologic, and virologic parameters. J Infect Dis 1994; 169:420-424.
176. Brinkman BM, Keet IP, Miedema F, Verweij CL, Klein MR. Polymorphisms within the human tumor necrosis factor-alpha promoter region in human immunodeficiency virus type 1-seropositive persons. J Infect Dis 1997; 175:188-190.
177. Knuchel MC, Spira TJ, Neumann AU, Xiao L, Rudolph DL, Phair J, Wolinsky SM, Koup RA, Cohen OJ, Folks TM, Lal RB. Analysis of a biallelic polymorphism in the tumor necrosis factor alpha promoter and HIV type 1 disease progression. AIDS Res Hum Retroviruses 1998; 14:305-309.
178. Khoo SH, Pepper L, Snowden N, Hajeer AH, Vallely P, Wilkins EG, Mandal BK, Ollier WE. Tumour necrosis factor c2 microsatellite allele is associated with the rate of HIV disease progression. AIDS 1997; 11:423-428.
179. Udalova IA, Nedospasov SA, Webb GC, Chaplin DD, Turetskaya RL. Highly informative typing of the human TNF locus using six adjacent polymorphic markers. Genomics 1993; 16:180-186.
180. Turner MW. Mannose-binding lectin: the pluripotent molecule of the innate immune system. Immunol Today 1996; 17:532-540.
181. Holmskov U, Malhotra R, Sim RB, Jensenius JC. Collectins: collagenous C-type lectins of the innate immune defense system. Immunol Today 1994; 15:67-74.
182. Epstein J, Eichbaum Q, Sheriff S, Ezekowitz RA. The collectins in innate immunity. Curr Opin Immunol 1996; 8:29-35.
183. Thiel S, Vorup-Jensen T, Stover CM, Schwaeble W, Laursen SB, Poulsen K, Willis AC, Eggleton P, Hansen S, Holmskov U, Reid KB, Jensenius JC. A second serine protease associated with mannan-binding lectin that activates complement. Nature 1997; 386:506-510.
184. Super M, Thiel S, Lu J, Levinsky RJ, Turner MW. Association of low levels of mannan-binding protein with a common defect of opsonisation. Lancet 1989; 2:1236-1239.
185. Garred P, Madsen HO, Hofmann B, Svejgaard A. Increased frequency of homozygosity of abnormal mannan-binding-protein alleles in patients with suspected immunodeficiency. Lancet 1995; 346:941-943.
186. Summerfield JA, Ryder S, Sumiya M, Thursz M, Gorchein A, Monteil MA, Turner MW. Mannose binding protein gene mutations associated with unusual and severe infections in adults. Lancet 1995; 345:886-889.
187. Taylor ME, Brickell PM, Craig RK, Summerfield JA. Structure and evolutionary origin of the gene encoding a human serum mannose-binding protein. Biochem J 1989; 262:763-771.
188. Sastry K, Herman GA, Day L, Deignan E, Bruns G, Morton CC, Ezekowitz RA. The human mannose-binding protein gene. Exon structure reveals its evolutionary relation-

ship to a human pulmonary surfactant gene and localization to chromosome 10. J Exp Med 1989; 170:1175-1189.

189. Lipscombe RJ, Sumiya M, Hill AV, Lau YL, Levinsky RJ, Summerfield JA, Turner MW. High frequencies in African and non-African populations of independent mutations in the mannose binding protein gene. Hum Mol Genet 1992; 1:709-715.
190. Madsen HO, Garred P, Kurtzhals JA, Lamm LU, Ryder LP,Thiel S, Svejgaard A. A new frequent allele is the missing link in the structural polymorphism of the human mannan-binding protein. Immunogenetics 1994; 40:37-44.
191. Sumiya M, Super M, Tabona P, Levinsky RJ, Arai T, Turner MW, Summerfield JA. Molecular basis of opsonic defect in immunodeficient children. Lancet 1991; 337:1569-1570.
192. Madsen HO, Garred P, Thiel S, Kurtzhals JA, Lamm LU, Ryder LP, Svejgaard A. Interplay between promoter and structural gene variants control basal serum level of mannan-binding protein. J Immunol 1995;155:3013-3020.
193. Ezekowitz RA, Kuhlman M, Groopman JE, Byrn RA. A human serum mannose-binding protein inhibits in vitro infection by the human immunodeficiency virus. J Exp Med 1989; 169:185-196.
194. Garred P, Madsen HO, Balslev U, Hofmann B, Pedersen C, Gerstoft J, Svejgaard A. Susceptibility to HIV infection and progression of AIDS in relation to variant alleles of mannose-binding lectin. Lancet 1997; 349:236-240.
195. Pastinen T, Liitsola K, Niini P, Salminen M, Syvanen AC. Contribution of the CCR5 and MBL genes to susceptibility to HIV type 1 infection in the Finnish population. AIDS Res Hum Retroviruses 1998; 14:695-698.
196. Maas J, de Roda Husman AM, Brouwer M, Krol A, Coutinho R, Keet I, van Leeuwen R, Schuitemaker H. Presence of the variant mannose-binding lectin alleles associated with slower progression to AIDS. Amsterdam Cohort Study. AIDS 1998; 12:2275-2280.

8

The Principles of Therapy for HIV-1 Infection

Thomas R. O'Brien and Eric A. Engels
National Cancer Institute, Rockville, Maryland

BACKGROUND

The availability of potent combination treatment regimens that suppress the replication of HIV-1 has led to dramatic changes in HIV-1-related morbidity and mortality where these therapies are available (1-7). Unfortunately these therapies are not curative and HIV-1 replication usually increases rapidly when treatment ceases. Therefore, with currently available therapies it is likely that most HIV-1-infected patients will require antiretroviral treatment throughout their lives. The drugs that are used in antiretroviral regimens often produce adverse effects that diminish the patient's quality of life. These adverse effects may also lead to poor compliance that, in turn, may increase the patient's risk of developing drug resistant viral strains. Because current therapies are not always adequate, new HIV-1 treatment options are needed. Therapies that act through novel mechanisms, such as interference with coreceptor binding (see Chapter 12), would be especially attractive.

The use of such new agents will likely be governed by the same principles that have been developed for currently available antiretroviral therapies. This chapter reviews those principles, but it is not meant to be a treatment guide. For that purpose, readers should refer to the latest recommendations from expert panels which can be found on various sites on the Internet [http://www.iasusa.org; http://www.hivatis.org]. Antiretroviral treatment is very complex and many aspects of treatment require considerable experience and excellent judgement.

Summary of the Principles of Therapy of HIV-1 Infection

In 1998, the NIH Panel to Define Principles of Therapy of HIV Infection summarized the principles by which treatment of HIV-1-infected patients should be undertaken (8). Although additional information about the benefits and risks of antiretroviral therapy has since become available, these principles remain generally valid for the treatment of non-pregnant adults who are chronically infected with HIV-1.

1. Ongoing HIV replication leads to immune system damage and progression to AIDS. HIV infection is always harmful, and true long-term survival free of clinically significant immune dysfunction is unusual.

2. Plasma HIV RNA levels indicate the magnitude of HIV replication and its associated rate of CD4+ T cell destruction, whereas CD4+ T cell counts indicate the extent of HIV-induced immune damage already suffered. Regular, periodic measurement of plasma HIV RNA levels and CD4+ T cell counts is necessary to determine the risk for disease progression in an HIV-infected person and to determine when to initiate or modify antiretroviral treatment regimens.

3. As rates of disease progression differ among HIV-infected persons, treatment decisions should be individualized by level of risk indicated by plasma HIV RNA levels and CD4+ T cell counts.

4. The use of potent combination antiretroviral therapy to suppress HIV replication to below the levels of detection of sensitive plasma HIV RNA assays limits the potential for selection of antiretroviral-resistant HIV variants, the major factor limiting the ability of antiretroviral drugs to inhibit virus replication and delay disease progression. Therefore, maximum achievable suppression of HIV replication should be the goal of therapy.

5. The most effective means to accomplish durable suppression of HIV replication is the simultaneous initiation of combinations of effective anti-HIV drugs with which the patient has not been previously treated and that are not cross-resistant with antiretroviral agents with which the patient has been treated previously.

6. Each of the antiretroviral drugs used in combination therapy regimens should always be used according to optimum schedules and dosages.

7. The available effective antiretroviral drugs are limited in number and mechanism of action, and cross-resistance between specific drugs has been documented. Therefore, any change in antiretroviral therapy increases future therapeutic constraints.

Treatment of pregnant women and children and prophylaxis of HIV-1-exposed individuals are beyond the scope of the present chapter. Treatment of acute HIV-1 infection will be discussed briefly.

SCIENTIFIC RATIONALE FOR TREATING HIV-1 INFECTION

HIV-1 RNA Levels and Clinical Progression

HIV-1 replication is the ultimate cause of the various conditions that constitute AIDS. HIV-1 appears to act both through the destruction of CD4+ lymphocytes and through direct effects of the virus. Although the time from initial infection to the development of AIDS varies widely, few HIV-1- infected people avoid the consequences of this infection in the absence of effective treatment (8).

The rate of HIV-1 replication, as reflected by plasma or serum HIV-1 RNA levels, is the most important determinant of clinical prognosis. In a natural history study of HIV-1-infected hemophiliacs, (9) HIV-1 RNA was measured in archived serum specimens that had been collected 12 to 36 months after the estimated date of HIV-1 seroconversion. The proportions of subjects with AIDS varied markedly by the number of HIV-1 RNA copies/ml (Figure 1). For example, the age-adjusted relative risk for AIDS for subjects with $\geq$10,000 copies/ml was 14.3 times greater than for the subjects with <1,000 copies/ml. There was also a strong trend between HIV-1 RNA level and the likelihood of long-term non-progression (Table 1). This study and work from other groups (10, 11) demonstrated that the early HIV-1 RNA level is a strong predictor of clinical outcome and that low HIV-1 RNA levels define persons with a high probability of long-term AIDS-free survival. Because the viral levels in these studies were measured many years before most of the subjects developed AIDS, these findings suggested that early events, perhaps occurring during primary infection, determine HIV-1 RNA levels and, thereby, long-term prognosis. The lack of a lower threshold in the relationship between HIV-1 RNA and the risk of AIDS lent support to a therapeutic goal of reducing circulating HIV-1 RNA to the lowest possible level.

HIV-1 replication leads to AIDS largely by causing destruction and sequestration of CD4+ lymphocytes. The HIV-1 RNA level predicts the rate of decline in circulating CD4+ lymphocyte counts (12), but HIV-1 RNA levels are not perfectly correlated with future rates of change in CD4+ lymphocyte levels, and individuals with similar HIV-1 RNA level can have different trends in CD4+ lymphocyte counts over time. Furthermore, the HIV-1 RNA level predicts the risk of developing AIDS independently of the CD4+ lymphocyte count. In the study of persons with hemophilia mentioned above, the relative risk of developing AIDS increased 2.6-fold with each one $\log_{10}$ increase in the HIV-1 RNA value even after controlling for the CD4+ lymphocyte count.

For some patients HIV-1 RNA levels are fairly constant for long periods of time, but most HIV-1-infected persons appear to lack a true long-term viral set point. In a longitudinal study of HIV-1-infected men who were enrolled during 1982-1992, HIV-1 RNA levels increased by a median of 0.08 $\log_{10}$ copies/ml/year (p=0.0001, compared to no change) during this period. HIV-1 RNA levels rose (either gradually or abruptly) for most subjects, although 41% had no increase.

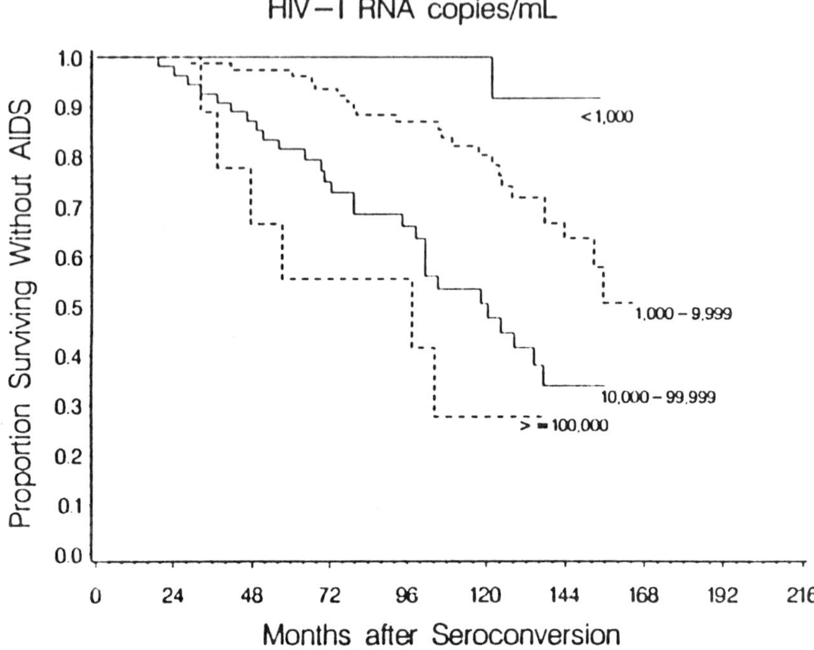

Figure 1 Proportion of subjects surviving without AIDS, by HIV-1 RNA level 12 to 36 months after the estimated date of HIV-1 seroconversion - Multicenter Hemophilia Cohort Study, 1979-1995 ($p < 0.001$). Adapted from Reference 9.

Table 1 Number of long-term non-progressors (LTNP) by serum HIV-1 RNA copies/ml measurements 12 to 36 months after the estimated date of seroconversion in the Multicenter Hemophilia Cohort Study, 1978-1995 ($p=0.002$, chi-square for linear trend). Adapted from Reference 9.

HIV-1 RNA	Number of Subjects	LTNP, No. (%)
≥100,000	6	0 (0.0%)
99,999-10,000	45	1 (2.2%)
9,999-1,000	66	7 (10.6%)
999-200	13	2 (15.4%)
<200	4	2 (50.0%)
Total	134	12

Long-term non-progressors are persons who, ten years after estimated date of seroconversion, are alive without a diagnosis of AIDS or an AIDS-related condition and who have a CD+ lymphocyte count of >500 cells/mm^3.

Among subjects surviving at least eight years, HIV-1 RNA levels were stable during the first four years after seroconversion, but rose in years five through eight. HIV-1 RNA levels measured at later time points are highly predictive of the risk of developing AIDS (12-14) even after controlling for multiple measures of CD4+ counts (14, 15). Because the failure to account for evolution of the viral level can lead to underestimation of the risk of progression, it is important that HIV-1 RNA levels, as well as CD4+ lymphocyte counts, be monitored regularly for patients in whom antiretroviral therapy has not yet been initiated.

Randomized clinical trials, which were originally designed to compare treatment regimens with regard to clinical outcome, also provided important information on the value of HIV-1 RNA level as a predictor of clinical endpoints. In the AIDS Clinical Trials Group 175 Study, (16) subjects with a CD4+ cell count of 200 to 500/mm^3 received reverse-transcriptase inhibitors as either monotherapy (zidovudine alone or didanosine alone) or dual therapy (zidovudine plus didanosine, or zidovudine plus zalcitabine). After eight weeks of treatment, the mean decrease from the initial HIV-1 RNA level was 0.26 ($\log_{10}$ copies/ml) for patients treated with zidovudine alone, 0.65 for didanosine alone, 0.93 for zidovudine plus didanosine, and 0.89 for zidovudine plus zalcitabine. The degree of suppression of HIV-1 RNA predicted the changes in CD4+ cell counts, as well as the risk of progression to AIDS and death. The clinical benefit of the suppression of HIV-1 replication was even more apparent in results from clinical trials of combination therapies with greater potency. The AIDS Clinical Trials Group 320 Study (17) compared patients treated with two reverse transcriptase inhibitors (zidovudine and lamivudine) plus the protease inhibitor indinavir to those treated with the two reverse transcriptase inhibitors alone. After 40 weeks of treatment, the three-drug regimen had reduced the HIV-1 RNA level by 2.8 $\log_{10}$ copies/ml compared to 0.6 $\log_{10}$ copies/ml for patients who had received the two reverse transcriptase inhibitors alone. The proportion of patients who progressed to AIDS or death was 6% for the three drug regimen compared to 11% with zidovudine and lamivudine alone ($p = 0.001$). Mortality in the two groups was 1.4 percent and 3.1 percent, respectively ($p = 0.04$) and the CD4+ lymphocyte count changes paralleled the clinical results. In another study, HIV-1-infected patients who had 50 to 400 CD4+ cells/mm^3 and $\geq$20,000 copies of HIV-1 RNA copies/ml were randomly assigned to one of three treatments: indinavir alone; zidovudine combined with lamivudine; or all three drugs (18). At week 24, RNA levels decreased to less than 500 copies/ml in 28 of 31 (90%) patients in the three-drug group, 12 of 28 (43%) patients in the indinavir group, and none of 30 patients in the zidovudine-lamivudine group. The increase in CD4+ cell counts over the first 24 weeks was greater in the two groups receiving indinavir than in the zidovudine-lamivudine group. A meta-analysis of clinical trial data confirmed that the decreased risk of clinical events was proportionate to the reduction in the HIV-1 RNA level (19). In sum, the data from clinical trials clearly demonstrate that reducing the HIV-1 replication rate with antiretroviral therapy can dramatically improve the prognosis for

HIV-1-infected patients and that the benefit of therapy correlates with the degree of suppression of HIV-1 replication.

IMMUNOLOGICAL RECOVERY AFTER ANTIRETROVIRAL THERAPY

Therapeutic regimens that markedly reduce the HIV-1 replication rate not only halt new damage to the immune system, but can also lead to immunological recovery (20-22). HIV-1 replication damages the immune system by causing decreases in the number of CD4+ lymphocytes, CD8+ lymphocytes, and other cells. A heightened state of activation of CD4+ and CD8+ lymphocytes appears to play an important role in the death of these cells and HIV-1 replication also leads to a functional deterioration of the immunological response. Immunological recovery after antiretroviral therapy consists of increases in the number of CD4+ lymphocytes and other cells, decreased activation of these cells, and a functional improvement in the immune system.

Immunological recovery occurs in phases for patients who have suffered extensive immunologic damage. The total number of peripheral blood CD4+ and CD8+ lymphocytes increases markedly during early treatment. In adults who were treated with potent therapy, total CD4+ lymphocytes increased at a rate of 5.3 cells/mm^3/ day during the first three weeks of therapy and at a rate of 0.3 cells/ mm^3/ day during the next 33 weeks. Total CD8+ lymphocytes also increased during the first six weeks of therapy, but not subsequently (23). Generally consistent results were obtained from the ACTG 315 Study which evaluated a regimen that consisted of zidovudine, lamivudine, and ritonavir. The median CD4+ lymphocyte count for treated patients increased from 189 cells/ mm^3 to 271 cells/ mm^3 after four weeks of treatment and to 297 cells/mm^3 after 12 weeks of treatment. After 48 weeks of treatment the CD4+ lymphocyte count for the ACTG 315 subjects had increased to 362/mm^3. The CD8+ lymphocyte counts at 4, 12 and 48 weeks were 726 cells/mm^3, 806 cells/mm^3, and 922 cells/ mm^3, respectively. (24, 25) In another study, patients were treated with two reverse transcriptase inhibitors and a protease inhibitor for one year. The median CD4+ lymphocyte count of these subjects increased from 26 cells/mm^3 to 200 cells/mm^3, although the CD4+ lymphocyte count did not increase in some patients despite a two-log reduction in the HIV-1 RNA level. (22) B lymphocytes also increase in numbers during the first phase of recovery, but natural killer cells do not appear to increase (24).

HIV-1 infection results in depletion of both naïve and memory cells, which can be differentiated on the basis of cell surface markers (21) (naïve CD4+ lymphocytes express CD45RA, while memory CD4+ lymphocytes express CD45RO). Naïve cells are newly generated cells with the potential to generate responses to newly encountered pathogens. After such exposure, naïve cells evolve into memory cells. Memory cells are capable of expression of cytokines and cytolysis in response to specific antigenic stimulation. In healthy adults about half of circulating cells are naïve cells and half are memory cells.

The marked increase in the number of both CD4+ lymphocytes and CD8+ lymphocytes in the blood during the first several weeks of effective therapy is chiefly due to an increase in the number of memory cells. This therapeutic response appears to result from a redistribution of memory cells from other compartments. Effective therapy also leads to a slow repopulation with newly produced naïve T cells. These new cells contribute relatively little to the initial increases in CD4+ lymphocytes, but produce the second, more gradual phase of CD4+ lymphocyte restoration (20, 23, 26). During the first year or more of therapy the number of circulating naïve CD4+ and CD8+ lymphocytes continue to increase, while circulating memory CD8+ lymphocytes may decrease. During the second phase of immunological recovery the diversity of the T-cell receptor repertoire may also improve.

Reduced Activation

HIV-1 infection results in inappropriate activation of both CD4+ and CD8+ lymphocytes (21). Among the CD4+ lymphocytes, it is predominately memory cells that are activated. Activated lymphocytes tend to function more poorly and be more susceptible to programmed cell death (apoptosis). Chronic activation may also cause CD4+ and CD8+ lymphocytes to become effectors of apoptosis, leading to the destruction of healthy activated HIV-1-uninfected cells through the premature induction of programmed cell death (27). Activated CD8+ lymphocytes are a highly predictive marker of the risk of AIDS and death (28).

Reduction in lymphocyte activation is part of both the early and late response to the suppression of HIV-1 replication. Among eight previously untreated patients with advanced HIV-1 infection, during the first twelve months of therapy there was a continuous decrease in the proportion of activated CD4+ and CD8+ lymphocytes that reached normal or near normal values (20). Data from other studies are consistent with these findings. Among 44 patients with moderately advanced HIV-1 infection, the percentage of CD4+ lymphocytes that coexpressed activation antigens (CD38 and HLA-DR) fell from 25% prior to treatment to 15% after four weeks of treatment and 12.5% after 12 weeks of therapy. The percentage of activated CD8+ lymphocytes fell from 59% initially to 44% at week 4 and 29% at week 12 (24). In 12 participants in the Multicenter AIDS Cohort Study, CD8+ lymphocyte activation significantly decreased after 48 weeks of combination therapy, and some T-cell activation markers decreased to levels observed in long-term non-progressors (29). Therefore, potent anti-retroviral therapies can decrease lymphocyte activation to normal levels, which may prevent premature apoptosis and contribute to restoration of the immune system.

Improved Immune Function

Effective suppression of HIV-1 replication can also yield functional improvements in the immunological response. Autran et al. (20) found that viral suppression due to highly active antiretroviral therapy (HAART) improved CD4+ T cell reactivity to recall antigens. In six previously untreated patients (mean CD4+ lymphocyte count, 176 cells/ mm^3) who had no detectable response to recall antigens from cytomegalovirus and Mycobacterium tuberculosis prior to therapy, CD4+ lymphocyte proliferation against these antigens was detected after one month of therapy, and improved further through 6 months of treatment. However, proliferation against the HIV-1 p24 antigen remained absent despite effective treatment. In an extension of this study, the investigators examined 20 patients (seven naive, 13 previously treated) who received potent therapy (30). CD4+ lymphocyte cell proliferation in response to cytomegalovirus and tuberculin antigens was measured and patients who had no antigen-specific reactivity at baseline, but who developed it during treatment, were classified as immunological responders. Four patients had antigen-specific reactivity at baseline compared with 14 at month 12 ($p < 0.001$). Immunological responders differed from non-responders in that their HIV-1 RNA reduction was sustained for 12 months, their CD4+ lymphocyte count increase was greater, and they showed an early increase in memory CD4+ lymphocytes. These data indicate that recovery of CD4+ T cell reactivity against opportunistic pathogens in immunosuppressed patients depends on the degree and duration of HIV-1 RNA reduction and the increase of memory CD4+ lymphocytes.

In the AIDS Clinical Trials Group 315 Study, (24, 25) the effects of potent therapy on immune reconstitution were evaluated in 34 HIV-1-infected patients. After 48 weeks of therapy, 59% of the subjects had <100 copies HIV-1 RNA/mL and the median CD4+ lymphocyte count had increased from 192 cells/mm^3 to 362 cells /mm^3. Lymphocyte proliferative responses to Candida normalized within 12 weeks, but responses to HIV-1 and tetanus remained depressed throughout therapy. Partial recovery of delayed-type hypersensitivity responses occurred after 12 weeks for Candida and after 48 weeks for mumps. The magnitude of virologic suppression was correlated with increases in the number of CD4+ lymphocytes, but not with measures of immune function reconstitution.

Immunological function was also evaluated in 21 AIDS patients (mean baseline CD4+ cell count, 20 cells/mm^3) who had received highly active antiretroviral therapy for 24 months (26). Most of the patients recovered lymphoproliferative responses to mitogens (phytohaemagglutinin, anti-CD3), but only four subjects showed a functional response to Candida mannoprotein. No patients showed a response to HIV-1 recombinant glycoprotein 160 or tetanus toxoid. These results provide further evidence that the functional recovery of the immune system may not be complete for patients who are severely immunocompromised at the initiation of potent therapy.

Immune function may improve after treatment with effective antiretroviral therapy even if the CD4+ lymphocyte count does not increase. Sondergaard et al. (31) studied 12 HIV-1-infected patients whose CD4+ counts did not change during treatment with HAART. With treatment, the patient's CD8+ lymphocytes expressed smaller amounts of the T-cell activation marker CD38 and proliferation increased in lymphocyte cell cultures stimulated with pokeweed mitogens or Candida. The production of interferon-gamma was also increased. These data are consistent with those from treatment trials in which a component of the clinical response to therapy can be attributable to HIV-1 RNA reduction, independent of change in CD4+ count (19, 32). Together these findings suggest that HIV-1 replication (or the actual HIV-1 virions) may interfere with immune function.

HIV-1-specific CD4+ lymphocyte function may be important in controlling HIV-1 infection. Individuals who control viremia in the absence of antiviral therapy exhibit vigorous, persistent, polyclonal CD4+ lymphocyte proliferative responses to HIV-1 antigens. These proliferative responses, which result in the elaboration of interferon-gamma and antiviral beta chemokines, are inversely related to the HIV-1 RNA level (33). However, studies mentioned above suggest that HIV-1-specific lymphoproliferative responses often remain absent after therapy, even though responses to other microbial antigens are restored. In contrast to these findings, Haslett et al. (34) observed strong HIV-1-specific CD4+ T cell responses of Th-1 phenotype in 11 of 22 chronically infected adults on HAART. The magnitude and frequency of these HIV-1-specific lymphoproliferative responses were strongly associated with previous interruptions in HAART, but the magnitude of CD8+ T cell responses to HIV-1 gag, pol, env, and nef was similar in patients who had and those who had not interrupted HAART. Similarly, Binley et al. (35) found that emergence of viral replication during short periods of intermittent therapy promoted generalized activation of T helper lymphocytes, manifested by increased T cell proliferative responses to HIV-1 gag antigens. Recovery of CD4+ T cell responses occurred in some individuals who initiated HAART years after infection and who were intermittently adherent to drug treatment.

These studies suggest that HIV-1-infected patients may be able to generate strong HIV-1-specific CD4+ and CD8+ T cell immunity and that interruptions in antiviral treatment may prime or boost HIV-1-specific CD4+ T-helper responses. Rosenberg and colleagures (36) administered one or two supervised treatment interruptions to eight subjects with treated acute infection. All eight subjects were able to achieve a viral level <5,000 HIV-1 RNA copies per ml off therapy and five of the eight subjects had <500 HIV-1 RNA copies per ml plasma after 5-8.7 months of follow-up. All of the subjects had increased virus-specific cytotoxic T lymphocytes and maintained T-helper-cell responses. For patients treated during chronic infection, it may also prove advantageous to schedule intermittent holidays from treatment to provide antigenic stimulation with HIV-1. However, treatment holidays expose the HIV-1-infected patient to repeated episodes of HIV-1-induced damage to the immune system and the risk for development of drug resistance. Furthermore, the overall long-term immunological benefits of scheduled treatment interuptions for chronically infected patients remain unclear. Treatment holidays are not currently recommended for any treated patients and should not be considered outside the trial setting.

Expansion of Constricted CD4+ T-Cell Repertoire

HIV-1 infection can disrupt the diversity of CD4+ T-cells and, thereby, limit a patient's responses to specific recall antigens. Connors et al. (37) used PCR-based techniques to examine 22 T-cell receptor β–chain, variable-region subfamilies in HIV-1-infected subjects and others. Constriction of the CD4+ T-cell repertoire was more common in HIV-1-infected subjects than among people who were not infected. Among HIV-1-infected patients, disruption of the CD4+ T cell repertoire was more profound among patients with lower CD4+ lymphocyte counts. In these patients the disruptions of the CD4+ T-cell repertoire were not immediately corrected by treatment with antiretroviral or immune-based (IL-2) therapies, but the antiretroviral regimen in these subjects was suboptimal according to current standards.

Gorochov et al. examined perturbations of both the CD4+ and CD8+ T-cell antigen receptor repertoires during different stages of HIV-1 infection by measuring the distribution of the lengths of the beta chain of the complementarity-determining region 3 (CDR3) in seven patients (38). For CD4+ T-cells, the repertoire was not decreased significantly for patients with CD4+ lymphocyte counts >200 cells/mm^3 and viral levels <100,000 HIV-1 RNA copies/ml, but it was perturbed in those patients who had either a low CD4+ lymphocyte count or a high HIV-1 RNA level. In contrast, the CD8+ T-cell repertoire was markedly restricted during all stages of HIV-1 infection. Gorochov and his colleagues also looked at the effect of potent antiretroviral therapy on these parameters (38). Among patients who had perturbations of the CD4+ T-cell repertoire before treatment, the CD4+ repertoire improved markedly for the patients who had a good response to therapy, but not for those who had a poor response. In contrast, the CD8+ T-cell repertoire perturbations persisted during the first six months of treatment for all of the patients who received potent combination therapy. This study indicates that suppression of HIV-1 replication may improve the CD4+ T-cell repertoire. However, Martinon et al (39) found persistent alterations in T-cell repertoire, cytokine and chemokine receptor gene expression after 1 year of highly active antiretroviral therapy. The CD8+ cell repertoire alterations were profound, whereas the CD4+ cell alterations were moderate. Both the CD4+ and the CD8+ cell repertoire alterations persisted unchanged even though the viral load was decreased by 2-3 $\log_{10}$ copies/ml.

Improvement in Immune Function Despite Incomplete Viral Suppression

Although the goal of antiretroviral therapy should be to suppress the HIV-1 RNA to an undetectable level, results from both epidemiologic cohort studies and clinical trials suggest that reducing a patient's HIV-1 RNA level may be beneficial, even if there is still measurable HIV-1 RNA and even if the CD4+ lymphocyte count fails to increase (19,40). The observation that higher HIV-1 RNA levels are associated with poorer immune function even after the CD4+ lymphocyte count is considered (14) suggests that the virus may interfere directly with immune function. Treatment-related benefits could result, in part, because circulating virus directly interferes with immune function or because viral strains that have mutated in response to selective pressures from drugs replicate poorly (41, 42) and are less pathogenic.

Long Term Restoration

It remains to be determined how often full recovery of the immune system can be achieved and how long a patient must be treated before a full recovery is made. In one of the longer studies reported to date, subjects were treated for two years with potent triple antiretroviral therapy (43). Treatment resulted in strong suppression of HIV-1 replication and increase in the median CD4+ lymphocyte count from 170 to 420 cells/ mm^3. In a number of these subjects the CD4+ lymphocytes did not increase further after 72 weeks of treatment even though that count had not yet reached a normal value. These data suggest that immunological recovery may not always be complete even for patients who are receiving therapy that successfully suppresses viral replication.

A second study of the immunological effects of two years of potent antiretroviral therapy involved patients who were more severely immunocompromised. These 21 patients had a mean baseline CD4+ cell count of 20 cells/μL and all of them had AIDS. In fourteen patients the decrease in HIV-1 RNA from the baseline value was at least 2 $\log_{10}$ copies/ml, yet the mean CD4+ lymphocyte count during treatment was 400 cells/ mm^3 (a good, but not complete CD4+ lymphocyte response). These data suggest that immune recovery is slow and incomplete in severely immunocompromised patients (26).

Clinical Benefits of Immunological Recovery

The implementation of more effective antiretroviral treatment regimens has led to dramatic decreases in the risk of AIDS and death among HIV-1-infected patients in the developed world (1-7). For example, Pallela et al. (1) looked at changes in mortality among patients with CD4+ lymphocyte counts <100 cells/mm^3 who were seen at HIV-1 treatment clinics in eight U.S. cities. During early 1995, mortality among these patients was 29.4%/year. In mid-1997, after the introduction of potent antiretroviral regimens, the mortality rate had fallen to 8.8%/year. These trends have continued with time (Figure 2). Similar data were reported from a London clinic (4), where the incidence of AIDS fell from 27.4%/year prior to 1992 to 6.9%/year during 1997. Furthermore, among the London clinic patients with CD4+ lymphocyte counts ≤200 cells/mm^3, the incidence of AIDS was 51.1%/year for patients taking no therapy and 6.1%/year for those receiving a potent regimen. It remains to be determined whether such improvements in HIV-1 clinical outcomes can be maintained over time.

Antimicrobial prophylaxis also contributes to decreased HIV-1-related morbidity and mortality among patients with low CD4+ lymphocyte counts, but these

Figure 2 Mortality and frequency of use of combination antiretroviral therapy including a protease inhibitor among HIV-1-infected patients with fewer than 100 CD4+ cells/mm^3, according to calendar quarter, from 1994 through 1999. Data updated from reference 1, courtesy of Dr. Scott Holmberg.

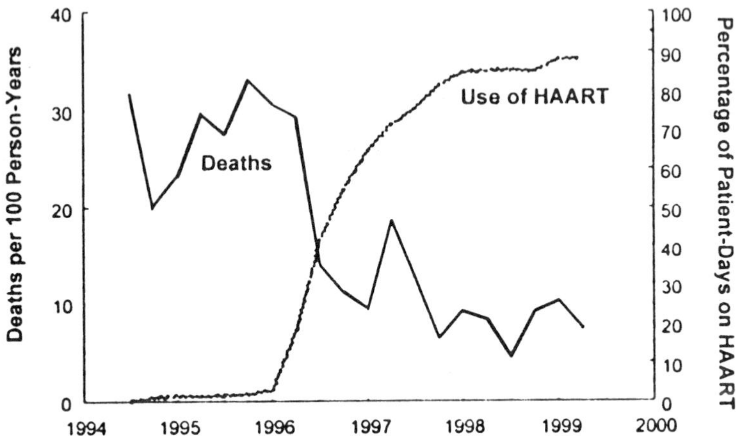

medications are not without adverse effects. Recent studies have shown that primary prophylaxis may be discontinued safely if the CD4+ lymphocyte count has increased in response to therapy (44, 45). Pneumocystis carinii pneumonia prophylaxis can be discontinued in patients with a sustained increase in CD4+ lymphocyte counts >200 cells/ mm^3, (46-49) and there is a low rate of disseminated infection with Mycobacterium avium complex among persons whose CD4+ T-lymphocyte count has increased to >100 cells/ mm^3 (50). Similarly, secondary prophylaxis against CMV retinitis often can be discontinued in patients whose CD4+ lymphocyte counts have increased to >100-150 cells/μL and whose HIV-1 plasma RNA levels have been suppressed in response to HAART (51-54).

When to Treat

Most experts recommend treatment for the small proportion of HIV-1-infected patients who are diagnosed during primary infection. HIV-1-specific CD4+ and CD8+ T-cell responses that appear to be important for controlling the virus may disappear during primary infection (55). If patients are treated with potent antiviral therapy during primary HIV-1 infection they may develop strong HIV-1-specific proliferative responses (33, 36). Initiation of antiretroviral therapy during primary HIV-1 infection may also prevent loss of the T-cell receptor beta chain repertoire (56). Maintenance of vigorous T-cell responses provides a strong rationale for aggressive treatment of the rare patient who is diagnosed during acute HIV-1 infection (57).

Table 2 Guidelines for initiation of antiretroviral therapy in chronically HIV-1-infected patients (Adapted from: Guidelines for the Use of Antiretroviral Therapy in HIV-Infected Adults and Adolescents, February, 2001; http://www.hivatis.org).

Clinical Category	CD4+ Lymphocyte Count	HIV RNA Level	Recommendation
Symptomatic	Any value	Any value	Treat
Asymptomatic	<200/mm^3	Any value	Treat
Asymptomatic	200-350/mm^3	Any value	Most experts would treat
Asymptomatic	>350/mm^3	>55,000 copies/ml (RT-PCR assay)	Some experts would treat, especially if HIV RNA level is very high
Asymptomatic	>350/mm^3	<55,000 copies/ml (RT-PCR assay)	Many experts would defer treatment

Most patients are diagnosed after HIV-1 infection has been well established and for these patients the benefits of treatment must be weighed against the cost and potential adverse effects of treatment regimens (57). Given that any level of HIV-1 replication may be harmful to the immune system and that immune reconstitution may be incomplete, there has been an extensive debate as to the optimal point at which to initiate therapy. The HIV-1 RNA level and the CD4+ lymphocyte count are the main parameters used for treatment decisions. The HIV-1 RNA level reflects the HIV-1 replication rate and is highly predictive of both the rate of CD4+ lymphocyte loss and clinical outcomes. The CD4+ lymphocyte count is the primary measure of the extent of current damage or dysfunction of the immune system. However, as noted above, the HIV-1 RNA level may also be an independent measure of immune dysfunction (14). Guidelines for initiating treatment are based on both of these parameters and the patient's symptoms. Current consensus guidelines recommend therapy for patients who are symptomatic, patients with low CD4+ lymphocyte counts, and patients with high HIV-1 RNA levels (Table 2). Therapy should be considered for other patients on an individual basis, recognizing that for some patients the adverse consequences of therapy may outweigh the benefits.

The goal of treatment should be to minimize HIV-1 replication (as reflected by the HIV-1 RNA level) in order to minimize further damage to the immune system, maximize immune reconstitution, and limit the development of HIV-1 strains that are resistant to antiretroviral therapies. Therefore, minimizing HIV-1 replication sets up a beneficial cycle, whereas continued viral replication in the face of treatment for HIV-1 may lead to resistant strains that decrease the effectiveness of the current treatment regimen and limit future treatment options.

Antiretroviral Therapies

There are a large number of individual drugs available for the treatment of HIV-1 infection, but most of these agents fall into one of three categories: nucleoside reverse transcriptase inhibitors (NRTIs), nonnucleoside reverse transcriptase inhibitors (NNRTIs), and protease inhibitors. NRTIs were the initial drugs developed for the treatment of HIV-1 and agents from this class are included in most HIV-1 treatment regimens. NRTIs are phosphorylated intracellularly to active triphosphate forms that are incorporated into newly synthesized HIV-1 DNA strands by the viral reverse transcriptase. The lack of a 3' hydroxyl results in termination of HIV-1 DNA synthesis (58). NRTIs include zidovudine (AZT), didanosine (ddI), lamivudine (3TC), stavudine (d4T), zalcitabine (ddC) and abacavir (57). The NNRTIs interact with a specific site of the HIV-1 reverse transcriptase protein that is closely associated with, but distinct from, the NRTI binding site (59). NNRTIs available in the United States include nevirapine, delaviridine, and efavirenz (57). Typical treatment regimens include one, two, or even three of these agents, and the availability of multiple NRTIs and NNRTIs offers numerous potential options for treatment combinations. However, overlapping drug toxicities prevent the use of some combinations, and their sequential use can be limited by cross-resistance.

The availability of protease inhibitors, a class of drug that interferes with the HIV-1 protease gene, opened up new treatment options for combination antiretroviral therapy, as protease inhibitor-containing regimens were instrumental to the development of potent antiretroviral regimens. Protease inhibitors that are approved for use in the United States include saquinavir, ritonavir, indinavir, nelfinavir, amprenavir, and lopinavir (57). Single or dual protease inhibitor regimens are often prescribed with combinations of NRTIs or an NNRTI, with the goal of achieving maximal suppression of viral replication through inhibition of two separate viral enzymes. Protease inhibitors inhibit or induce hepatic P450 enzymes, strongly affecting the metabolism of other medications including other antiretrovirals. This effect on drug metabolism can be used advantageously. For example, several effective combinations of dual protease inhibitors (e.g., ritonavir/indinavir, ritonavir/saquinavir) allow dosing at longer intervals for the separate drugs, with augmented drug levels, because one agent (ritonavir) slows metabolism of the other. Lopinavir, a newer protease inhibitor, was approved for use in the United States in a formulation with ritonavir; in this combination, ritonavir acts to slow metabolism of lopinavir.

Treatment Regimens

Theoretically, the aforementioned individual drugs could be combined to form a very large number of possible treatment regimens. However, practical considerations of cross-resistance and adverse effects limit the number of potential regimens. As of the year 2000, several different types of treatment regimens were in

Table 3 Potential antiretroviral treatment regimens. (Adapted from reference 57.)

Currently Recommended Regimens
Two Nucleoside Reverse Transcriptase Inhibitors and One Protease Inhibitor
Two Nucleoside Reverse Transcriptase Inhibitors and One Non-Nucleoside Reverse Transcriptase Inhibitor
Two Nucleoside Reverse Transcriptase Inhibitors and Two Protease Inhibitors
Regimens Under Evaluation
Three Nucleoside Reverse Transcriptase Inhibitors
One Nucleoside Reverse Transcriptase Inhibitor and One Non-Nucleoside Reverse Transcriptase Inhibitor and One Protease Inhibitor

use and other regimens were under evaluation. All regimens use at least three different drugs because single or dual drug regimens lead to high rates of virologic failure due to frequent mutations. Most regimens include drugs from at least two different classes in order to minimize cross-resistance, but regimens consisting of three NRTIs are also in use (Table 3).

Although it was initially hoped that treatment for HIV-1 might be curative, it is now clear that despite prolonged treatment the virus remains integrated within resting CD4+ lymphocytes in host DNA as latent provirus and that this reservoir of virus may persist for life (60-62). Even small amounts of HIV-1 replication can replenish this pool of latently infected cells (62). Virus from these latent pools can reactivate when treatment is stopped, leading to replenished infection of other cell compartments. As a result, cessation of treatment usually leads to rapid virologic relapse, and it is anticipated that treatment must be administered indefinitely. Attempts to shift to less intensive one or two drug maintenance regimens after successful viral suppression with triple combination therapy were unsuccessful (63). However, studies are underway to determine whether totally stopping treatment periodically may yield equivalent or even better virologic control than continuous treatment.

Monitoring Therapy

The HIV-1 RNA level is the key measure of therapeutic success. Most current HIV-1 RNA assays have a lower limit of detection of 40 to 50 HIV-1 RNA copies/ml. The goal of therapy is to suppress viral replication so that HIV-1 RNA is undetectable (57). The HIV-1 RNA level declines rapidly with effective treatment and there should be at least a 1.5 log decline during the first month of therapy. Suppression of the HIV-1 RNA level within the first 8 weeks of treatment predicts a good long-term response (57) and the HIV-1 RNA nadir also predicts the subsequent risk of treatment failure (64). The failure to suppress the HIV-1 RNA below the level of detection by 24 weeks suggests poor adherence, inadequate drug absorption, or drug resistance (57). The HIV-1 RNA level should be monitored every 2 to 3 months after viral suppression is achieved and an increase in the HIV-1 RNA level should be confirmed by a test on a second specimen before the treatment regimen is altered (57).

Suppression of HIV-1 RNA levels below the level of detection is the goal of antiretroviral therapy and these treatment-induced declines usually lead to notable increases in the CD4+ lymphocyte count. As noted above, sustained increases in CD4+ lymphocyte counts during treatment represent true improvements in immune function. Even in the absence of CD4+ count increase, successful suppression of HIV-1 replication confers clinical benefit in that there is reduced risk for opportunistic illnesses (19), and in these cases therapy is usually continued unchanged. Thus, during therapy, monitoring of CD4+ lymphocyte counts is a useful adjunct to monitoring of HIV-1 RNA levels, providing information on level of immune dysfunction, but CD4+ response is secondary to HIV-1 RNA level response in guiding therapy.

Recent studies suggest that polymorphisms in chemokine receptor genes may explain some of the heterogeneity in therapeutic response observed among patients receiving potent antiretroviral therapy. As discussed in detail in Chapter 7, polymorphisms in chemokine receptor genes modulate the natural history of HIV-1 infection. Compared to subjects with other genotypes, the prognosis for HIV-1-infected *CCR5-Δ32* heterozygotes or those who carry the *CCR2-64I* allele is more favorable, while homozygotes for the *CCR5* promoter allele *59029A* have a less favorable natural history. Valdez and colleagues studied 293 HIV-1-infected patients who were treated with a regimen that included a protease inhibitor. They found that 81% of *CCR5-Δ32* heterozygotes achieved an HIV-1 RNA level <400 copies/ml, as compared to 57% of subjects who had two normal alleles at this locus (p=.04) (65). Another study examined the predictive value of several chemokine receptor gene polymorphisms among subjects enrolled in the ACTG 343 trial (HIV-1-infected adults with a CD4+ lymphocyte count $\geq$200 cells/mm^3 and a plasma HIV RNA level $\geq$1000 copies/ml who were treated with indinavir, zidovudine and lamivudine for 6 months). In this study *CCR5-Δ32* heterozygotes did not have a significantly different therapeutic response, but viral suppression failure was more common among patients with the *CCR5-59029* A/A genotype (28%) than among other subjects (relative risk, 2.0; p=0.06). After 24 weeks of therapy, patients with the *CCR5-59029* A/A genotype had a mean reduction from baseline the HIV RNA level of 2.12 $\log_{10}$ copies/ml compared to 2.64 $\log_{10}$ copies/ml for other subjects (p=0.02) (66). If additional studies confirm that chemokine receptor genes polymorphisms can predict the response to therapy for HIV-1, then genotyping for these alleles may eventually play a part in therapeutic decision making.

Reasons for Treatment Failure

Treatment failure has been generally defined as either inadequate viral suppression (failure to achieve an undetectable RNA level), a decreasing CD4+ lymphocyte count, or clinical progression (57), but no more specific definition is in common use. For example, although suppression of the HIV-1 RNA level to undetectable levels is the primary goal of therapy, there is no generally accepted level above this at which therapy should be changed. Most often, treatment failure occurs with incompletely suppressed HIV-1 RNA level, with or without decreases in CD4+ lymphocyte count or clinical progression (weight loss, development of thrush or opportunistic illness). It is unusual for a patient to progress clinically with fully suppressed HIV-1 replication. Reasons for treatment failure (detectable HIV-1 replication) can be classified as either poor compliance or drug failure.

Compliance

Poor compliance to the treatment regimen is probably the biggest reason for failure in regimens for naive patients (58, 67). The proportion of patients who achieve viral suppression on a potent antiretroviral regimen is lower in a clinic setting than in patients who are enrolled in clinical trials (40, 67). There are many reasons for lack of compliance. HIV-1 treatment regimens are complex and require frequent dosing, strict timing, and food restrictions. In addition to these inconveniences, antiretroviral treatments frequently cause adverse effects (58) and these effects may lead the patient to stop or alter the regimen without consulting the prescribing physician. Finally, some HIV-1-infected patients abuse drugs or alcohol, and for that reason may be less likely to adhere to treatment (67). Physicians need to monitor and encourage compliance for patients who are receiving antiretroviral treatment.

Drug Failure

A treatment regimen may also fail because one or more of the medications in the regimen is ineffective for that patient. A medication may be ineffective due to poor absorption, drug-drug interactions, other pharmacologic factors, or viral resistance. Data on drug level testing for antiretroviral regimens are very limited and this testing is not currently in wide clinical use (57). For some drugs, serum levels may not reflect levels inside the cell, where the drugs act. Nonetheless, drug level testing for some agents may prove useful in the future.

Viral resistance testing is becoming readily available (68) and should be considered for treated patients who fail to suppress the virus to undetectable levels. In the setting of ineffective therapy, virus circulating in the patient can be assessed for resistance to specific antiretroviral medications. There are two types of resistance assays: genotype assays, which sequence viral reverse transcriptase and protease genes to detect specific resistance mutations; and phenotype assays, which characterize the ability of virus circulating in the patient to replicate *in vitro* in the presence of the various antiretroviral agents.

In a randomized study of the utility of genotype resistance testing in HIV-1-infected patients who failed combination therapy, 32% of those who were treated with new regimens on the basis of a viral genotyping achieved an HIV-1RNA level <200 copies/ml, compared with 14% of patients who had their new regimens selected without the benefit of resistance testing (69). Similarly, Cohen and colleagues have presented preliminary data that appropriate use of phenotype resistance testing can improve treatment success rates for patients failing a first protease inhibitor-containing regimen (70). In a randomized trial comparing therapy guided by phenotype resistance testing with standard of care (no resistance testing), RNA responses after 16 weeks on the newly selected regimen were better for subjects randomized to phenotype testing (mean decrease from baseline 1.25 $\log_{10}$ copies/ml compared to 0.56 $\log_{10}$ copies/ml, $p=0.01$). Also, more subjects randomized to phenotype testing had an HIV-1 RNA level <400 copies/ml (62% vs. 33%).

Nonetheless, further work is needed to improve these resistance assays, since both types have limitations. A limitation of genotype assays is that a treated patient will often have a circulating strain with multiple mutations, and the effects of combinations of mutations on virus resistance are difficult to interpret. For example, the M184V mutation associated with lamivudine resistance partially reverses zidovudine resistance conferred by other mutations (71). Phenotypic assay results are also difficult to interpret, because it remains unclear what level of phenotypic (i.e., laboratory) resistance actually corresponds to clinical resistance. A limitation of both types of assays is the need for sufficient circulating virus (typically an HIV-1 RNA level of at least 1000 copies/ml), which makes it difficult to obtain results for patients only beginning to fail therapy. Also, both assays detect resistance only in the dominant circulating strains of HIV-1, and patients may have alternative resistance patterns in minority strains. Finally, neither type of assay can reliably detect resistance to drugs that the patient is not currently taking. Detectable resistance occurs only for a strain reaching high replication levels, which usually occurs only under selective pressure from the medication itself. Thus, at present resistance testing might best be viewed as informative regarding which of the patient's current medications are *not* working, and less informative for which medications *will* work. Furthermore, improved quality control of HIV-1 drug resistance testing is needed before such testing can be implemented widely (72). A multicenter study on the quality of DNA sequencing approaches for identifying HIV-1 drug resistance mutations revealed large interlaboratory differences in the quality of the results that in some cases would lead to incorrect diagnostic results (73).

Drug Toxicity

Drug toxicity is another major reason for alteration of therapeutic regimens. The major adverse effects that are associated with current antiretroviral drugs include mitochondrial toxicity, lipodystrophy, and hypersensitivity (see reference 58 for a review). Adverse effects thought to be related to mitochondrial toxicity are common with NRTIs and range in severity from mild to life threatening. These conditions include myopathy, neuropathy, hepatic steatosis, pancreatitis, and lactic acidosis. The prevalence and severity of these conditions are related to the duration of therapy, and both the rate and frequency of recovery varies by condition. These effects are thought to be caused by inhibition of the mitochodrial DNA polymerase γ and resultant impaired synthesis of mitochondrial enzymes that generate ATP by oxidative posphorylation, but the conditions are, nonetheless, somewhat drug specific. Estimates of the frequency of NRTI-associated peripheral neuropathy (mainly due to ddI, d4T, and ddC) range up to 30%, but hepatic and pancreatic complications are less frequent. There are currently no assays that can predict who will develop these mitochondrial toxicities.

A lipodystrophy syndrome occurs in many HIV-1-infected patients who are receiving long term protease inhibitor therapy (58). Clinically the syndrome consists of fat loss in peripheral anatomic areas, such as the face and limbs, combined with fat accumulation in central areas, such as the abdomen, chest and upper back. The syndrome also includes metabolic abnormalities, including hypertriglyceridemia, hypercholesterolemia, insulin resistance, impaired glucose tolerance, and lactic acidemia. It has been hypothesized that the syndrome might result from homology between the protease inhibitor binding site (on HIV-1 protease), and lipid and adipocyte regulatory proteins (74). The finding that protease inhibitors inhibit lipogenesis *in vitro* (75) supports this theory, but other explanations have been suggested. Some clinical features of the lipodystrophy syndrome have been found in patients who were receiving NRTIs (especially d4T) without protease inhibitors (76, 77), which suggests that in some cases these findings may be due to mitochondrial toxicity.

Antiretroviral agents can also cause a host of other adverse effects. Drug hypersensitivity that results in rash (with or without fever) is fairly common in patients receiving NNRTIs and a few other antiretroviral therapies. About half of these cases resolve without cessation of therapy, but more severe cases (e.g., Stevens-Johnson syndrome) require termination of the agent (58). The pathogenesis of this hypersensitivity is unknown. A number of drugs have been associated with gastrointestinal symptoms (i.e., nausea, vomiting, diarrhea) or hepatitis (58). In addition, some adverse effects are specific for certain drugs. Such associations include zidovudine and anemia, efavirenz and central nervous system symptoms, and indinavir and renal calculi.

Changing Therapy

The appropriate clinical response to treatment failure is often not clearcut. In considering when and if to change failing therapy, physicians must consider the cause of treatment failure and the therapeutic options that are available to the specific patient. A first antiretroviral treatment regimen is most likely to successfully suppress viral replication, because viral resistance evolving in the setting of repeated treatment failures reduces the potency of many agents. Second regimens are less effective than first regimens, and beyond second regimens success rates are very poor. Therefore, if treatment failure occurs, a new regimen should be contemplated with careful consideration for the reasons that the current regimen is failing. If poor adherence is the underlying problem, the reason for lack of compliance must be determined. For example, if substance abuse, depression, or social issues (e.g., homelessness, lack of medical insurance) prevent a patient from filling prescriptions or taking medications properly, these issues should be addressed prior to initiating another regimen. Otherwise, the patient will likely fail the subsequent regimen, leading to development of high-level antiretroviral resistance and rapid depletion of therapeutic options. As noted above, viral resistance testing is useful in selecting successive drug regimens, especially for selecting a second regimen, where undetectable resistance mutations arising from prior therapies would not be present. Selection of successive regimens is complex and should best be undertaken with input from an expert in HIV-1 clinical care.

SUMMARY

HIV-1 replication causes the immune system damage that leads to AIDS. Plasma HIV-1 RNA levels reflect the rate of viral replication and, therefore, are the strongest predictors of long term prognosis in untreated patients and of therapeutic response in treated patients. The CD4+ lymphocyte count also predicts prognosis and response to therapy. For the rare HIV-1-infected patient who is diagnosed during primary infection, immediate treatment is generally recommended in order to preserve HIV-1 specific immune responses. For chronically infected patients, initiation of treatment is based on the HIV-1 RNA level and the CD4+ lymphocyte count, which measures the current extent of immunological function. Potent combination antiretroviral regimens are used with a goal of suppressing the HIV-1 RNA level below the level of detection. Successful therapy decreases the risk of AIDS, reconstitutes the immune system, and avoids selection for drug-resistant HIV-1 strains. The availability of potent combination treatment regimens that supress the replication of HIV-1 has led to dramatic changes in HIV-1-related morbidity and mortality, but current regimens are complex, expensive, and associated with a number of adverse outcomes. Furthermore, for many patients these regimens do not yield lasting viral suppression. New HIV-1 therapies that work through novel mechanisms are needed to increase the armamentarium of antiretroviral drugs.

ACKNOWLEDGMENT

The authors thank Dr. Michael Lederman for his helpful comments on an earlier version of this chapter.

REFERENCES

1. Palella FJ Jr, Delaney KM, Moorman AC, Loveless MO, Fuhrer J, Satten GA, Aschman DJ, Holmberg SD. Declining morbidity and mortality among patients with advanced human immunodeficiency virus infection. N Engl J Med 1998;338:853-60.
2. Gebhardt M, Rickenbach M, Egger M. Impact of antiretroviral combination therapies on AIDS surveillance reports in Switzerland. Swiss HIV Cohort Study. AIDS 1998;12:1195-201.
3. Chiasson MA, Berenson L, Li W, Schwartz S, Singh T, Forlenza S, Mojica BA, Hamburg MA. Declining HIV/AIDS mortality in New York City. J Acquir Immune Defic Syndr 1999;21:59-64.
4. Mocroft A, Sabin CA, Youle M, Madge S, Tyrer M, Devereux H, Deayton J, Dykhoff A, Lipman MC, Phillips AN, Johnson MA. Changes in AIDS-defining illnesses in a London Clinic, 1987-1998. J Acquir Immune Defic Syndr 1999;21:401-7.
5. Moore RD, Chaisson RE. Natural history of HIV infection in the era of combination antiretroviral therapy. AIDS 1999;13:1933-42.
6. Vittinghoff E, Scheer S, O'Malley P, Colfax G, Holmberg SD, Buchbinder SP. Combination antiretroviral therapy and recent declines in AIDS incidence and mortality. J Infect Dis 1999;179:717-20.
7. Kaplan JE, Hanson D, Dworkin MS, Frederick T, Bertolli J, Lindegren ML, Holmberg S, Jones JL. Epidemiology of human immunodeficiency virus-associated opportunistic infections in the United States in the era of highly active antiretroviral therapy. Clin Infect Dis 2000;30 Suppl 1:S5-14.
8. Report of the NIH Panel to Define Principles of Therapy of HIV Infection. Ann Intern Med. 1998;128(12 Pt 2):1057-78.
9. O'Brien TR, Blattner WA, Waters D, Eyster E, Hilgartner MW, Cohen AR, Luban N, Hatzakis A, Aledort LM, Rosenberg PS, Miley WJ, Kroner BL, Goedert JJ. Serum HIV-1 RNA levels and time to development of AIDS in the Multicenter Hemophilia Cohort Study. JAMA 1996;276:105-110.
10. Mellors JW, Kingsley LA, Rinaldo CR Jr, Todd JA, Hoo BS, Kokka RP, Gupta P. Quantitation of HIV-1 RNA in plasma predicts outcome after seroconversion. Ann Intern Med 1995;122:573-9.
11. Mellors JW, Rinaldo CR Jr, Gupta P, White RM, Todd JA, Kingsley LA. Prognosis in HIV-1 infection predicted by the quantity of virus in plasma. Science 1996;272:1167-70.
12. Mellors JW, Munoz A, Giorgi JV, Margolick JB, Tassoni CJ, Gupta P, Kingsley LA, Todd JA, Saah AJ, Detels R, Phair JP, Rinaldo CR Jr.Plasma viral load and CD4+ lymphocytes as prognostic markers of HIV-1 infection. Ann Intern Med 1997;126:946-54.
13. Vlahov D, Graham N, Hoover D, Flynn C, Bartlett JG, Margolick JB, Lyles CM, Nelson KE, Smith D, Holmberg S, Farzadegan H. Prognostic indicators for AIDS and infectious disease death in HIV-infected injection drug users: plasma viral load and CD4+ cell count. JAMA 1998;279:35-40.
14. Engels EA, Rosenberg PS, O'Brien TR, Goedert JJ. Plasma HIV viral load in patients with hemophilia and late-stage HIV disease: a measure of current immune suppression. Multicenter Hemophilia Cohort Study. Ann Intern Med 1999;131:256-64.
15. O'Brien TR, Rosenberg PS, Yellin F, Goedert JJ. Longitudinal HIV-1 RNA levels in a cohort of homosexual men. J Acquir Immune Defic Syndr Hum Retrovirol 1998;18:155-161.

16. Katzenstein DA, Hammer SM, Hughes MD, Gundacker H, Jackson JB, Fiscus S, Rasheed S, Elbeik T, Reichman R, Japour A, Merigan TC, Hirsch MS. The relation of virologic and immunologic markers to clinical outcomes after nucleoside therapy in HIV-infected adults with 200 to 500 CD4 cells per cubic millimeter. New Eng J Med 1996;335:1091-8.
17. Hammer SM, Squires KE, Hughes MD, Grimes JM, Demeter LM, Currier JS, Eron JJ Jr, Feinberg JE, Balfour HH Jr, Deyton LR, Chodakewitz JA, Fischl MA. A controlled trial of two nucleoside analogues plus indinavir in persons with human immunodeficiency virus infection and CD4 cell counts of 200 per cubic millimeter or less. N Engl J Med 1997; 337:725-33.
18. Gulick RM, Mellors JW, Havlir D, Eron JJ, Gonzalez C, McMahon D, Richman DD, Valentine FT, Jonas L, Meibohm A, Emini EA, Chodakewitz JA. Treatment with indinavir, zidovudine, and lamivudine in adults with human immunodeficiency virus infection and prior antiretroviral therapy. N Engl J Med 1997;337:734-9.
19. Marschner IC, Collier AC, Coombs RW, D'Aquila RT, DeGruttola V, Fischl MA, Hammer SM, Hughes MD, Johnson VA, Katzenstein DA, Richman DD, Smeaton LM, Spector SA, Saag MS. Use of changes in plasma levels of human immunodeficiency virus type 1 RNA to assess the clinical benefit of antiretroviral therapy. J Infect Dis 1998;177:40-7.
20. Autran B, Carcelain G, Li TS, Blanc C, Mathez D, Tubiana R, Katlama C, Debre P, Leibowitch J. Positive effects of combined antiretroviral therapy on CD4+ T cell homeostasis and function in advanced HIV disease. Science 1997;277:112-6.
21. Powderly WG, Landay A, Lederman MM. Recovery of the immune system with antiretroviral therapy: the end of opportunism? JAMA 1998;280:72-7.
22. Autran B, Carcelaint G, Li TS, Gorochov G, Blanc C, Renaud M, Durali M, Mathez D, Calvez V, Leibowitch J, Katlama C, Debre P. Restoration of the immune system with anti-retroviral therapy. Immunol Lett 1999;66:207-11.
23. Pakker NG, Notermans DW, de Boer RJ, Roos MT, de Wolf F, Hill A, Leonard JM, Danner SA, Miedema F, Schellekens PT. Biphasic kinetics of peripheral blood T cells after triple combination therapy in HIV-1 infection: a composite of redistribution and proliferation. Nat Med 1998;4:208-14.
24. Lederman MM, Connick E, Landay A, Kuritzkes DR, Spritzler J, St. Clair M, Kotzin BL, Fox L, Chiozzi MH, Leonard JM, Rousseau F, Wade M, Roe JD, Martinez A, Kessler H. Immunologic responses associated with 12 weeks of combination antiretroviral therapy consisting of zidovudine, lamivudine, and ritonavir: results of AIDS Clinical Trials Group Protocol 315. J Infect Dis 1998;178:70-9.
25. Connick E, Lederman MM, Kotzin BL, Spritzler J, Kuritzkes DR, St Clair M, Sevin AD, Fox L, Chiozzi MH, Leonard JM, Rousseau F, D'Arc Roe J, Martinez A, Kessler H, Landay A. Immune reconstitution in the first year of potent antiretroviral therapy and its relationship to virologic response. J Infect Dis 2000;181:358-63.
26. Mezzaroma I, Carlesimo M, Pinter E, Alario C, Sacco G, Muratori DS, Bernardi ML, Paganelli R, Aiuti F. Long-term evaluation of T-cell subsets and T-cell function after HAART in advanced stage HIV-1 disease. AIDS 1999;13:1187-93.
27. Gougeon ML, Montagnier L. Programmed cell death as a mechanism of CD4 and CD8 T cell deletion in AIDS. Molecular control and effect of highly active antiretroviral therapy. Ann N Y Acad Sci 1999;887:199-212.
28. Liu Z, Cumberland WG, Hultin LE, Prince HE, Detels R, Giorgi JV. Elevated CD38 antigen expression on CD8+ T cells is a stronger marker for the risk of chronic HIV disease progression to AIDS and death in the Multicenter AIDS Cohort Study than

CD4+ cell count, soluble immune activation markers, or combinations of HLA-DR and CD38 expression. J Acquir Immune Defic Syndr Hum Retrovirol 1997;16:83-92.
29. Giorgi JV, Majchrowicz MA, Johnson TD, Hultin P, Matud J, Detels R. Immunologic effects of combined protease inhibitor and reverse transcriptase inhibitor therapy in previously treated chronic HIV-1 infection. AIDS 1998;12:1833-44.
30. Li TS, Tubiana R, Katlama C, Calvez V, Ait Mohand H, Autran B. Long-lasting recovery in CD4 T-cell function and viral-load reduction after highly active antiretroviral therapy in advanced HIV-1 disease. Lancet 1998;351:1682-6.
31. Sondergaard SR, Aladdin H, Ullum H, Gerstoft J, Skinhoj P, Pedersen BK. Immune function and phenotype before and after highly active antiretroviral therapy. J Acquir Immune Defic Syndr 1999;21:376-83.
32. O'Brien WA, Hartigan PM, Martin D, Esinhart J, Hill A, Benoit S, Rubin M, Simberkoff MS, Hamilton JD. Changes in plasma HIV-1 RNA and CD4+ lymphocyte counts and the risk of progression to AIDS. N Engl J Med. 1996;334:426-31.
33. Rosenberg ES, Billingsley JM, Caliendo AM, Boswell SL, Sax PE, Kalams SA, Walker BD. Vigorous HIV-1-specific CD4+ T cell responses associated with control of viremia. Science 1997;278:1447-50.
34. Haslett PA, Nixon DF, Shen Z, Larsson M, Cox WI, Manandhar R, Donahoe SM, Kaplan G. Strong human immunodeficiency virus (HIV)-specific CD4+ T cell responses in a cohort of chronically infected patients are associated with interruptions in anti-HIV chemotherapy. J Infect Dis 2000;181:1264-72.
35. Binley JM, Schiller DS, Ortiz GM, Hurley A, Nixon DF, Markowitz MM, Moore JP. The relationship between T cell proliferative responses and plasma viremia during treatment of human immunodeficiency virus type 1 infection with combination antiretroviral therapy. J Infect Dis 2000;181:1249-63.
36. Rosenberg ES, Altfeld M, Poon SH, Phillips MN, Wilkes BM, Eldridge RL, Robbins GK, D'Aquila RT, Goulder PJ, Walker BD. Immune control of HIV-1 after early treatment of acute infection. Nature. 2000;407:523-6.
37. Connors M, Kovacs JA, Krevat S, Gea-Banacloche JC, Sneller MC, Flanigan M, Metcalf JA, Walker RE, Falloon J, Baseler M, Feuerstein I, Masur H, Lane HC. Nat Med 1997;3:533-40.
38. Gorochov G, Neumann AU, Kereveur A, Parizot C, Li T, Katlama C, Karmochkine M, Raguin G, Autran B, Debre P. Perturbation of CD4+ and CD8+ T-cell repertoires during progression to AIDS and regulation of the CD4+ repertoire during antiviral therapy. Nat Med 1998;4:215-21.
39. Martinon F, Michelet C, Peguillet I, Taoufik Y, Lefebvre P, Goujard C, Guillet JG, Delfraissy JF, Lantz O. Persistent alterations in T-cell repertoire, cytokine and chemokine receptor gene expression after 1 year of highly active antiretroviral therapy. AIDS 1999;13:185-94.
40. Ledergerber B, Egger M, Opravil M, Telenti A, Hirschel B, Battegay M, Vernazza P, Sudre P, Flepp M, Furrer H, Francioli P, Weber R. Clinical progression and virological failure on highly active antiretroviral therapy in HIV-1 patients: a prospective cohort study. Swiss HIV Cohort Study. Lancet. 1999;353:863-8.
41. Martinez-Picado J, Savara AV, Sutton L, D'Aquila RT. Replicative fitness of protease inhibitor-resistant mutants of human immunodeficiency virus type 1. J Virol 1999;73:3744-52.
42. Harrigan PR, Bloor S, Larder BA. Relative replicative fitness of zidovudine-resistant human immunodeficiency virus type 1 isolates in vitro. J Virol. 1998;72:3773-8.

43. Notermans DW, Pakker NG, Hamann D, Foudraine NA, Kauffmann RH, Meenhorst PL, Goudsmit J,Roos MT, Schellekens PT, Miedema F, Danner SA. Immune reconstitution after 2 years of successful potent antiretroviral therapy in previously untreated human immunodeficiency virus type 1-infected adults. J Infect Dis 1999;180:1050-6.
44. 1999 USPHS/IDSA guidelines for the prevention of opportunistic infections in persons infected with human immunodeficiency virus. MMWR 1999; 48(RR10):1-59.
45. Kovacs JA, Masur H. Prophylaxis against opportunistic infections in patients with human immunodeficiency virus infection. N Engl J Med 2000;342:1416-29.
46. Furrer H, Egger M, Opravil M, Bernasconi E, Hirschel B, Battegay M, Telenti A, Vernazza PL, Rickenbach M, Flepp M, Malinverni R. Discontinuation of primary prophylaxis against Pneumocystis carinii pneumonia in HIV-1-infected adults treated with combination antiretroviral therapy. N Engl J Med 1999;340:1301-6.
47. Schneider MME, Borleffs JCC, Stolk RP, Jaspers CAJJ, Hoepelman AIM. Discontinuation of Pneumocystis carinii pneumonia prophylaxis in HIV-1 infected patients treated with highly active antiretroviral therapy. Lancet 1999;353:201-3.
48. Weverling GJ, Mocroft A, Ledergerber B, Kirk O, Gonzales-Lahoz J, d'Arminio Monforte A, Proenca R, Phillips AN, Lundgren JD, Reiss P. Discontinuation of Pneumocystis carinii pneumonia prophylaxis after start of highly active antiretroviral therapy in HIV-1 infection. Lancet 1999;353:1293-8.
49. Yangco BG, Von Bargen JC, Moorman AC, Holmberg SD. Discontinuation of chemoprophylaxis against Pneumocystis carinii pneumonia in patients with HIV infection. Ann Intern Med 2000;132:201-5.
50. El-Sadr WM, Burman WJ, Grant LB, Matts JP, Hafner R, Crane L, Zeh D, Gallagher B, Mannheimer SB, Martinez A, Gordin F. Discontinuation of prophylaxis for Mycobacterium avium complex disease in HIV-infected patients who have a response to antiretroviral therapy. N Engl J Med 2000;342:1085-92.
51. MacDonald JC, Torriani FJ, Morse LS, Karavellas MP, Reed JB, Freeman WR. Lack of reactivation of cytomegalovirus (CMV) retinitis after stopping CMV maintenance therapy in AIDS patients with sustained elevations in CD4 T cells in response to highly active antiretroviral therapy. J Infect Dis 1998;177:1182-7.
52. Tural C, Romeu J, Sirera G, Andreu D, Conejero M, Ruiz S, Jou A, Bonjoch A, Ruiz L, Arno A, Clotet B. Long-lasting remission of cytomegalovirus retinitis without maintenance therapy in human immunodeficiency virus-infected patients. J Infect Dis 1998;177:1080-3.
53. Vrabec TR, Baldassano VF, Whitcup SM. Discontinuation of maintenance therapy in patients with quiescent cytomegalovirus retinitis and elevated CD4+ counts. Ophthalmology 1998; 105:1259-64.
54. Whitcup SM, Fortin E, Lindblad AS, Griffiths P, Metcalf JA, Robinson MR, Manischewitz J, Baird B, Perry C, Kidd IM, Vrabec T, Davey RT Jr, Falloon J, Walker RE, Kovacs JA, Lane HC, Nussenblatt RB, Smith J, Masur H, Polis MA. Discontinuation of anticytomegalovirus therapy in patients with HIV infection and cytomegalovirus retinitis. JAMA 1999;282:1633-7.
55. Pantaleo G, Soudeyns H, Demarest JF, Vaccarezza M, Graziosi C, Paolucci S, Daucher M, Cohen OJ, Denis F, Biddison WE, Sekaly RP, Fauci AS. Evidence for rapid disappearance of initially expanded HIV-specific CD8+ T cell clones during primary HIV infection. Proc Natl Acad Sci U S A 1997;94:9848-53.
56. Soudeyns H, Campi G, Rizzardi GP, Lenge C, Demarest JF, Tambussi G, Lazzarin A, Kaufmann D, Casorati G, Corey L, Pantaleo G. Initiation of antiretroviral therapy during primary HIV-1 infection induces rapid stabilization of the T-cell receptor beta

chain repertoire and reduces the level of T-cell oligoclonality. Blood. 2000;95:1743-1751.

57. Carpenter CC, Cooper DA, Fischl MA, Gatell JM, Hammer SM, Hirsch MS, Jacobsen DM, Katzenstein DA, Montaner JS, Richman DD, Saag MS, Schechter M, Schooley RT, Thompson MA, Vella S, Yeni PG, Volberding PA. Antiretroviral therapy in adults: updated recommendations of the International AIDS Society-USA Panel. JAMA 2000;283:381-390.
58. Carr A, Cooper DA. Adverse effects of antiretroviral therapy. Lancet 2000;356:1423-30.
59. De Clercq E. The role of non-nucleoside reverse transcriptase inhibitors (NNRTIs) in the therapy of HIV-1 infection. Antiviral Res 1998;38:153-79.
60. Finzi D, Blankson J, Siliciano JD, Margolick JB, Chadwick K, Pierson T, Smith K, Lisziewicz J, Lori F, Flexner C, Quinn TC, Chaisson RE, Rosenberg E, Walker B, Gange S, Gallant J, Siliciano RF. Latent infection of CD4+ T cells provides a mechanism for lifelong persistence of HIV-1, even in patients on effective combination therapy. Nat Med. 1999;5:512-7.
61. Siliciano RF. Latency and reservoirs for HIV-1. AIDS 1999;13 Suppl A:S49-58.
62. Ramratnam B, Mittler JE, Zhang L, Boden D, Hurley A, Fang F, Macken CA, Perelson AS, Markowitz M, Ho DD. The decay of the latent reservoir of replication-competent HIV-1 is inversely correlated with the extent of residual viral replication during prolonged anti-retroviral therapy. Nat Med. 2000;6:82-5.
63. Havlir DV, Marschner IC, Hirsch MS, Collier AC, Tebas P, Bassett RL, Ioannidis JP, Holohan MK, Leavitt R, Boone G, Richman DD. Maintenance antiretroviral therapies in HIV-infected subjects with undetectable plasma HIV RNA after triple-drug therapy. N Engl J Med 1998;339:1261-8.
64. Raboud JM, Montaner JS, Conway B, Rae S, Reiss P, Vella S, Cooper D, Lange J, Harris M, Wainberg MA, Robinson P, Myers M, Hall D. Suppression of plasma viral load below 20 copies/ml is required to achieve a long-term response to therapy. AIDS 1998;12:1619-24.
65. Valdez H, Purvis SF, Lederman MM, Fillingame M, Zimmerman PA. Association of the CCR5delta32 mutation with improved response to antiretroviral therapy. JAMA. 1999;282:734.
66. O'Brien TR, McDermott DH, Ioannidis JP, Carrington M, Murphy PM, Havlir DV, Richman DD. Effect of chemokine receptor gene polymorphisms on the response to potent antiretroviral therapy. AIDS 14:821-826, 2000.
67. Lucas GM, Chaisson RE, Moore RD. Highly active antiretroviral therapy in a large urban clinic: risk factors for virologic failure and adverse drug reactions. Ann Intern Med. 1999;131:81-7.
68. Hirsch MS, Brun-Vezinet F, D'Aquila RT, Hammer SM, Johnson VA, Kuritzkes DR, Loveday C, Mellors JW, Clotet B, Conway B, Demeter LM, Vella S, Jacobsen DM, Richman DD. Antiretroviral drug resistance testing in adult HIV-1 infection: recommendations of an International AIDS Society-USA Panel. JAMA 2000;283:2417-26.
69. Durant J, Clevenbergh P, Halfon P, Delgiudice P, Porsin S, Simonet P, Montagne N, Boucher CA, Schapiro JM, Dellamonica P. Drug-resistance genotyping in HIV-1 therapy: the VIRADAPT randomised controlled trial. Lancet 1999;353:2195-9.
70. Cohen C, Hunt S, Sension M, Farthing C, Conant S, Jacobson J, Nadler J, Verbiest W, Hertogs K, Ames M, Rinehart A, Graham N. Phenotypic resistance testing significantly improves response to therapy: a randomized trial (VIRA3001). Presented at the

7th Conference on Retroviruses and Opportunistic Infections, San Francisco, January 31, 2000.

71. Larder BA, Kemp SD, Harrigan PR. Potential mechanism for sustained antiretroviral efficacy of AZT-3TC combination therapy. Science. 1995;269:696-9.
72. Hirsch MS, Conway B, D'Aquila RT, Johnson VA, Brun-Vezinet F, Clotet B, Demeter LM, Hammer SM, Jacobsen DM, Kuritzkes DR, Loveday C, Mellors JW, Vella S, Richman DD. Antiretroviral drug resistance testing in adults with HIV infection: implications for clinical management. JAMA 1998;279:1984-91.
73. Schuurman R, Demeter L, Reichelderfer P, Tijnagel J, de Groot T, Boucher C. Worldwide evaluation of DNA sequencing approaches for identification of drug resistance mutations in the human immunodeficiency virus type 1 reverse transcriptase. J Clin Microbiol 1999;37:2291-6.
74. Carr A, Samaras K, Thorisdottir A, Kaufmann GR, Chisholm DJ, Cooper DA. Diagnosis, prediction, and natural course of HIV-1 protease-inhibitor-associated lipodystrophy, hyperlipidaemia, and diabetes mellitus: a cohort study. Lancet. 1999;353:2093-9.
75. Zhang B, MacNaul K, Szalkowski D, Li Z, Berger J, Moller DE. Inhibition of adipocyte differentiation by HIV protease inhibitors. J Clin Endocrinol Metab 1999;351:1881-83.
76. Saint-Marc T, Partisani M, Poizot-Martin I, Bruno F, Rouviere O, Lang JM, Gastaut JA, Touraine JL. A syndrome of peripheral fat wasting (lipodystrophy) in patients receiving long-term nucleoside analogue therapy. AIDS 1999;13:1359-67.
77. Carr A, Miller J, Law M, Cooper DA. A syndrome of lipoatrophy, lactic acidaemia and liver dysfunction associated with HIV nucleoside analogue therapy: contribution to protease inhibitor-related lipodystrophy syndrome. AIDS 2000;14:F25-32.

9

Limitations of Current Therapies for HIV-1 Infection

Douglas D. Richman
San Diego VA Healthcare System and University of California, San Diego and La Jolla, California

INTRODUCTION

Studies evaluating combinations of antiretroviral drugs introduced the new treatment paradigm for HIV infection -- the suppression of plasma HIV RNA below detectable levels (1,2). This strategy has become the standard for patient management and the criterion by which new drugs and new drug combinations are evaluated (3,4). Moreover the implementation of these potent combination regimens has resulted in a remarkable impact on morbidity and mortality in developed countries in Europe and the Americas (5). However, the use of the term HAART (for highly active antiretroviral therapy) is to be eschewed because it implies both that all regimens are equivalent and that current regimens are sufficiently potent (6). Neither implication can be supported.

The introduction of potent suppressive therapy also permitted investigations of viral dynamics, providing insights into rates and magnitude of viral production, parameters of the viral replication cycle in vivo, and the lymphatic source of plasma virus (7-10). The analysis by Perelson et al. characterizing two phases of viral decay led to the speculation that prolonged treatment might result in the extinction of virus infected cells and the cure of HIV infection (11). The documentation of long lived latently infected CD4 lymphocytes from patients with undetectable plasma HIV RNA doused this optimism (12-14).

This chapter will summarize the evidence why current regimens, despite the remarkable achievements that have been accomplished, are still inadequately potent and require significant improvements. The strategies to design such improvements will also be summarized.

EVIDENCE THAT CURRENT REGIMENS ARE NOT SUFFICIENTLY POTENT

A significant minority of patients initiating antiretroviral therapy with wild type virus at baseline fail to suppress HIV RNA to undetectable levels. An initial study proposing undetectability as a treatment endpoint was the Merck 035 study which described an 85% rate of undetectability at 1 year on zidovudine/lamivudine/indinavir and a rate of 78% after 100 weeks of such treatment (1,15). The INCAS study reported a 51% rate of undetectability at 1 year on zidovudine/didanosine/nevirapine (2). Most studies have fallen somewhere in between with lower rates of success associated with higher baseline plasma HIV RNA levels and lower CD4 levels. Of importance, the lack of rigorous, blinded randomized comparisons of various patient regimens has precluded fair assessments of their relative potency and tolerability in equivalent situations and patient populations. The point to be made, however, is that even 90% efficacy is not good enough. Clinical progression and accumulating drug resistance are the inevitable consequences of failing regimens.

Evidence of Residual Replication

There is histological evidence of residual replication in lymphoid tissue of patients with undetectable HIV RNA. Nucleic acid extracts of lymph node biopsies from patients with undetectable HIV RNA after 6-12 months of suppressive treatment showed 4 $\log_{10}$ reductions (from approximately 10^8 copies HIV RNA/gram tissue) (16). Of note, this value stabilized, showing no further reductions after an additional year of suppression (17). Studies of RNA in lymphoid tissue of such patients using in situ hybridization showed remarkable reductions of a similar magnitude; however, rare lymphocytes with high copy number indicating active replication are occasionally discerned (18) and with more prolonged development times additional cells with lower copy number are seen (19). It is not clear whether these cells represent latently infected CD4 cells or a smoldering low level replication; nevertheless, recent studies indicate that these cells are non-activated lymphocytes and represent the predominant population of infected cells in the body during potent suppressive therapy (19).

Several studies of patients on suppressive therapy have also shown the accumulation of either HIV RNA (20) or HIV p24 antigen (21) associated with the follicular dendritic cells in the germinal centers of lymph nodes. These studies are labor intensive and can only be performed on limited numbers of patients. It is always difficult to document rigorously whether such patients have experienced intermittent failures of suppression or have always been below the levels of detection. Günthard et al. showed that the occasional patient with intermittent levels of detectable HIV RNA exhibits nucleotide diversity and expresses multiply spliced transcripts of HIV RNA (22) even if the HIV RNA level is low (~100 copies/ml).

HIV-1 Continues to Evolve

The RNA in HIV-1 from some patients with suppressive therapy continues to evolve. Evolution is the inevitable consequence of HIV replication. Two studies of the nucleotide sequence of clones of the most variable region of the HIV genome, the third variable loop (V3) of gp120, indicate that some patients show no evidence of evolution, indicating no HIV replication or extremely low rates of replication in vivo (18,23). However, many patients receiving suppressive therapy, especially those exhibiting low intermittent levels ("blips") of HIV RNA, exhibit continuing nucleotide diversity and divergence from the "ancestral" baseline sequence (18,23). Most recently Günthard et al. made similar observations of ongoing evolution in nucleotide sequences derived from HIV RNA in lymphoid tissue. The rate of this evolution correlated with the amount of residual measurable RNA in plasma and in lymphoid tissue (17, 24).

Virus Emerging After Treatment Failure is Sensitive

The virus emerging after failure of previously suppressive treatment with protease inhibitors remains sensitive to those drugs. The loss of viral suppression in HIV-infected patients receiving potent antiretroviral therapy has been attributed to the outgrowth of drug resistant virus (25,26). This principle had been well documented with monotherapy failures with nevirapine and lamivudine for which a single nucleotide change confers high level resistance (27-29).

A recent study characterized the drug susceptibility of virus recovered from HIV-infected patients failing to sustain viral suppression on an indinavir-containing antiretroviral regimen. Indinavir resistance was not detected in 9 subjects with viral rebound during indinavir monotherapy or in 17 subjects during triple drug therapy despite HIV RNA levels ranging from 10^2 to 10^5 copies/mL plasma (30). In contrast, lamivudine resistance was detected by the phenotypic assay in viral rebound isolates from 14 of 17 subjects on triple therapy. Genotypic analyses demonstrated changes at codon 184 of reverse transcriptase in these 14 isolates.

Additional studies have generated similar data with other protease inhibitors (31,32). Of note, the studies of protease inhibitor regimens containing efavirenz, analogous to those containing lamivudine, demonstrated the emergence of the K103N mutation in reverse transcriptase conferring resistance to efavirenz without mutations in protease (33).

These data are consistent with the explanation that, in contrast to resistance mutations with lamivudine and non-nucleoside reverse transcriptase inhibitors, the first mutation in protease confers only a small resistance advantage to the virus but also confers a fitness cost with regard to enzyme activity and replicative capacity

(34-38). An important implication of this explanation is that the potency of current protease containing regimens are often at the threshold of activity to suppress wild type virus, a conclusion also made simply by observing the suboptimal proportions of patients who adequately suppress HIV RNA below detectable levels.

The mathematical modeling of the ACTG 343 study by Wein et al. predicted failure in those patients who experienced the largest increment of CD4 cells, based on the assumption that these potential target cells would provide more prey for the predatory virus (26). The multivariate analysis of risks for failure in the ACTG 343 study supported this model (39).

Host Genetics And Treatment Failure.

The genetics of the host affect the likelihood of treatment failure. CC-chemokine receptor 5 (CCR5) is the major coreceptor for macrophage-tropic HIV-1 strains. Homozygosity for a 32 base pair deletion (*Δ32*) of the *CCR5* gene provides strong relative protection against HIV-1 infection, (40-44) and HIV-1-infected *CCR5-Δ32* heterozygotes have a more favorable natural history than people with two wild type alleles. (42,44,45). Variants of other chemokine receptor genes also may alter the course of HIV-1 infection. Heterozygosity or homozygosity for the *CCR2-64I* allele of the minor HIV coreceptor CCR2b has been associated with better prognosis; (45,50) and homozygosity for *CCR5* promoter alleles *59029 A* (47) and *P1* (46) has been associated with worse prognosis. The *59029 A* and *P1* alleles appear to define the same haplotype (48). Certain human leukocyte antigen (HLA) haplotypes, as well as homozygosity of HLA genotypes, also predisposed to more rapid disease progression, presumably as a consequence of diminished effectiveness of CTL immunity (49).

The participants in the ACTG 343 protocol, described above, were genotyped with regard to the known chemokine receptor polymorphisms affecting disease progression to assess whether these would also affect response to potent antiretroviral chemotherapy (50). Time to first HIV RNA 200 copies/ml was not predicted by genotype. Among 272 Caucasian patients, viral suppression failure was more common among patients with the *CCR5 +/+* | *CCR2+/+* | *CCR5-59029* A/A genotype (28%) than among all other subjects combined (relative risk, 2.0; p=0.06) or *CCR5* Δ32 heterozygotes (relative risk, 2.1; p=0.10). After 24 weeks of therapy, the genotype groups differed in the reduction of the HIV RNA level from baseline (p=0.02); patients with the *CCR5 +/+* | *CCR2+/+* | *CCR5-59029* A/A genotype had a mean reduction of 2.12 $\log_{10}$ copies/ml compared to 2.64 $\log_{10}$ copies/ml among all other groups combined. Thus, polymorphisms in chemokine receptor genes may explain some of the heterogeneity in sustaining viral suppression observed among patients receiving potent antiretroviral therapy.

These observations are relevant to the issue of treatment potency. Since patients cannot select their parents and since physicians will want to treat without performing chemokine receptor genotyping, antiretroviral treatment regimens must be identified that are not further jeopardized by the genotype of the patient.

STRATEGIES TO INCREASE TREATMENT EFFICACY

The evidence generated above argue for more effective treatment regimens. The challenge is to identify strategies to help develop such regimens.

Improve Ratio of Free Drug Concentration to Level of Virus Susceptibility

It is likely that antiretroviral drug activity will prove to be a function of the ratio of drug exposure to viral susceptibility. Parameters requiring better characterization include: 1) what magnitude that ratio needs to be to assure suppression; 2) whether susceptibility should be defined as IC_{50}, IC_{90}, IC_{95} etc; and 3) whether the concentration used should be the trough level (most likely) or some other pharmacokinetic parameter. For nucleosides, exposure determinations are complicated by the fact the concentrations of the triphosphates of the drug, as well as the physiologic deoxynucleosides within the infected cells is what is important. For compounds not anabolized to active drugs like non-nucleoside reverse transcriptase inhibitors and protease inhibitors, exposure is probably defined by free drug concentration which is determined by plasma level and protein binding. Intracellular transport and efflux, however, may also pose important hurdles (51-53).

If this formulation is valid, then a number of aspects of drug design require specific targeting. First design more potent drugs. Everything else being equal, if an IC_{50} of 10 nM is good, then one of 1 nM is better. Second, minimize protein binding that reduces levels of active free drug. Drug bound to albumin or alpha1, acid glycoprotein (AAG) with high affinity is drug not available for the viral target, even though the drug is measurable in the blood (54-56). Third, prolong plasma half-life. More rapid excretion of drug results in steeper decay curves and lower trough levels. More data are needed; however, preliminary evidence supports the contention that the trough levels are an important correlate of activity (or its loss) with non-nucleoside inhibitors and protease inhibitors. In addition and as discussed below, prolonged half lives confer significant adherence benefits.

Contend with HIV Drug Resistance

There are two fundamental approaches to contend with HIV drug resistance – to prevent it and to treat it. Prevention can be accomplished by more intelligent prescribing of antiretroviral drugs by health care providers, by better adherence to regimens by patients and to more effective suppressive drug regimens. Physician education is beyond the scope of this review, but strategies to improve adherence and potency are discussed elsewhere.

One approach to the treatment of resistant virus, and the standard one in antimicrobial drug development, is to identify drugs active against drug resistant virus. Candidate compounds with activity against virus resistant to each of the classes of antiretroviral drugs are in development.

Reduce Poor Adherence

To take many pills several times a day dependably for years is difficult for any patient. Educational efforts to improve awareness and effectiveness in dealing with this problem both on the parts of healthcare providers and of patients are continuing. Nevertheless, drug development can address several aspects that will improve adherence. First, almost all antiretroviral drugs are associated with toxicities and side effects which discourage patients. The more benign the drug the less difficulty with adherence. Second, pill counts should be reduced. Even seemingly trivial approaches like combining zidovudine and lamivudine in a single tablet appeals to consumers. However pill counts can also be reduced by identifying drugs that are more potent and that have longer half lives, thus reducing the amount of compound that needs to be administered.

Identifying drugs with long half lives confers significant benefits other than the prospect of reducing pill burden. A long half life permits less frequent dosing which enhances adherence. Perhaps even more important, flattened plasma decay curves with less depressed trough levels provide a more forgiving regimen with regard to erratic pill administration. Delayed or missed doses are less likely to subject the patient to suboptimal drug levels. These characteristics may account for some of the success of nevirapine and efavirenz which have plasma half–lives of greater than 24 hours.

Invade Pharmacologic Sanctuaries

Unlike in vitro conditions, the body is not a well mixed vessel. It contains anatomic complexity and cellular heterogeneity, with implications for pathogenesis, transmission and treatment failure. Virus in the genital tract is critical for transmission and virus in the central nervous system causes neuropathology. There may be additional important targets as well.

In general, the response of HIV RNA in these compartment parallels that in the circulation; however, discordance does exist (57-59). This is especially true in the central nervous system where P glycoprotein pumps and other mechanisms significantly reduce the proportion of protease inhibitors that penetrate the blood-brain barrier (51,60). As proved a hurdle with the chemotherapy for leukemia, effective antiretroviral chemotherapy of all potential pharmacologic sanctuaries will be critical for the sustained long-term suppression of HIV replication in vivo. The potential contribution of these compartments to treatment failure has been mathematically modeled (61).

Develop Therapies Against Novel Targets

Drugs with activity against novel targets would permit both more broadly effective regimens for new patients and new opportunities for effective treatment of patients failing currently available drugs. Such targets include enzymes other than protease and reverse transcriptase like integrase and ribonuclease H. They include the various "accessory" proteins like nef, vpr, vif, tat and rev. They also include inhibitors of viral entry, so-called fusion inhibitors.

Two classes of compounds targeting viral fusion have been reported. Clinical proof of activity has been documented for T-20, a polypeptide that binds to gp41 and prevents the "spring-loaded" conformational change from mediating membrane fusion and viral entry (62). More practical small molecule inhibitors of this proven target are the long term goal. Elegant structural studies dissecting this target have been conducted (63). The second target is chemokine receptors which are essential for viral entry. Small molecule inhibitors that are effective in vitro have been reported for both CXCR4 (64,65) and CCR5 (66). Neither of these is orally bioavailable; nevertheless, extensive discovery programs are underway in a number of pharmaceutical companies and their success is eagerly awaited. The next chapter of this book provides a detailed review of research on potential therapies to block or inhibit chemokine receptor expression.

Enhance HIV Specific Immunity

A number of lines of evidence have emerged to support the contention that HIV specific immunity, especially that mediated by cytotoxic CD8 T cells, contribute to the control of HIV replication [briefly summarized by Richman (67)]. Critical questions are: 1) Which T-cell functions are critical for the control of HIV replication? 2) Which immunologic assays best measure the T-cell functions of interest? 3) Which immunizing strategies elicit these desired functions? Approaches to induce immunity are therapeutic vaccines with HIV antigens or "autoimmunization" by drug withdrawal, called strategic treatment interruption (68-70). These approaches have generated hope and anecdotes, but rigorous documentation of their utility is needed.

SUMMARY

Despite the remarkable and encouraging reductions in morbidity and mortality that have been achieved with potent antiretroviral chemotherapy, a number of lines of evidence support the contention that more effective regimens are need. Several strategies that could be pursued to design more effective regimens have been described.

ACKNOWLEDGMENTS

This work was supported by grants AI 27670, AI 38858, and AI 36214 (Center for AIDS Research) and grant AI 29164 from the National Institutes of Health. It was also supported by the Research Center for AIDS and HIV Infection of the San Diego Veterans Affairs Medical Center.

REFERENCES

1. Gulick RM, Mellors JW, Havlir D, Eron JJ, Gonzalez C, McMahon D, Richman DD, Valentine FT, Jonas L, Deutsch P, Meibohm A, Holder D, Schleif WA, Condra JH, Emini EA, Chodakewitz JA. Treatment with indinavir, zidovudine, and lamivudine in adults with human immunodeficiency virus infection and prior antiretroviral therapy. N Engl J Med 337:734-739, 1997.
2. Montaner JSG, Reiss P, Cooper D, Vella S, Harris M, Conway B, Wainberg MA, Smith D, Robinson P, Hall D, Myers M, Lange JMA. A randomized, double-blind trial comparing combinations of nevirapine, didanosine, and zidovudine for HIV-infected patients: the INCAS trial. JAMA 279:930-937, 1998.
3. Carpenter CCJ, Fischl MA, Hammer SM, Hirsch MS, Jacobsen DM, Katzenstein DA, Montaner JSG, Richman DD, Saag MS, Schooley RT, Thompson MA, Vella S, Yeni PG, Volberding PA. Antiretroviral therapy for HIV infection in 1998: updated recommendations of the International AIDS Society-USA panel. JAMA 280:78-86, 1998.
4. US Department of Health and Human Services Panel on Clinical Practices for Treatment of HIV Infection, Guidelines for the use of antiretroviral agents in HIV-1 infected adults and adolescents. MMWR 47:42-82, 1998.
5. Palella FJ, Delaney KM, Moorman AC, Loveless MO, Fuhrer J, Satten GA, Aschman DJ, Holmberg SD. Declining morbidity and mortality among patients with advanced human immunodeficiency virus infection. N Engl J Med 338:853-860, 1998.
6. Lange JMA and Richman DD. Retroviruses and opportunistic infections '99. Antiviral Therapy 4:5, 1999.
7. Ho DD, Neumann AU, Perelson AS, Chen W, Leonard JM, Markowitz M. Rapid turnover of plasma virions and CD4 lymphocytes in HIV-1 infection. Nature 373:123-126, 1995.
8. Wei X, Ghosh SK, Taylor ME, Jonson VA, Emini EA, Deutsch P, Lifson JD, Bonhoeffer S, Nowak MA, Hahn BH, Saag MS, Shaw GM. Viral dynamics in human immunodeficiency virus type 1 infection. Nature 373:117-122, 1995.
9. Haase AT, Henry K, Zupancic M, Sedgewick G, Faust RA, Melroe H, Cavert W, Gebhard K, Staskus K, Zhang Z-Q, Dailey PJ, Balfour HH, Jr., Erice A, Perelson AS. Quantitative image analysis of HIV-1 infection in lymphoid tissue. Science 274:985-989, 1996.
10. Perelson AS, Neumann AU, Markowitz M, Leonard JM, Ho DD. HIV-1 dynamics in vivo: virion clearance rate, infected cell lifetime, and viral generation time. Science 271:1582-1586, 1996.
11. Perelson AS, Essunger P, Cao Y, Vesanen M, Hurley A, Saksela K, Markowitz M, Ho DD. Decay characteristics of HIV-1-infected compartments during combination therapy. Nature 387:188-191, 1997.
12. Wong JK, Hezareh M, Günthard H, Havlir DV, Ignacio CC, Spina CA, Richman DD. Recovery of replication-competent HIV despite prolonged suppression of plasma viremia. Science 278:1291-1294, 1997.
13. Finzi D, Hermankova M, Pierson T, Carruth LM, Chaisson RE, Quinn TC, Brookmeyer R, Gallant J, Markowitz M, Ho DD, Richman DD, Siliciano RF. Identification of a reservoir for HIV-1 in patients on highly active antiretroviral therapy. Science 278:1295-1300, 1997.

14. Chun T-W, Stuyver L, Mizell SB, Ehler LA, Mican JM, Baseler M, Lloyd AL, Nowak MA, Fauci AS. Presence of an inducible HIV-1 latent reservoir during highly active antiretroviral therapy. Proc Natl Acad Sci USA 94:13193-13197, 1997.
15. Gulick RM, Mellors JW, Havlir D, Eron JJ, Gonzalez C, McMahon D, Jonas L, Meibohm A, Holder D, Schleif WA, Condra JH, Emini EA, Isaacs R, Chodakewitz JA, Richman DD. Simultaneous vs sequential intitiation of therapy with indinavir, zidovudine, and lamivudine for HIV-1 infection. JAMA 280:35-41, 1998.
16. Wong JK, Gunthard H, Havlir DV, Zhang Z-Q, Haase AT, Ignacio CC, Kwok S, Emini E, Richman DD. Reduction of HIV-1 in blood and lymph nodes following potent anti-retroviral therapy and the virologic correlates of treatment failure. Proc Natl Acad Sci USA 94:12574-12579, 1997.
17. Gunthard HF, Havlir DV, Fiscus S, Zhang ZQ, Eron J, Mellors J, Gulick R,Frost SD, Brown AJ, Schleif W, Valentine F, Jonas L, Meibohm A, Ignacio CC, Isaacs R, Gamagami R, Emini E, Haase A, Richman DD, Wong JK. Residual human immunodeficiency virus (HIV) type 1 RNA and DNA in lymph nodes and HIV RNA in genital secretions and in cerebrospinal fluid after suppression of viremia for 2 years. J Infect Dis. 183:1318-1327, 2001.
18. Zhang L, Ramratnam B, Tenner-Racz K, He Y, Vesanen M, Lewin S, Talal A, Racz P, Perelson AS, Korber BT, Markowitz M, Ho DD, Guo Y, Duran M, Hurley A, Tsay J, Huang Y-C. Quantifying residual HIV-1 replication in patients receiving combinatin antiretroviral therapy. N Engl J Med 340:1605-1613, 1999.
19. Zhang Z-Q, Schuler T, Zupancic M, Wietgrefe SW, Reimann KA, Reinhart TA, Rogan M, Cavert W, Miller CJ, Veazey RS, Notermans D, Little S, Danner SA, Richman DD, Havlir D, Wong J, Jordan HL, Schacker TW, Racz P, Tenner-Racz K, Letvin NL, Wolinsky S, Haase AT. Sexual transmission and propagation of simian and human immunodeficiency viruses in resting and activated $CD4^+$ T cells, Science 286:1353-7, 1999.
20. Ruiz L, van Lunzen J, Arno A, Stellbrink H-J, Schneider C, Rull M, Castella E, Ojanguren I, Richman DD, Clotet B, Tenner-Racz K, Racz P. Protease inhibitor-containing regimens compared with nucleoside analogues alone in the suppression of persistent HIV-1 replication in lymphoid tissue. AIDS 13:F1-F81999.
21. Cohen Stuart JWT, De Boer R, Borleffs JCC, Boucher CAB, Visser C. Persistence of HIV antigens in lymphoid tissue despite 18 months of HAART may explain the slow decay of activated CD4 cells, Antiviral Therapy 4[Suppl. 1]:107(1999) (Abstract).
22. Günthard HF, Wong JK, Ignacio CC, Guatelli JC, Riggs NL, Havlir DV, Richman DD. Human immunodeficiency virus replication and genotypic resistance in blood and lymph nodes after a year of potent antiretroviral therapy. J Virol 72:2422-2428, 1998.
23. Günthard HF, Frost SDW, Leigh Brown AJ, Ignacio CC, Kee K, Perelson AS, Spina CA, Havlir DV, Hezareh M, Looney DJ, Richman DD, Wong JK. Evolution of envelope sequences of human immunodeficiency virus type 1 in cellular reservoirs in the setting of potent antiviral therapy. J Virol 73:9404-9412, 1999.
24. Günthard H, Wong J, Havlir D, Richman D. Evolution of HIV-1 V3 envelope sequences from residual lymph node RNA from patients on potent antiretroviral therapy with undetectable plasma viraemia for up to 2 years, Antiviral Therapy 4[Suppl. 1]:118(1999) (Abstract).
25. Coffin JM, HIV population dynamics in vivo: implications for genetic variation, pathogenesis and therapy. Science 267:483-489, 1995.

26. Wein LM, D'Amato RM, Perelson AS. Mathematical analysis of antiretroviral therapy aimed at HIV-1 eradication or maintenance of low viral loads. J Theor Biol 192:81-89, 1998.
27. Richman DD, Havlir D, Corbeil J, Looney D, Ignacio C, Spector SA, Sullivan J, Cheeseman S, Barringer K, Pauletti D, Shih C-K, Myers M, Griffin J. Nevirapine resistance mutations of human immunodeficiency virus type 1 selected during therapy. J Virol 68:1660-1666, 1994.
28. Havlir DV, Gamst A, Eastman S, Richman DD. Nevirapine-resistant human immunodeficiency virus: kinetics of replication and estimated prevalence in untreated patients. J Virology 70:7894-7899, 1996.
29. Schuurman R, Nijhuis M, van Leeuwen R, Schipper P, Collis P, Danner S, Mulder J, Loveday C, Christopherson C, Kwok S, Sninsky J, Boucher CAB. Rapid changes in human immunodeficiency virus type 1 RNA load and appearance of drug-resistant virus populations in persons treated with lamivudine. J Infect Dis 171:1431-1437, 1995.
30. Havlir DV, Hellmann NS, Petropoulos CJ, Whitcomb JM, Collier AC, Hirsch MS, Tebas P, Sommadossi J-P, Richman DD. Drug susceptibility in HIV isolates obtained after viral rebound from patients receiving an indinavir containing regimen, JAMA 283:229-34, 2000.
31. Descamps D, Peytavin G, Calvez V, Flandre P, Meiffredy V, Raffi F, Pialoux G, Aboulker JP, Brun-Vezinet F, the Trilège study group-France. Virologic failure, resistance and plasma drug measurements in induction maintenance therapy trial (Anrs 072, Trilege), 6th Conference on Retroviruses and Opportunistic Infections Chicago, IL:January 31-February 4, (1999) (Abstract).
32. de Pasquale P, Murphy R, Kuritzkes D, Martinez-Picado J, Sommadossi J-P, Gulick R, Smeaton L, DeGruttola V, Caliendo A, Sutton L, Savara AV, D'Aquila RT. Resistance during early virological rebound on amprenavir plus zidovudine plus lamivudine triple therapy or amprenavir monotherapy in ACTG protocol 347. Antiviral Therapy 3[Suppl 1]:50, 1998 (Abstract).
33. Holder D, Condra JH, Schleif WA, Chodakewitz J, Emini EA. Virologic failure during combination therapy with crixivan and RT inhibitors is often associated with expression of resistance-associated mutations in RT only, 6th Conference on Retroviruses and Opportunistic Infections Chicago, IL:Jan 31-Feb 4(1999) (Abstract).
34. Nijhuis M, Boucher C, de Jong D, Gustchina E, Schuurman R, Erickson J, Gulnik S. Enzymatic basis for increased replication kinetics of ritonavir resistant HIV-1 protease. Antiviral Therapy 3[Suppl 1]:76(1998) (Abstract).
35. Ho DD, Toyoshima T, Mo H, Kempf DJ, Norbeck D, Chen C-M, Wideburg NE, Burt SK, Erickson JW, Singh MK. Characterization of human immunodeficiency virus type 1 variants with increased resistance to a C_2-symmetric protease inhibitor. J Virol 68:2016-2020, 1994.
36. Condra JH, Holder DJ, Schleif WA, Blahy OM, Danovich RM, Gabryelski LJ, Graham DJ, Laird D, Quintero JC, Rhodes A, Robbins HL, Roth E, Shivaprakash M, Yang T, Chodakewitz JA, Deutsch PJ, Leavitt RY, Massari FE, Mellors JW, Squires KE, Steigbigel RT, Teppler H, Emini EA. Genetic correlates of in vivo viral resistance to indinavir, a human immunodeficiency virus type 1 protease inhibitor. J Virol 70:8270-8276, 1996.
37. Erickson JW, Gulnik SV, Markowitz M. Protease inhibitors: resistance, cross-resistance, fitness and the choice of initial and salvage therapies. AIDS Suppl A:S189-S204, 1999.

38. Martinez-Picado J, Savara A, Sutton L, D'Aquila R. Replicative fitness of protease inhibitor resistant mutants of human immunodeficiency virus type 1. J Virol 73:3744-3752, 1999.
39. Havlir DV, Marschner IC, Hirsch MS, Collier AC, Tebas P, Bassett RL, Ioannidis JPA, Holohan MK, Leavitt R, Boone G, Richman DD. Maintenance antiretroviral therapies in HIV-infected subjects with undetectable plasma HIV RNA after triple-drug therapy. N Engl J Med 339:1261-1268, 1998.
40. Samson M, Libert F, Doranz BJ, Rucker J, Liesnard C, Farber CM, Saragosti S, Lapoumeroulie C, Cognaux J, Forceille C, Muyldermans G, Verhofstede C, Burtonboy G, Georges M, Imai T, Rana S, Yi Y, Smyth RJ, Collman RG, Doms RW, Vassart G, Parmentier M. Resistance to HIV-1 infection in caucasian individuals bearing mutant alleles of the CCR-5 chemokine receptor gene. Nature 382:722-725, 1996.
41. Liu R, Paxton WA, Choe S, Ceradini D, Martin SR, Horuk R, MacDonald ME, Stuhlmann H, Koup RA, Landau NR. Homozygous defect in HIV-1 coreceptor accounts for resistance of some multiply-exposed individuals to HIV-1 infection. Cell 86:367-377, 1996.
42. Dean M, Carrington M, Winkler C, Huttley GA, Smith MW, Allikmets R, Goedert JJ, Buchbinder SP, Vittinghoff E, Gomperts E, Donfield S, Vlahov D, Kaslow R, Saah A, Rinaldo C, Detels R, O'Brien SJ. Genetic restriction of HIV-1 infection and progression to AIDS by a deletion allele of the CKR5 structual gene. Science 273:1856-1862, 1996.
43. O'Brien TR, Winkler C, Dean M, Nelson JA, Carrington M, Michael NL, White. HIV-1 infection in a man homozygous for CCR5 delta 32. Lancet 349:1219-1219, 1997.
44. Zimmerman PA, Buckler-White A, Alkhatib G, Spalding T, Kubofcik J, Coimbadiere C, Weissman D, Cohen O, Rubbert A, Lam G, Vaccarezza M, Kennedy PE, Kumaraswami V, Giorgi JV, Detels R, Hunter J, Chopek M, Berger EA, Fauci AS, Nutman TB, Murphy R. Inherited resistance to HIV-1 conferred by an inactivating mutation in CC chemokine receptor 5: Studies in populations with contrasting clinical phenotypes, defined racial background, and quantified risk. Molecular Medicine 3:23-36, 1997.
45. Ioannidis JPA, O'Brien TR, Rosenberg PS, Contopoulous-Ioannidis DG, Goedert JJ. Meta-analysis of host genetic effects on HIV disease progression. Nature Medicine 4:53-61, 1998.
46. Martin MP, Dean M, Smith MW, Winkler C, Gerrard B, Michael NL, Lee B, Doms RW, Margolick J, Buchbinder S, Goedert JJ, O'Brien TR, Hilgartner MW, Vlahov D, O'Brien SJ, Carrington M. Genetic acceleration of AIDS progression by a promoter variant of CCR5. Science 282:1907-1911, 1998.
47. McDermott DH, Zimmerman PA, Guignard F, Kleeberger CA, Leitman SF, Murphy PM. CCR5 promoter polymorphism and HIV-1 disease progression. Lancet 352:866-870, 1998.
48. Mummidi S, Ahuja SS, Gonzalez E, Anderson SA, Santiago EN, Stephan KT, Craig FE, O'Connell P, Tryon V, Clark RA, Dolan MJ, Ahuja SK. Genealogy of the CCR5 locus and chemokine system gene variants associated with altered rates of HIV-1 disease progression. Nature Med 4:786-793, 1998.
49. Carrington M, Nelson GW, Martin MP, Kissner T, Vlahov D, Goedhert JJ, Kaslow R, Buchbinder S, Hoots K, O'Brien SJ. HLA and HIV-1: heterozygote advantage and B*35-Cw*04 disadvantage. Science 283:1748-1752, 1999.
50. O'Brien TR, McDermott DH, Ioannidis JPA, Carrington M, Murphy PM, Havlir DV, Richman DD. Effect of chemokine receptor gene polymorphisms on the response to potent antiretroviral therapy. AIDS 14:821-6, 2000.

51. Kim RB, Fromm MF, Wandel C, Leake B, Woods AJJ, Roden DM, Wilkinson GR. The drug transporter P-glycoprotein limits oral absorption and brain entry of HIV-1 protease inhibitors. J Clin Invest 101:289-294, 1998.
52. Lee CG, Gottesman MM, Cardarellir CO, Ramachandra M, Jeang K-T, Ambudkar SV, Pastan I, Dey S. HIV-1 protease inhibitors are substrates for the MDR1 multidrug transporter. Biochemistry 37:3594-3601, 1998.
53. Schuetz JD, Connelly MC, Sun D, PaiBir SG, Flynn PM, Srinivas RV, Kumar A, Fridland A. MRP4: A previously unidentified factor in resistance to nucleoside-based antiviral drugs. Nature Med 5:1048-1051, 1999.
54. Molla A, Vasavanonda S, Kumar G, Sham HL M, Johnson M, Grabowski B, Denis-senvJF, Kohlbrenner W, Plattner JJ, Norbeck DW, Kempf DJ. Human serum attenuates the activity of protease inhibitors toward wild-type and mutant human immunodeficiency virus. Virology 250:255-262, 1998.
55. Kageyama S, Anderson BD, Hoesterey BL, hayashi H, Kiso Y, Flora KP, Mitsuya H. Protein binding of human immunodeficiency virus protease inhibitor NKI-272 and alteration of its in vitro antiretroviral activity in the presence of high concentrations of proteins, Antimicrob Agents Chemother 38:1107-1111 (1994) (Abstract).
56. Bilello JA, Drusano GL, Prichard M, Robins T, Drusano G. Reduction of the in vitro activity of A77003, an inhibitor of human immunodeficiency virus protease, by human serum $_1$ acid glycoprotein. J Infect Dis 171:546-551, 1995.
57. Wong JK, Ignacio CC, Torriani F, Havlir D, Fitch NJS, Richman DD. *In vivo* compartmentalization of HIV: evidence from the examination of *pol* sequences from autopsy tissues. J Virol 70:2059-2071, 1997.
58. Byrn RA and Kiessling AA. Analysis of human immunodeficiency virus in semen: indications of a genetically distinct virus reservoir. J Reprod Immunol 41:161-176, 1998.
59. Eron JJ, Vernazza PL, Johnston DM, Seillier-Moiseiwitsch F, Alcorn TM, Fiscus SA, Cohen MS. Resistance of HIV-1 to antiretroviral agents in blood and seminal plasma: implications for transmission. AIDS 12:F181-F189, 1998.
60. Enting RH, Hoetelmans RMW, Lange JMA, Burger DM, Beijnen JH, Protegies P. Antiretroviral drugs and the central nervous system. AIDS 12:1941-55, 1998.
61. Kepler TB and Perelson AS. Drug concentration heterogeneity facilitates the evolution of drug resistance. Proc Natl Acad Sci USA 95:11514-11519, 1998.
62. Kilby JM, Hopkins S, Venetta TM, DiMassimo B, Cloud GA, Lee JY, Alldredge L, Hunter E, Lambert D, Bolognesi D, Matthews T, Johnson MR, Nowak MA, Shaw GM, Saag MS. Potent suppression of HIV-1 replication in humans by T-20, a peptide inhibitor of gp41-mediated virus entry. Nature Med 4:1302-1307, 1998.
63. Eckert DM, Malashkevich VN, Hong LH, Carr PA, Kim PS. Inhibiting HIV-1 entry: discovery of D-peptide inhibitors that target the gp41 coiled-coil pocket. Cell 99:103-115, 1999.
64. Donzella GA, Schols D, Lin SW, Este JA, Nagashima KA, Maddon PJ, Allaway GP, Sakmar TP, Hensen G, De Clercq E, Moore JP. AMD3100, a small molecule inhibitor of HIV-1 entry via the CXCR4 co-receptor. Nature Med 4:72-77, 1999.
65. Rieko Arakaki, Hirokazu Tamamura, Mariappan Premanathan, Kenji Kanbara, Sivasundaram Ramanan, Katsura Mochizuki, Masanori Baba, Nobutaka Fujii, and Hideki Nakashima. T134, a Small-Molecule CXCR4 Inhibitor, Has No Cross-Drug Resistance with AMD3100, a CXCR4 Antagonist with a Different Structure. J. Virol. 73: 1719-1723, 1999.

66. Baba M, Nishimura O, Kanzaki N, Okamoto M, Sawada H, Iizawa Y, Shiraishi M, Aramaki Y, Okonogi K, Ogawa Y, Meguro K, Fujino M. A small-molecule, nonpeptide CCR5 antagonist with highly potent and selective anti-HIV-1 ativity. *Proc Natl Acad Sci USA* 96:5698-5703, 1999.
67. Richman DD, The challenge of immune control of immunodeficiency virus. J Clin Invest 104:677-678, 1999.
68. Ortiz GM, Nixon DF, Trkola A, Binley J, Jin X, Bonhoeffer S, Kuebler PJ, Donahoe SM, Demoitie M-A, Kakimoto WM, Ketas T, Clas B, Heymann JJ, Zhang L, Cao Y, Hurley A, Moore JP, Ho DD, Markowitz M. HIV-1-specific immune responses in subjects who temporarily contain virus replication after discontinuation of HAART. J Clin Invest 104:R13-R181999.
69. Lisziewicz J, Jessen H, Finzi D, Siliciano RF, Lori F. HIV-1 suppression by early treatment with hydroxurea, didanosine, and a protease inhibitor. Lancet 352:199-200, 1998.
70. Vila J, Nugier F, Barguaes G, Vallett T, Peyramond D, Hamedi-Sangsari F, Seigneurin JM. Absence of viral rebound after treatment of HIV-infected patients with didanosine and hydroxycarbamide. Lancet 350:635-636, 1997.

10

Origin and Phenotypic Expressions of the *CCR5-Δ32* Allele

Thomas R. O'Brien and Michael Dean
National Cancer Institute, Rockville and Frederick, Maryland

BACKGROUND

Because *CCR5-Δ32* homozygotes are highly resistant to infection by HIV-1 and HIV-1-infected *CCR5-Δ32* heterozygotes have delayed progression to AIDS (Chapter 7), therapies that might blockade or downregulate CCR5 are under serious consideration for treating HIV-1 infection (Chapter 12). Before such therapies are implemented it is important to determine whether any deleterious effects are associated with the *CCR5-Δ32* allele, such as might result from the absence of CCR5 or from increased levels of β-chemokines. The β-class (CC) chemokines play a critical role in the inflammatory process through recruitment or activation of lymphocytes, monocytes, mast cells, and eosinophils. Lymphocytes from *CCR5-Δ32* homozygotes produce elevated levels of CCR5 ligand β-chemokines *in vitro* (1), and these proteins can bind chemokine receptors other than CCR5 (Chapter 1). Studies in genetically altered mice indicate that the absence of CCR5 or higher levels of β-chemokines may have phenotypic expressions. Mice lacking CCR5 had impaired macrophage function and an enhanced T-cell dependent immune response (2). Higher levels of MIP-1α are associated with Coxsackievirus-induced myocarditis in mice (3).

Conversely, the *CCR5-Δ32* allele may have beneficial phenotypic expressions besides those related to HIV-1 infection. Observations regarding the origin of the *CCR5*-Δ32 allele suggest that it may offer protection against one or more potentially deadly infectious agents that predate the emergence of HIV-1. In addition, chemokines and their receptors are known to play important roles in a number of chronic diseases, especially those involving inflammation (Chapter 1). These links offer the possibility that novel therapies directed against CCR5 expression may prove useful in the treatment of diseases other than HIV-1 infection. In this chapter we explore the origin of the *CCR5-Δ32* allele and its possible phenotypic expressions.

POPULATION DISTRIBUTION OF THE *CCR5-Δ32* ALLELE

Initial investigations of the *CCR5-Δ32* allele indicated that it is relatively common in Caucasians, but rare or absent in other populations (4-7). Subsequent, more extensive, surveys of the population distribution of the *CCR5-Δ32* allele have included a total of more than 12,000 subjects (8-11). The results of the various studies are generally consistent. The *CCR5-Δ32* allele appears to be restricted to Caucasian populations, including those residing in western Asia (8, 9), and to populations in which there has been genetic inflow from Caucasian populations. The allele is rarely found in indigenous African, American, or Far Eastern Asian populations (8, 9). Among populations residing in Europe the allele has an overall frequency of about 10% with a strong cline (i.e., geographic gradient). A north to south latitudinal correlation (r = 0.73) with *CCR5-Δ32* allele frequency has been formally demonstrated (11). The highest allele frequencies have been found in Scandinavian and Celtic populations, as well as in populations from northeastern Europe. Low frequencies of the *CCR5-Δ32* allele have been observed in populations from the Mediterranean region, such as Greeks (8), Sardinians (10), and Corsicans (11). Some exceptions to this pattern have been reported. Libert and colleagues (10) found an allele frequency of 8.3% in Saamis (who reside in the north of Sweden) and a frequency of 14.2% in Swedes residing further south. However, the Saamis are known to be genetically distinct from other Swedes (10). Relatively high frequencies of the *CCR5-Δ32* allele have been observed in Ashkenazi Jews (range 20.9% to 9.7%) (8, 9). The population distribution of the *CCR5-Δ32* allele indicates that the mutational event which gave rise to this allele was a relatively recent event in evolutionary history, having occurred after Caucasians separated from African ancestors (5).

ORIGIN AND EXPANSION OF THE *CCR5-Δ32* ALLELE

Several groups have attempted to date the origin of the *CCR5-Δ32* allele. Libert et al. (10) examined two highly polymorphic microsatellites (i.e., tandem repeats of simple DNA sequences that occur with a range of frequencies) located near the site of *CCR5-Δ32* allele on the p21.3 region of chromosome 3. They determined the haplotype (i.e., linked alleles found on a single maternal or paternal chromosome) of the chromosomes that carry the *CCR5-Δ32* allele and found evidence of strong linkage disequilibrium (i.e., non-random assortment of alleles) between the

CCR5-Δ32 allele and specific microsatellite alleles. Among the chromosomes that carried *CCR5-Δ32*, more than 95% also carried the IRI3.1-0 allele (located 11 kb upstream from *CCR5-Δ32*) and 88% carried the IRI3.2-0 allele (located 68 kb downstream from *CCR5-Δ32*). In contrast, these alleles were found in only 1.5-2% of the chromosomes carrying a wild-type *CCR5* gene. On that basis the investigators inferred that most, if not all *CCR5-Δ32* alleles originated from a single mutation event. The investigators then estimated the date of the origin of the *CCR5-Δ32* allele by calculating the recombination frequency expected between the *CCR5-Δ32* allele and the IRI3.1 locus (on the basis of their distance apart on chromosome 3), and then estimating the number of generations that would have occurred since that event. On this basis Libert et al. calculated that the mutation which produced the *CCR5-Δ32* allele occurred 3500 years ago, but their estimate had a very wide 95% confidence interval of 400 to 13,000 years.

Stephens et al. dated the origin of the *CCR5-Δ32* allele to the earlier portion of this span by using microsatellite markers and coalescence analysis. In this study, the recombination distance between *CCR5* and adjacent microsatellite markers was imputed from a regression radiation hybrid physical distance and recombination distances (9). The origin of the *CCR5-Δ32*-containing ancestral haplotype was estimated to be about 700 years ago, with a range of 275-1,875 years.

Maayan et al. (12) genotyped Ashkenazi and Sephardic Jews residing in Israel in order to estimate the original date of the *CCR5-Δ32* allele. Among 922 HIV seronegative blood donors the alelle frequency was 13.8% in Ashkenazi Jews and 4.9% in Sephardic Jews. Using the Island model, they calculated that a minimal genetic migration rate of 3% per generation would have been necessary to fully explain the higher *CCR5-Δ32* allele frequency in Ashkenazi Jews by their genetic mixture with the indigenous northern European populations. This putative genetic migration rate is 20-fold higher than that currently estimated from other genes, and would correspond to a non-realistic current admixture of 80% or more for Ashkenazi Jews. Maayan et al. concluded that a positive selection process for *CCR5-Δ32* occurred in northern Europe at most 1000 years ago, after Ashkenazi Jews had separated from Sephardic Jews and moved to north Europe.

The high frequency and geographic cline of the *CCR5-Δ32* allele, along with the evidence that it originated from a single, relatively recent mutational event, suggest that the allele increased in frequency due to positive genetic selection. Because chemokine receptors are known to be receptors for infectious agents (e.g., HIV-1) and because CCR5 is the ligand for several immune response signaling molecules, an epidemic of a pathogen that, like HIV-1, utilizes CCR5, may have increased the frequency of the *CCR5-Δ32* allele in ancestral Caucasian populations.

PHENOTYPIC EXPRESSIONS OF THE *CCR5-Δ32* ALLELE

Mortality

The *CCR5-Δ32* allele is in Hardy-Weinberg equilibrium (i.e., *CCR5-Δ32* genotype frequencies are consistent with the *CCR5*-Δ32 allele frequency) (6), which indicates that the *CCR5-Δ32* allele has no drastic impact on genetic fitness (i.e., the ability to survive and reproduce successfully). Nguyễñ et al. (13) looked at mortality among 15 HIV-1-uninfected *CCR5*-Δ32 homozygotes who were enrolled in prospective epidemiologic studies of HIV-1 incidence. They found no evidence of increased mortality in these subjects, but the number of enrolled *CCR5*-Δ32 homozygotes was too small for a meaningful analysis of genotype specific mortality.

Infectious Diseases

Because the *CCR5-Δ32* allele may offer protection from an infectious agent that predates the recently emergent HIV-1, Nguyễñ et al. (13) also looked for evidence of infection with common viruses among the *CCR5-Δ32* homozygotes who were enrolled in epidemiologic studies. Thirteen of these subjects were men with hemophilia and two were homosexual males. For 9 common viruses (cytomegalovirus, Epstein-Barr virus, varicella zoster virus, respiratory syncytial virus, herpes simplex virus, influenza A virus, influenza B virus, mumps, rubella), antibody prevalence was similar for *CCR5-Δ32* homozygous subjects and a reference population. Antibody to measles virus was found less commonly than expected among these subjects, but that finding was not confirmed in an analysis of 14 U.S. blood donors who were homozygous for *CCR5-Δ32*. In addition, *in vitro* studies indicated that CCR5 was not required for infection with measles virus (13).

Consistent with the high prevalence of blood borne infections that are found among persons with hemophilia, antibody was detected in all 11 *CCR5-Δ32* homozygotes with hemophilia who were tested for hepatitis B virus and 10 of 12 (83.3%) who were tested for hepatitis C virus (HCV) (13). Among patients with hemophilia who were infected with HCV, mean alanine aminotransferase levels were 117% higher among *CCR5-Δ32* homozygotes ($p < .05$). Because lymphocytes are an important component of the hepatic infiltrates found in chronic HCV infection (14), the finding of elevated transaminase levels among HCV-infected *CCR5-Δ32* homozygotes might be related to an increase in the number of lymphocytes or an enhanced T-cell dependent immune response, as reported in mice who lack CCR5 (2). Regardless, this study found no evidence that the *CCR5-Δ32* homozygous genotype was clinically deleterious or beneficial with regard to HCV infection: none of these men developed hepatic failure and serum HCV levels did not differ by genotype. There was also no evidence of conditions that might be due to impaired macrophage function, such as have been observed in mice that lack CCR5.

Many infectious diseases that caused significant mortality in the past are no longer common in Caucasian populations. There is evidence that poxviruses can use chemokine receptors to infect leukocytes (15), which suggests the possibility that the *CCR5-Δ32* allele might provide resistance to variola (smallpox) virus. Organisms which, like HIV-1, target macrophages are especially attractive candidates for increasing the frequency of the *CCR5-Δ32* allele (9). Bubonic plague caused significant mortality in Europe during the 14th century and *Yersinia pestis*, the plague bacillus, targets macrophages, as do *Shigella*, *Salmonella*, and *Mycobacterium tuberculosis*. Further research is required to determine if the *CCR5-Δ32* allele offers protection against these or other infectious agents.

Lymphocyte Counts

In the study by Nguyen et al. (13), *CCR5-Δ32* homozygotes were compared to CCR5 wild-type subjects for a wide range of hematologic measures. The results were generally similar among the genotypes, but total lymphocyte counts were approximately 20% higher in *CCR5-Δ32* homozygous study subjects than in CCR5 wild type subjects ($p < .05$). Each individual count for the *CCR5-Δ32* homozygotes, however, fell within the reference range for the assay. As β-chemokines regulate lymphocyte trafficking, it is plausible that *CCR5-Δ32* homozygotes, who may have elevated levels of β-chemokines, could tend to have slightly elevated lymphocyte counts.

Rheumatoid Arthritis and Related Diseases

Rheumatoid arthritis is a chronic multisystem disease of unknown etiology in which chemokines and chemokine receptors appear to play an important role. CCR5 expression on CD4+ and CD8+ leukocytes (lymphocytes, monocytes, and natural killer cells) from the synovial fluid of patients with rheumatic joint diseases is considerably higher than that from the same patients' peripheral blood leukocytes (16). This finding suggests a role for CCR5 in the process of joint inflammation. Several groups have examined whether *CCR5-Δ32* genotypes are associated with rheumatoid arthritis or related diseases.

The frequency of the *CCR5-Δ32* allele was lower in 163 Danish patients (10%) who had rheumatoid arthritis than in a control group of 151 Danish Caucasians (14%), but the difference was not statistically significant (p=0.4) (17). Similarly, in a study from Spain (18), the frequency of the *CCR5-Δ32* allele did not differ significantly between patients with rheumatoid arthritis (5.8%; n=673) and controls (7.1%; n=815). None of the Spanish patients with rheumatoid arthritis had the homozygous *CCR5-Δ32* genotype (compared with 0.9% of the controls, p=0.04), but *CCR5-Δ32* homozygotes with rheumatoid arthritis were found in other studies at expected frequencies (17, 19), which indicates that this genotype does not strongly protect against rheumatoid arthritis, if at all. The frequency of the *CCR5-Δ32* allele among 113 Spanish patients with systemic lupus erythematosus (9.3%) was somewhat higher than the frequency in controls, but the difference was not statistically significant (18). The frequency of the *CCR5-Δ32* allele was 4.5% in 88 Italian patients with polymyalgia rheumatica and 6.9% in healthy blood donors from the same geographic area, (20) a difference that was not statistically significant. On the basis of these studies, there is little evidence that *CCR5-Δ32* genotype alters susceptibility to rheumatoid diseases.

The *CCR5-Δ32* allele may be associated, however, with less severe manifestations of rheumatoid arthritis. Among the Danish patients with rheumatoid arthritis (17), 35% of those with the *CCR5-Δ32* allele had swollen joints compared 58% of patients that were homozygous for the normal allele (p=0.03). The median duration of morning stiffness was 0 minutes for *CCR5-Δ32* allele carriers and 60 minutes for wild type patients (p = 0.0002). In addition, 29% of the rheumatoid arthritis patients who carried the deletion allele were negative for IgM rheumatoid factor compared to 9% of those that were homozygous for the normal allele (p = 0.007). These findings suggest that CCR5 could be a target for therapeutic intervention against rheumatoid arthritis, especially in light of the finding that a RANTES derivative [aminooxypentane (AOP)-RANTES] completely down-modulated CCR5 expression on synovial fluid leukocytes in *in vitro* studies (16).

Inflammatory Bowel Disease

Crohn's disease and ulcerative colitis appear to have a genetic component. The *CCR5-Δ32* allele is an attractive candidate to explain susceptibility to these inflammatory bowel diseases, because the chromosomal location of the CCR5 gene on 3p21 coincides with an identified inflammatory bowel disease susceptibility locus (21) and because studies have shown the important role of chemokines, including the CCR5 ligand RANTES, in inflammatory bowel disease (22).

Rector et al. (21) investigated the presence of the *CCR5-Δ32* allele in a large cohort of inflammatory bowel disease patients. Blood samples were obtained from 538 inflammatory bowel disease patients and 135 unaffected first-degree family members. Of the patients, 36% had familial inflammatory bowel disease with at least two affected family members. There were no significant differences in the *CCR5-Δ32* allele frequency between patients and controls. Furthermore, there was no correlation between the *CCR5-Δ32* genotype and age at diagnosis, frequency of surgical intervention, or disease localization. Analysis by the transmission/disequilibrium test showed no significant transmission distortion to patients or to unaffected siblings. Similarly, Martin et al. (23) examined the role of the *CCR5-Δ32* allele in 101 patients with Crohn's disease, and 99 patients with ulcerative colitis, and 120 healthy unrelated controls. The frequency of the *CCR5-Δ32* allele was not significantly different in patients with Crohn's disease or ulcerative colitis when compared to the controls (P 0.2 or more). Therefore, it appears unlikely that the *CCR5-Δ32* allele alters the predisposition to Crohn's disease or ulcerative colitis.

Multiple Sclerosis

Multiple sclerosis is a T-cell-dependent chronic inflammatory disease of the central nervous system which is characterized by myelin loss and progressive neurological dysfunction. Genetic susceptibility appears to play a role in the etiology of multiple sclerosis (24), likely acting in concert with an undefined environmental exposure, possibly an infectious agent. Genome screening of families in which multiple members have multiple sclerosis identified several potential susceptibility regions, including evidence for weak linkage in the region of chromosome 3 that includes *CCR5* (25). The *CCR5-Δ32* allele is also a candidate loci for genetic susceptibility to multiple sclerosis because increased levels of the CCR5 ligand MIP-1α have been demonstrated in the cerebrospinal fluid of patients with multiple sclerosis (26). In addition, MIP-1α levels are increased in mice with experimental autoimmune encephalomyelitis (EAE-an animal model for multiple sclerosis) and anti-MIP-1α alpha antibodies can prevent EAE (27).

To determine if *CCR5* genotype plays a role in multiple sclerosis, Bennetts et al. (28) compared 120 unrelated Australians with relapsing remitting multiple sclerosis to 168 unrelated control subjects. There was no significant difference in the allele frequency of *CCR5-Δ32* allele between the multiple sclerosis patients (11.3%) and the control population (9.2%). The presence of two *CCR5-Δ32* homozygotes in the multiple sclerosis patients indicated that the absence of CCR5 is not protective against multiple sclerosis. Barcellos et al. (25) examined the chromosome 3p21-24 region in 125 multiple sclerosis families (322 total affected and 200 affected sib-pairs), and performed genetic analyses of *CCR5* and *CCR2B* loci and two nearby markers (D3S1289 and D3S1300) using both linkage- and association-based tests. They found no evidence that the *CCR5-Δ32* allele (or any of the other tested markers) decreased the risk of multiple sclerosis risk, but the age of onset of multiple sclerosis was about 3 years later in patients with the *CCR5* deletion (p=0.02). Sellebjerg et al. (29) found that the *CCR5-Δ32* allele did not confer protection from multiple sclerosis, but was associated with a lower risk of recurrent clinical disease activity. These data suggest that the absence of CCR5 does not protect against the development of multiple sclerosis, but that the level of CCR5 expression may alter the severity of the disease for some patients. If so, CCR5 may be a target for therapies directed against multiple sclerosis.

Asthma and Allergy

Chemokines, including the CCR5 ligand RANTES, may play an important role in allergic diseases. Several studies have examined whether the *CCR5-Δ32* allele alters the risk of asthma or allergy. In a study of Scottish children (30), 11.2% of asthmatics were reported to carry the *CCR5-Δ32* allele compared to 26.2% of children without asthma (p=0.003). This result suggested a protective effect for the *CCR5-Δ32* allele, but the finding was not confirmed by Mitchell et al. (31). They investigated the *CCR5-Δ32* allele for linkage and association to asthma and atopy among 1284 individuals that comprised two panels of families. No statistically significant linkage to asthma or atopy was observed in either panel. Similarly, there was no evidence of a link between the *CCR5-Δ32* allele and allergic diseases found among Hungarian children (32): allele frequencies were 9.5% in the allergic children (n=121) and 11.0% in the controls (n=295). Therefore, there is no consistent evidence that the *CCR5-Δ32* polymorphism is associated with an increased risk of either allergy or asthma.

Insulin-Dependent Diabetes Mellitus

Although no genetic locus for insulin-dependent diabetes mellitus has been identified near the p21 region of chromosome 3, studies have shown that proinflammatory cytokines may play a role in this disease. Szalai et al. (33) determined the frequency of the *CCR5-Δ32* and *CCR2-64I* alleles in 115 Hungarian children with insulin-dependent diabetes mellitus and 280 nondiabetic children of similar age. *CCR5-Δ32* allele frequencies were similar in both groups of children, but the *CCR2-64I* allele frequency in children with insulin-dependent diabetes mellitus was 22.6% compared to 11.4% in controls (p = 0.001). This study suggests that the *CCR5-Δ32* allele plays no role in insulin-dependent diabetes mellitus. The potential role of the *CCR2-64I* allele in this disease deserves further examination.

Hypertension

Nguyen et al. (13) compared 15 *CCR5-Δ32* homozygotes with 201 CCR5 wild type subjects for a wide range of clinical conditions ascertained during prospective cohort studies and routine clinical care. They found that hypertension and conditions attributable to hemophilia were the only diagnoses frequently found in clinical records of *CCR5-Δ32* homozygotes study subjects. Based on blood pressure measurement and treatment history, *CCR5-Δ32* homozygotes had a 2.8-fold higher prevalence of hypertension than age-matched *CCR5* wild type study subjects (95% confidence interval, 1.2-6.4; p=.01); none of the homozygotes had severe hypertension. This finding gains plausibility by the fact that AT1, the major angiotensin receptor, is a seven-transmembrane G protein-coupled receptor (34) that shares about 60% amino acid homology with CCR5. Confirmatory investigations are needed to determine whether hypertension represents a true phenotypic expression of the *CCR5-Δ32* homozygous genotype.

CONCLUSION

The *CCR5-Δ32* allele originated relatively recently in a Caucasian population and increased in frequency due to positive genetic selection. Protection against a fatal infectious disease is the most likely cause of this selection, but the specific agent or agents involved have not been identified. People who are homozygous for the

CCR5-Δ32 allele appear to suffer little or no adverse consequences, perhaps due to the redundancy of the chemokine/chemokine receptor system. Certainly, there is no evidence of any effects of the *CCR5-Δ32* allele that are sufficiently deleterious to preclude therapeutic CCR5 blockade or downregulation, if such treatment proves to be effective for HIV-1 infection. There is preliminary evidence that the clinical benefit of the *CCR5-Δ32* allele may extend beyond patients who are infected with HIV-1, to include patients with certain inflammatory diseases (i.e., rheumatoid arthritis and multiple sclerosis). Further work is needed to confirm those relationships, which offer hope of a broad utility for future therapies that are directed toward CCR5.

REFERENCES

1. Dragic T, Litwin V, Allaway GP, Martin SR, Huang Y, Nagashima KA, Cayanan C, Maddon PJ, Koup RA, Moore JP, Paxton WA. HIV-1 entry into CD4+ cells is mediated by the chemokine receptor CC-CKR5. Nature 1996;381:667-73.
2. Zhou Y, Kurihara T, Ryseck RP, Yang Y, Ryan C, Loy J, Warr G, Bravo R. Imparied macrophage function and enhanced T cell-dependent immune response to mice lacking CCR5, the mouse homologue of the major HIV-1 coreceptor. J Immunol 1998;160:4018-25.
3. Cook DN, Beck MA, Coffman TM, Kirby SL, Sheridan JF, Pragnell IB, Smithies O. Requirement of MIP-1α for an inflammatory response to viral infection. Science 1995;269:1583-5.
4. Liu R, Paxton WA, Choe S, Ceradini D, Martin SR, Horuk R, MacDonald ME, Stuhlmann H, Koup RA, Landau NR. Homozygous defect in HIV-1 coreceptor accounts for resistance of some multiply-exposed individuals to HIV-1 infection. Cell 1996;86:367-77.
5. Dean M, Carrington M, Winkler C, Huttley GA, Smith MW, Allikmets R, Goedert JJ, Buchbinder SP, Vittinghoff E, Gomperts E, Donfield S, Vlahov D, Kaslow R, Saah A, Rinaldo C, Detels R, Hemophilia Growth and Development Study, Multicenter AIDS Cohort Study, Multicenter Hemophilia Cohort Study, San Francisco City Cohort, ALIVE Study, O'Brien SJ. Genetic restriction of HIV-1 infection and progression to AIDS by a deletion allele of the CKR5 structural gene. Science 1996;273:1856-62.
6. Samson M, Frédérick L, Doranz B, Rucker J, Liesnard C, Farber C-M, Saragosti S, Lapouméroulie C, Cognaux J, Forceille C, Muyldermans G, Verhofstede C, Burtonboy G, Georges M, Imai T, Rana S, Yi Y, Smyth RJ, Collman RG, Doms RW, Vassart G, and Parmentier M. Resistance to HIV-1 infection in Caucasian individuals bearing mutant alleles of the CCR-5 chemokine receptor gene. Nature 1996;382:722-5.
7. Zimmerman PA, Buckler-White A, Alkhatib G, Spalding T, Kubofcik J, Combadiere C, Weissman D, Cohen O, Rubbert A, Lam G, Vaccarezza M, Kennedy PE, Kumaraswami V, Giorgi JV, Detels R, Hunter J, Chopek M, Berger EA, Fauci AS, Nutman TB, Murphy PM. Inherited resistance to HIV-1 conferred by an inactivating mutation in CC chemokine receptor 5: studies in populations with contrasting clinical phenotypes, defined racial background, and quantified risk. Mol Med 1997;3:23-36.
8. Martinson JJ, Chapman NH, Rees DC, Liu Y-T, Clegg, J.B. Global distribution of the CCR5 gene 32-basepair deletion. Nature Genet. 1997;16:100-3.

9. Stephens JC, Reich DE, Goldstein DB, Shin HD, Smith MW, Carrington M, Winkler C, Huttley GA, Allikmets R, Schriml L, Gerrard B, Malasky M, Ramos MD, Morlot S, Tzetis M, Oddoux C, di Giovine FS, Nasioulas G, Chandler D, Aseev M, Hanson M, Kalaydjieva L, Glavac D, Gasparini P, Dean M, et al. Dating the origin of the CCR5-Delta32 AIDS-resistance allele by the coalescence of haplotypes. Am J Hum Genet. 1998;62:1507-15.
10. Libert F, Cochaux P, Beckman G, Samson M, Aksenova M, Cao A, Czeizel A, Claustres M, de la Rua C, Ferrari M, Ferrec C, Glover G, Grinde B, Guran S, Kucinskas V, Lavinha J, Mercier B, Ogur G, Peltonen L, Rosatelli C, Schwartz M, Spitsyn V, Timar L, Beckman L, Vassart G. The *Δccr5* mutation conferring protection against HIV-1 in Caucasian populations has a single and recent origin in Northeastern Europe. Hum Mol Genet. 1998;7:399-406.
11. Lucotte G, Mercier G. Distribution of the CCR5 gene 32-bp deletion in Europe. J Acquir Immune Defic Syndr Hum Retrovirol. 1998;19:174-7.
12. Maayan S, Zhang L, Shinar E, Ho J, He T, Manni N, Kostrikis LG, Neumann AU. Evidence for recent selection of the CCR5-delta 32 deletion from differences in its frequency between Ashkenazi and Sephardi Jews. Genes Immun. 2000;1:358-61.
13. Nguyen GT, Carrington M, Beeler JA, Dean M, Aledort LM, Blatt PM, Cohen AR, DiMichele D, Eyster ME, Kessler CM, Konkle B, Leissinger C, Luban N, O'Brien SJ, Goedert JJ, O'Brien TR. Phenotypic expressions of CCR5-delta32/delta32 homozygosity. J Acquir Immune Defic Syndr. 1999;22:75-82.
14. Houghton M. Hepatitis C viruses. Field's Virology. Third edition. Fields BN, Knipe DM, Howley PM, et al. Lippincott - Raven Publishers, Philadelphia 1996:1035-58.
15. Lalani AS, Masters J, Zeng W, Barrett J, Pannu R, Everett H, Arendt CW, McFadden G. Use of chemokine receptors by poxviruses. Science 1999;286:1968-71.
16. Mack M, Bruhl H, Gruber R, Jaeger C, Cihak J, Eiter V, Plachy J, Stangassinger M, Uhlig K, Schattenkirchner M, Schlondorff D. Predominance of mononuclear cells expressing the chemokine receptor CCR5 in synovial effusions of patients with different forms of arthritis. Arthritis Rheum. 1999;42:981-8.
17. Garred P, Madsen HO, Petersen J, Marquart H, Hansen TM, Freiesleben Sorensen S, Volck B, Svejgaard A, Andersen V. CC chemokine receptor 5 polymorphism in rheumatoid arthritis. J Rheumatol. 1998;25:1462-5.
18. Gomez-Reino JJ, Pablos JL, Carreira PE, Santiago B, Serrano L, Vicario JL, Balsa A, Figueroa M, de Juan MD. Association of rheumatoid arthritis with a functional chemokine receptor, CCR5. Arthritis Rheum. 1999;42:989-92.
19. Cooke SP, Forrest G, Venables PJ, Hajeer A. The delta32 deletion of CCR5 receptor in rheumatoid arthritis. Arthritis Rheum. 1998;41:1135-6.
20. Salvarani C, Boiardi L, Timms JM, Silvestri T, Ranzi A, Macchioni PL, Pulsatelli L, di Giovine FS. Absence of the association with CC chemokine receptor 5 polymorphism in polymyalgia rheumatica. Clin Exp Rheumatol. 2000;18:591-5.
21. Rector A, Vermeire S, Thoelen I, Keyaerts E, Struyf F, Vlietinck R, Rutgeerts P, Van Ranst M. Analysis of the CC chemokine receptor 5 (CCR5) delta-32 polymorphism in inflammatory bowel disease. Hum Genet. 2001;108:190-3.
22. Mazzucchelli L, Hauser C, Zgraggen K, Wagner HE, Hess MW, Laissue JA, Mueller C. Differential in situ expression of the genes encoding the chemokines MCP-1 and RANTES in human inflammatory bowel disease. J Pathol. 1996;178:201-6.
23. Martin K, Heinzlmann M, Borchers R, Mack M, Loeschke K, Folwaczny C. Delta 32 mutation of the chemokine-receptor 5 gene in inflammatory bowel disease. Clin Immunol. 2001;98:18-22.

24. Bell JI, Lathrop GM. Multiple loci for multiple sclerosis. Nat Genet. 1996;13:377-8.
25. Barcellos LF, Schito AM, Rimmler JB, Vittinghoff E, Shih A, Lincoln R, Callier S, Elkins MK, Goodkin DE, Haines JL, Pericak-Vance MA, Hauser SL, Oksenberg JR. CC-chemokine receptor 5 polymorphism and age of onset in familial multiple sclerosis. Multiple Sclerosis Genetics Group. Immunogenetics. 2000;51:281-8.
26. Miyagishi R, Kikuchi S, Fukazawa T, Tashiro K. Macrophage inflammatory protein-1 alpha in the cerebrospinal fluid of patients with multiple sclerosis and other inflammatory neurological diseases. J Neurol Sci. 1995;129:223-7.
27. Karpus WJ, Lukacs NW, McRae BL, Strieter RM, Kunkel SL, Miller SD. An important role for the chemokine macrophage inflammatory protein-1 alpha in the pathogenesis of the T cell-mediated autoimmune disease, experimental autoimmune encephalomyelitis. J Immunol. 1995;155:5003-10.
28. Bennetts BH, Teutsch SM, Buhler MM, Heard RN, Stewart GJ. The CCR5 deletion mutation fails to protect against multiple sclerosis. Hum Immunol. 1997;58:52-9.
29. Sellebjerg F, Madsen HO, Jensen CV, Jensen J, Garred P. CCR5 delta32, matrix metalloproteinase-9 and disease activity in multiple sclerosis. J Neuroimmunol. 2000;102:98-106.
30. Hall IP, Wheatley A, Christie G, McDougall C, Hubbard R, Helms PJ. Association of CCR5 delta32 with reduced risk of asthma. Lancet. 1999;354:1264-5.
31. Mitchell TJ, Walley AJ, Pease JE, Venables PJ, Wiltshire S, Williams TJ, Cookson WO. Delta 32 deletion of CCR5 gene and association with asthma or atopy. Lancet. 2000;356:1491-2.
32. Szalai C, Bojszko A, Beko G, Falus A. Prevalence of *CCR5Δ32* in allergic diseases. Lancet. 2000;355:66.
33. Szalai C, Csaszar A, Czinner A, Szabo T, Panczel P, Madacsy L, Falus A. Chemokine receptor CCR2 and CCR5 polymorphisms in children with insulin-dependent diabetes mellitus. Pediatr Res. 1999;46:82-4.
34. Curnow KM, Pascoe L, White PC. Genetic analysis of the human type-1 angiotensin II receptor. Molec Endocrinol 1992;6:1113-8.

11

HIV-1 Infection in Patients with the *CCR5-Δ32* Homozygous Genotype

Thomas R. O'Brien
National Cancer Institute, Rockville, Maryland

Nelson L. Michael
Walter Reed Army Institute of Research, Rockville, Maryland

Haynes W. Sheppard
California Department of Health Services, Berkeley, California

Susan Buchbinder
San Francisco Department of Health, San Francisco, California

"Treasure your exceptions"
–*William Bateson (1861-1926)*
leading early 20th century geneticist

BACKGROUND

Although about 1% of Caucasians are homozygous for the *CCR5-Δ32* allele, initial studies, totaling several thousand HIV-1 infected persons, found no infected people with this genotype (1-5). These results suggested that a functional CCR5 protein might be an absolute requirement for HIV-1 infection. Subsequent reports of HIV-1 infection in *CCR5-Δ32* homozygotes demonstrated that HIV-1 could be acquired in the absence of CCR5 expression on cell surfaces (6-8), but HIV-1 infection has been documented in only nine people with the *CCR5-Δ32* homozygous genotype to date. These rare patients offer unique insights into HIV-1 transmission and virology that may be informative for the potential use of therapies designed to block CCR5.

RESISTANCE TO HIV-1 INFECTION AND CORECEPTOR USAGE

Risk of Infection

Known HIV-1-infected *CCR5-Δ32* homozygotes consist of seven homosexual or bisexual men, one man with hemophilia, and one man who reportedly became infected through heterosexual intercourse (references 6-13; Table 1). Because the total number of persons who have been tested for the *CCR5-Δ32* homozygous genotype is unknown, it is difficult to gauge the exact strength of the relative protection that is afforded by the *CCR5-Δ32* homozygous genotype. An estimate of this protective effect may be obtained from epidemiologic cohort studies that were initiated early in the HIV-1 epidemic and that are, therefore, less subject to survivorship biases. In Chapter 5, Michael Dean reports data obtained by combining subjects from five such studies, including cohorts of homosexual men and persons with hemophila. Dean found that the *CCR5-Δ32* homozygous genotype provided about a thirty-fold decreased risk of infection with HIV-1.

The strength of the protection afforded by *CCR5-Δ32* homozygosity was also gauged among the subjects with hemophilia. During the late 1970s and early 1980s, patients with hemophilia were exposed to blood products made from blood that was pooled from thousands of donors (14). Some of these patients remained uninfected despite very heavy treatment with blood products that were likely to have been contaminated with HIV-1 (7). In one study, the *CCR5-Δ32* homozygous genotype was present in five (29%) of 17 heavily treated patients, which is 29 times higher than the 1% genotype frequency generally found in Caucasians (2). Furthermore, there is no evidence that any *CCR5-Δ32* homozygotes became infected with HIV-1 via a contaminated blood transfusion (15). Thus, *CCR5-Δ32* homozygosity provides very strong resistance to HIV-1 infection through both sexual and blood-borne routes of infection.

Viral Characteristics

As detailed in Chapter 4, chemokine receptors are essential coreceptors for HIV-1 cell entry and CCR5 is the major coreceptor for the strains that are usually present during early infection. Viruses that use CCR5 as a coreceptor (R5 strains) are typically, macrophage-tropic and non-syncytium inducing (NSI) strains. As infection progresses, some patients develop HIV-1 strains that can use CXCR4 or other coreceptors. Viruses that use CXCR4 (X4 strains) are syncytium inducing (SI) and typically more pathogenic than R5 strains. One very important implication of the observation that *CCR5-Δ32* homozygotes can become infected with HIV-1 is that the virus is able to initiate infection by using a coreceptor or coreceptors other than

CCR5. Therefore, if novel measures that are designed to prevent HIV-1 infection by blocking CCR5 are developed, these approaches might not be 100% effective even if used properly.

Investigators have characterized the viral strains recovered from HIV-1-infected *CCR5-Δ32* homozygotes by using three types of assays. These assays are: viral phenotyping assays, which determine whether a strain induces syncytia in MT-2 cells; viral genotyping assays, which detect sequences of the HIV-1 V3 loop that have been associated with SI viruses; and HIV-1 infectivity assays, which determine the coreceptors that a specific virus can use to infect cells *in vitro*. Viral strains from seven of the nine HIV-1-infected *CCR5-Δ32* homozygotes have been evaluated by at least one of these three types of assays.

Viruses from subjects 2 and 8 (Table 1) have been studied extensively, including coreceptor typing. Michael and colleagues examined samples that had been collected longitudinally from patient 2, who was a man with hemophilia (9). The earliest analyzed sample from this patient was collected about four years after initial infection and the last sample was collected nine and one half years later. The viruses from these samples were of the SI type on the basis of both phenotype and genotype. Heteroduplex mobility assay results (a measure of viral diversity) showed that the viruses from this subject were genetically homogenous and that the virus did evolve significantly over time. HIV-1 strains that were collected from this patient over a nine and one half-year period were also examined for coreceptor use with an infectivity assay. All of these strains used the CXCR4 coreceptor exclusively. The persistent and exclusive use of the CXCR4 coreceptor in viruses from this patient was in sharp contrast to the usual pattern of HIV-1 coreceptor usage. In most cases, initial viral strains use the CCR5 coreceptor and, over time, coreceptor use may broaden to include CXCR4 or minor coreceptors. However, because no early specimens were available from this patient, it was impossible to determine the coreceptor use of the virus at the initiation of infection.

Specimens from very early in the course of infection were available from patient 8, who was enrolled in the HIVNET Vaccine Preparedness study (16), which is an epidemiological study of people at risk for HIV-1 infection. Patient 8 engaged in frequent unprotected anal intercourse with HIV-1-infected men. He developed antibodies to HIV-1 sometime between May 1995, when he was last documented to be antibody negative, and October 1995, when he was first shown to be antibody positive. An HIV-1 RNA level >200,000 copies/ml was obtained from the May 1995 serum sample and that result is consistent with primary HIV-1 infection. Additionally, the patient had symptoms that were consistent with acute retroviral syndrome during June 1995. On the basis of this laboratory and clinical information, it is likely that this man became infected with HIV-1 during April or May of 1995. Genetic sequence analysis of the V3 loop portion of HIV-1 *env* gene from the June 1995 serum sample revealed an SI genotype. A virus isolate with an SI phenotype was obtained from a specimen that was collected in October 1995. In addition, four other specimens that were obtained during the first two

Table 1 HIV-1-infected patients with the *CCR5-Δ32* homozygous genotype.

Subject/ Risk Group	Viral Phenotype/ Genotype	HIV-1 Co-receptor	Clinical Course and Response to Therapy	Ref
1 Homosexual man	NR/NR	NR	Seroconversion in 1992; five years later patient was asymptomatic and untreated with a CD4+ count 460 cells/mm^3 and HIV-1 RNA level 19,000 copies/mL	6
2 Man with hemophilia	SI / SI	CXCR4	Infected ~1982 (~12 years of age); ~ 4 years later CD4+ count <200 cells/mm^3 (7th percentile for cohort) and HIV-1 RNA level ~5,000 copies/mL (~50th percentile); developed AIDS ~14 years after infection (42nd percentile); died of hepatitis C virus related liver failure 1996	7, 9
3 Homosexual man	NR / SI	NR	Infected in 1989; CD4 count decreased rapidly and remained persistently below 150 cells/mm^3 despite 'very low' HIV-1 RNA level.	8
4 Homosexual man	SI / NR	CCR5 and CXCR4	Became infected sometime before 1988; HIV RNA 14,664 copies/mL and CD4+ lymphocytes 87 cells/mm^3 in 1994	10*
5 Heterosexual man	NR / SI	NR	Date of infection unknown; CD4+ counts initially in normal range, but declined rapidly after HIV-1 diagnosis; HIV-1 RNA decreased from 20,000 to <50 copies/mL after initiation of potent therapy.	11
6 Homosexual man	NR / SI	NR	Seroconverted between 1994 and 1995; HIV-1 RNA level 93,050 copies/mL one year after infection. CD4+ count 'low' at diagnosis and <200 cells/mm^3 within 2.5 years; HIV-1 RNA <400 copies/mL after potent therapy initiated	12
7 Homosexual man	SI / NR	NR	Seroconverted 1992; initial CD4+ count 280 cells/mm^3, falling to <100 cells/mm^3 ~5 years after seroconversion; HIV RNA level <400 copies/mL after initiation of potent therapy	13

8 Homosexual man	SI / SI	CXCR4	Seroconverted 1995; CD4+ count ~200-300 cells/mm^3 during 28 months after seroconversion; HIV RNA level fell from 125,500 to <400 copies/mL after initiation of potent therapy	13
9 Bisexual man	NR. / NR	NR	Date of initial infection unknown; CD4+ count 180-270 cells/mm^3 in 1991-92 while on AZT alone; CD4+ count nadir of 27 cells/mm^3 and HIV-1 RNA peak of 218,776 copies/mL in 1996; HIV RNA 11,000-30,000, CD4 cell count >200 cells/mm^3 on potent therapy	**

NR, not reported; SI, synctium inducing
*Also personal communication, Dr. Claudia Balotta
**Personal communication, Dr. Martyn French

years of this patient's HIV-1 infection also proved to be SI isolates. All five SI isolates replicated well in peripheral blood mononculear cells (PBMCs), and PCR-amplified env sequences from the PBMCs were homogeneous by heteroduplex mobility assay. The earliest isolate, which was collected in October 1995, used the CXCR4 coreceptor exclusively, thereby providing very strong evidence for acquisition of infection through that receptor. Taken together, the data from these two extensively studied patients suggest that HIV-1 infection can be initiated and maintained by viral strains that use CXCR4 alone.

HIV-1 obtained from subject 4 also was studied with an *in vitro* chemokine receptor infection assay (personal communication, Dr. Claudia Balotta). This patient became infected with HIV-1 sometime before 1988 (10). Low $TCID_{50}$/mL concentrations of a 1994 isolate from this subject were exposed to U87MG.CD4 cells expressing either CCR2, CCR3, CCR5, CXCR4, or no chemokine receptor. In contrast to coreceptor assay results from subjects 2 and 8, the isolate from subject 4 was able to use both CCR5 and CXCR4 as a coreceptor; similar to the results from the other two subjects the isolate from subject 4 did not use either CCR2b or CCR3 for cell entry. Viral SI phenotype results for subject 4 were consistent with the coreceptor findings - HIV-1 isolates obtained in 1994 and in 1997 had the SI phenotype (10). The demonstration of a "dual tropic" HIV-1 strain obtained from a *CCR5-Δ32* homozygote at least 6 years after the onset of infection indicates that HIV-1 may not lose the ability to use CCR5 as a coreceptor even if it infects a host who does not express this protein.

Data on viral phenotype or genotype, but not coreceptor use, are available for subjects 3, 5, 6, and 7 (Table 1). Results from these four HIV-1-infected *CCR5-Δ32* homozygotes are consistent with those from the more intensively studied subjects - all viruses obtained from these subjects were SI strains. Therefore, all viruses obtained to date from HIV-1-infected *CCR5-Δ32* homozygotes appear capable of using CXCR4 as a coreceptor for cell entry.

Implications

CCR5-Δ32 homozygosity confers protection against both sexual and blood-borne transmission of HIV-1. As noted above, this protection was extended to persons with hemophilia who were repeatedly treated with blood products that were pooled from thousands of blood donors. These *CCR5-Δ32* homozygotes were presumably exposed to HIV-1 strains that could use CXCR4 for cell entry. The protection they experienced suggests that initiation of HIV-1 infection via the CXCR4 coreceptor may be inefficient.

Initial HIV-1 infection theoretically could occur through coreceptors other than CCR5 or CXCR4, but that has not been observed thus far among HIV-1-infected *CCR5-Δ32* homozygotes. Instead it appears that "minor" HIV-1 coreceptors, including CCR2 which is expressed on macrophages (see Chapter 1, table 1), rarely, if ever, facilitate initial HIV-1. The lack of use of other coreceptors by HIV-1 reinforces the importance of the major coreceptors (CCR5 and CXCR4) in HIV-1 infection.

CLINICAL COURSE OF HIV-1 INFECTION IN *CCR5-Δ32* HOMOZYGOTES

Natural History

Because HIV-1-infected *CCR5-Δ32* heterozygotes have a more favorable clinical course than patients with two normal copies of this gene (see Chapter 7), HIV-1-infected *CCR5-Δ32* homozygotes might be expected to have a more favorable response to infection than patients with other genotypes. The small number of HIV-1-infected *CCR5-Δ32* homozygotes and the limited data on disease outcomes restrict the ability to generalize about the clinical course of HIV-1 infection in these patients. However, information on HIV-1 RNA levels and CD4+ lymphocyte counts, which are the most important prognostic markers of HIV-1 infection, are informative for these cases.

HIV-1 RNA levels are the strongest known predictor of the long-term course of HIV-1 infection and higher levels lead to a markedly increased risk of developing AIDS (Chapter 8). Pre-treatment HIV-1 RNA measurements were reported for eight of the nine HIV-1-infected *CCR5-Δ32* homozygotes, but the results were not consistent. Four patients (1, 2, 4, and 5) had HIV RNA levels between 5,000–20,000 copies/mL [values that are within the average range for early chronic infection (17)], one subject (number 3) had an HIV RNA level that was reported only as "very low," and three subjects (6, 8, and 9) had high HIV

RNA values. From these reports, it appears that HIV-1 RNA levels in *CCR5-Δ32* homozygotes may be low, medium, or high.

The CD4+ lymphocyte count reflects the current degree of immunological damage for HIV-1-infected patients and is a more proximate predictor of the risk of AIDS than the HIV-1 RNA level. Because CD4+ lymphocytes are lost over time in almost all HIV-1-infected patients, knowledge of the duration of infection is required to interpret CD4+ lymphocyte counts. The date of infection can be estimated by the date of seroconversion (usually defined as the mid-point between the date of last HIV-1 antibody test that was negative and the date of the first HIV-1 antibody test that was positive) or by observing primary HIV-1 infection. As noted in Chapter 3, primary HIV-1 infection usually resolves within 4 weeks after the initial HIV-1 infection. Information on the date of HIV-1 infection is available for subjects 1-3, and subjects 6-8. Five years after seroconversion, subject 1 had a CD4+ lymphocyte count of 460 cells/mm^3, which is within the expected range for a patient with that duration of infection. In contrast, the other five *CCR5-Δ32* homozygotes with well-characterized dates of infection appear to have lost CD4+ lymphocytes rapidly. Subject 2 had hemophilia and he was enrolled in a long-term epidemiologic study of HIV-1 infection. Compared to other subjects in that cohort, his rate of CD4+ lymphocyte loss was at the lowest 7th percentile. For subject 3, the CD4+ lymphocyte count decreased rapidly and remained persistently below 150 cells/mm^3 despite a 'very low' HIV-1 RNA level. The CD4+ lymphocyte count for subject 6 was noted to be 'low' at diagnosis and <200 cells/mm^3 within 2.5 years after infection. Similarly, both subject 7 and subject 8 had relatively low CD4+ lymphocyte counts soon after seroconversion.

CD4+ lymphocyte data for the three *CCR5-Δ32* homozygotes that lacked good information on the date of initial infection were consistent with the observations for the patients in whom duration of infection was known. For subject 4, the CD4+ lymphocyte count had fallen to 87 cells/mm^3 within 6 years after HIV-1 infection was discovered. CD4+ lymphocyte counts for subject 5 were within the normal range at the time of diagnosis of HIV-1 infection, but declined rapidly thereafter. The CD4+ lymphocyte count for subject 9 was relatively low on initial presentation. In sum, information from these 9 case reports suggests that HIV-1-infected *CCR5-Δ32* homozygotes tend to lose CD4+ lymphocytes relatively rapidly. The rapid loss of CD4+ lymphocytes by these patients may result from primary infection with SI strains that deplete CD4+ lymphocytes through syncytia formation.

Treatment Response

Although HIV-1-infected *CCR5-Δ32* homozygotes may lose CD4+ lymphocytes rapidly, they appear to respond well to treatment with potent antiretroviral therapy. Patients 5-8 had a sustained reduction in the HIV RNA level to undetectable levels in response to treatment. Patient 9 was at high risk for treatment failure because his CD4+ lymphocyte count was 27 cells/mm^3 at the time triple combination therapy was initiated, and because he had received a number of drugs in single and dual drug treatment regimens prior to the availability of protease inhibitors. Nevertheless, he achieved partial immunological recovery (CD4+ lymphocyte count >200 cells/mm^3) and a fairly good virological response (about one log reduction in HIV RNA) after treatment with a potent regimen (two reverse transcriptase inhibitors and a protease inhibitor) consisting of drugs that he had not received previously (personal communication, Dr. Martyn French).

Implications for the Development of Novel Agents

What do these findings imply for the development of novel prophylactic or therapeutic agents that block CCR5? The strong relative resistance to HIV-1 infection among people who do not express CCR5 because they are *CCR5-Δ32* homozygotes suggests that a preventative agent that effectively blocked CCR5 (see Chapter 12) might reduce the risk of acquiring HIV-1 substantially, perhaps thirty-fold. An agent offering that degree of risk reduction could have a marked effect on an individual's risk of acquiring HIV-1 infection. Given the continued spread of HIV-1 throughout the world and the ineffectiveness of spermicidal agents in preventing its transmission, the use of agents that block CCR5 should be explored, especially in vehicles that might be used by women who are at high risk of acquiring the infection.

As detailed in Chapter 12, potential therapies that might block or down-regulate CCR5 have generated considerable interest. The apparent rapid depletion of CD4+ lymphocytes among *CCR5-Δ32* homozygotes who have been infected with viruses that use CXCR4 reinforces concerns that CCR5 blockade could lead to the emergence of more pathogenic HIV-1 strains and, therefore, that therapeutic blockade of both CXCR4 and CCR5 might be required (18). On the other hand, the excellent therapeutic response to potent antiretroviral therapy seen in HIV-1 infected homozygotes suggests that blockade of CCR5, in conjunction with combination treatments that decrease viral replication, may suffice. In either case, chemokine receptor blockade eventually may offer an attractive new approach for treating HIV-1 infection that should be rigorously examined in controlled clinical trials.

REFERENCES:

1. Samson M, Libert F, Doranz BJ, Rucker J, Liesnard C, Farber C-M, Saragosti S, Lapouméroulie C, Cognaux J, Forceille C, Muyldermans G, Verhofstede C, Burtonboy G, Georges M, Imai T, Rana S, Yi Y, Smyth R, Collman RG, Doms RW, Vassart G, Parmentier M. Resistance to HIV-1 infection in caucasian individuals bearing mutant alleles of the CCR-5 chemokine receptor gene. Nature 1996;382:722-725.
2. Dean M, Carrington M, Winkler C, Huttley GA, Smith MW, Allikmets R, Goedert JJ, Buchbinder SP, Vittinghoff E, Gomperts E, Donfield S, Vlahov D, Kaslow R, Saah A, Rinaldo R, Detels R, Hemophilia Growth and Development Study, Multicenter AIDS Cohort Study, Multicenter Hemophilia Cohort Study, San Francisco City Cohort,

Cohort Study, Multicenter Hemophilia Cohort Study, San Francisco City Cohort, ALIVE Study, O'Brien SJ. Genetic restriction of HIV-1 infection and progression to AIDS by a deletion allele of the CKR5 structural gene. Science 1996;273:1856-1862.

3. Liu R, Paxton WA, Choe S, Ceradini D, Martin SR, Horuk R, MacDonald ME, Stuhlmann H, Koup RA, Landau NR. Homozygous defect in HIV-1 coreceptor accounts for resistance of some multiply-exposed individuals to HIV-1 infection. Cell 1996;86:367-377.
4. Huang Y, Paxton WA, Wolinsky SM, Neumann AU, Zhang L, He T, Kang S, Ceradini D, Jin Z, Yazdanbakhsh K, Kunstman K, Erickson D, Dragon E, Landau NR, Phair J, Ho DD, Koup RA. The role of a mutant CCR5 allele in HIV-1 transmission and disease progression. Nature Medicine 1996;2:1240-1243.
5. Zimmerman PA, Buckler-White A, Alkhatib G, et al. Inherited resistance to HIV-1 conferred by an inactivating mutation in CC chemokine receptor 5: studies in populations with contrasting clinical phenotypes, defined racial background, and quantified risk. Mol Med 1997;3:23-36.
6. Biti R, French R, Young J, Bennetts B, Stewart G, Liang T. HIV-1 infection in an individual homozygous for the CCR5 deletion allele. Nature Med 1997;3:252-253.
7. O'Brien TR, Winkler C, Dean M, et al. HIV-1 infection in a man homozygous for CCR5 Δ32. Lancet 1997;349:1219.
8. Theodorou I, Meyer L, Magierowska M, Katlama C, Rouzioux, and the Seroco Study Group. HIV-1 infection in an individual homozygous for CCR5Δ32. Lancet 1997;349:1219-1220.
9. Michael NL, Nelson JA, KewalRamani VN, Chang G, O'Brien SJ, Mascola JR, Volsky B, Louder M, White GC, II, Littman DR, Swanstrom R, O'Brien TR: Exclusive and persistent use of the entry coreceptor CXCR4 by human immunodeficiency virus type 1 from a subject homozygous for CCR5 delta32. J Virol 1998;72:6040-6047.
10. Balotta C, Bagnarelli P, Violin M, Ridolfo AL, Zhou D, Berlusconi A, Corvasce S, Corbellino M, Clementi M, Clerici M, Moroni M, Galli M. Homozygous Δ32 deletion of the CCR-5 chemokine receptor gene in an HIV-1-infected patient. AIDS 1997;11:F67-71.
11. Heiken H, Becker S, Bastisch I, Schmidt RE. HIV-1 infection in a heterosexual man homozygous for CCR-5 Δ32. AIDS;13:529-30.
12. Kuipers H, Workman C, Dyer W, Geczy A, Sullivan J, Oelrichs R. An HIV-1-infected individual homozygous for the CCR-5 Δ32 allele and the SDF-1 3'A allele. AIDS. 1999;13:433-4.
13. Sheppard H, Celum C, Michael N, O'Brien S, Dean M, Carrington M, Dondero D, Buchbinder S. HIV-1 infection in individuals with the CCR5-Δ32/Δ32 genotype: acquisition of syncytium inducing virus at seroconversion. Submitted.
14. Kroner BL, Rosenberg PS, Aledort LM, Alvord WG, Goedert JJ. HIV-1 infection incidence among persons with hemophilia in the United States and western Europe, 1978-1990. J Acquir Immune Defic Syndr 1994;7:279-86.
15. Wilkinson DA, Operskalski EA, Busch MP, Mosley JW, Koup RA. A 32-bp deletion within the CCR5 locus protects against transmission of parenterally acquired human immunodeficiency virus but does not affect progression to AIDS-defining illness. J Infect Dis 1998;178:1163-6.
16. Koblin BA, Heagerty P, Sheon A, Buchbinder S, Celum C, Douglas JM, Gross M, Marmor M, Mayer K, Metzger D, Seage G. Readiness of high-risk populations in the

HIV Network for Prevention Trials to participate in HIV vaccine efficacy trials in the United States. AIDS 1998;12:785-93

17. O'Brien TR, Blattner WA, Waters D, Eyster E, Hilgartner MW, Cohen AR, Luban N, Hatzakis A, Aledort LM, Rosenberg PS, Miley WJ, Kroner BL, Goedert JJ. Serum HIV-1 RNA levels and time to development of AIDS in the Multicenter Hemophilia Cohort Study. JAMA 1996;276:105-110.
18. Michael NL, Moore JP. HIV-1 entry inhibitors: evading the issue. Nat Med. 1999;5:740-742.

12

Therapies to Prevent or Inhibit Chemokine Receptor Expression

J. Scott Cairns and M. Patricia D'Souza
National Institute of Allergy and Infectious Diseases, Bethesda, Maryland

INTRODUCTION

The availability of drugs that target HIV-1 reverse transcriptase and protease gene products represents an important therapeutic advance that has dramatically improved the prognosis for HIV-infected people. Although these agents do not eradicate the virus, combinations of these drugs are capable of profound suppression of HIV-1 replication for long periods, and have been referred to as highly active antiretroviral therapy (HAART). However, a number of pharmacologic, immunologic and virologic issues challenge the ultimate success of highly active retroviral therapy. These include the inability of patients to tolerate the toxic effects associated with HAART, the pharmacologic complexity of multiple drug regimens, and poor adherence to complicated and expensive regimens. Further, the ability of HIV to integrate its genetic information into host cells, the capacity for the integrated proviral DNA to remain latent and refractory to antiretroviral therapy, and the ability of the proviral DNA to re-activate, create additional problems, such as life-long dependence on HAART therapy. Moreover, in cases of incomplete viral suppression or suboptimal compliance with drug regimens, the rapid kinetics of viral replication combined with the high rate of transcriptional errors made by viral reverse transcriptase virtually guarantee the emergence of drug resistant virus.

Despite the fact that 15 antiviral drugs are now licensed for therapy in the United States, the treatment options for patients who have failed antiretroviral therapy remain limited. Therapeutic agents that target the steps involved in viral entry, including the interaction between the virus envelope and chemokine receptors, represent novel opportunities to block viral infection (1,2). Strategies targeted to these steps would be welcome additions to the antiretroviral armamentarium.

CHEMOKINE RECEPTORS SERVE AS CRITICAL COMPONENTS OF HIV-1 ENTRY

HIV replication is initiated by the high affinity binding of the HIV envelope glycoprotein subunit, gp120, to its primary cellular receptor, the CD4 molecule (3,4), followed by an interaction with a cellular coreceptor. HIV coreceptors are seven-transmembrane G-protein-coupled chemokine receptors, and the coreceptor function of these proteins is inhibited by their natural chemokine ligands. Chemokines are small pro-inflammatory proteins that serve to recruit and activate specific types of leukocytes. Most chemokines can be classified into two major classes: CC- (β) or CXC- (α) based on the number of amino acids between conserved cysteine residues. The α-chemokine receptor, CXCR4, was identified as the fusion cofactor or second receptor for laboratory-adapted CD4+ T cell line tropic (T-tropic) strains of HIV (5), whereas the β-chemokine receptor, CCR5, was identified as the analogous cofactor used by primary macrophage-tropic (M-tropic) HIV-1 isolates (6-10).

A linkage between HIV and chemokine receptors was established by the discovery that three β-chemokines, RANTES, MIP-1α, and MIP-1β, suppressed infection by M-tropic HIV isolates by inhibiting envelope mediated membrane fusion and viral entry (11). These factors constitute the natural ligands for CCR5. Similarly, SDF-1, the ligand for CXCR4, demonstrated an analogous inhibitory effect on T-tropic HIV isolates (12,13). A model for HIV coreceptor usage and the strain-specific inhibition of HIV binding by coreceptor ligands is shown in Figure 1.

The differential use of CCR5 and CXCR4 by HIV strains coupled with the expression patterns of these receptors in primary cells largely explains viral tropism. M-tropic or non-syncytium-inducing (NSI) viruses are designated R5 viruses since they utilize CCR5, a chemokine receptor present on CD4+ macrophages and CD4+ T lymphocytes (14-16). T-tropic or syncytium-inducing (SI) viruses utilize CXCR4 and are designated X4 viruses. CXCR4 is present on CD4+ T cell lines and many other types of primary human cells (17-19). Dual tropic strains of HIV are designated R5X4 since they are capable of infecting CD4+ macrophages and lymphocytes as well as immortalized CD4+ T cell lines that express both CCR5 and CXCR4 (20).

Although CXCR4 and CCR5 serve as the major coreceptors for HIV, other chemokine receptors, such as CCR2b (9), CCR3 (9,10), CCR8 (21), and CX_3CR1 (22), as well as orphan receptors for which the ligand is unknown, including Apj (23), STRL33 (BONZO) (24,25), and BOB (GPR15) (24), can also function

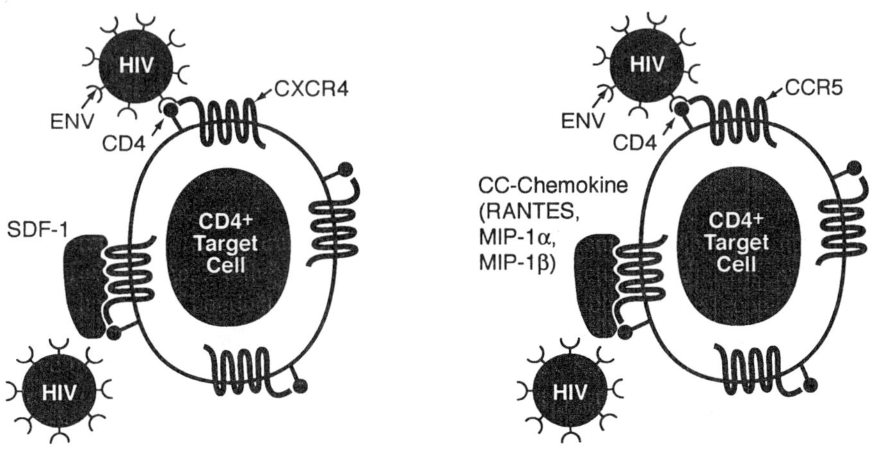

Figure 1 Model of CCR5 and CXCR4 usage and strain-specific inhibition of HIV binding by coreceptor ligands on CD4+ T cells. Entry of R5 strains of HIV is blocked by the CCR5 ligands MIP-1α, MIP-1β and RANTES. Entry of X4 viruses is blocked by the CXCR4 ligand SDF-1. [Adapted with permission from (133)].

as fusion cofactors for HIV entry in laboratory assays. Clearly, proteins belonging to this family have biochemical properties that promote HIV membrane fusion. However, most of the above mentioned secondary coreceptors are not very efficient and function only with certain strains of HIV-1, HIV-2 or SIV. Their relevance in transmission and pathogenesis *in vivo* is unknown.

CHEMOKINE RECEPTORS AS TARGETS FOR ANTI-HIV THERAPIES

The chemokine receptors provide an attractive target for drug development because they belong to the seven-transmembrane domain family of proteins that have historically proven to be highly susceptible to inhibition by small molecule antagonists. Coreceptor-based strategies target relatively invariant host determinants in contrast to anti-HIV agents that are directed against rapidly mutating viral components. A summary of the viral life cycle, including the targets for currently available anti-viral agents, is shown in Figure 2.

The CCR5 chemokine receptor is a particularly viable drug target because it is the principle coreceptor for transmission of NSI R5 isolates (26). Most individuals who die of AIDS have R5 variants exclusively, demonstrating that these isolates are lethal. However, in approximately 40% of infected humans, viruses arise that can use CXCR4 in addition to, or instead of CCR5 (27,28). The use of CXCR4 signals accelerated CD4+ T cell loss and disease progression (26,28).

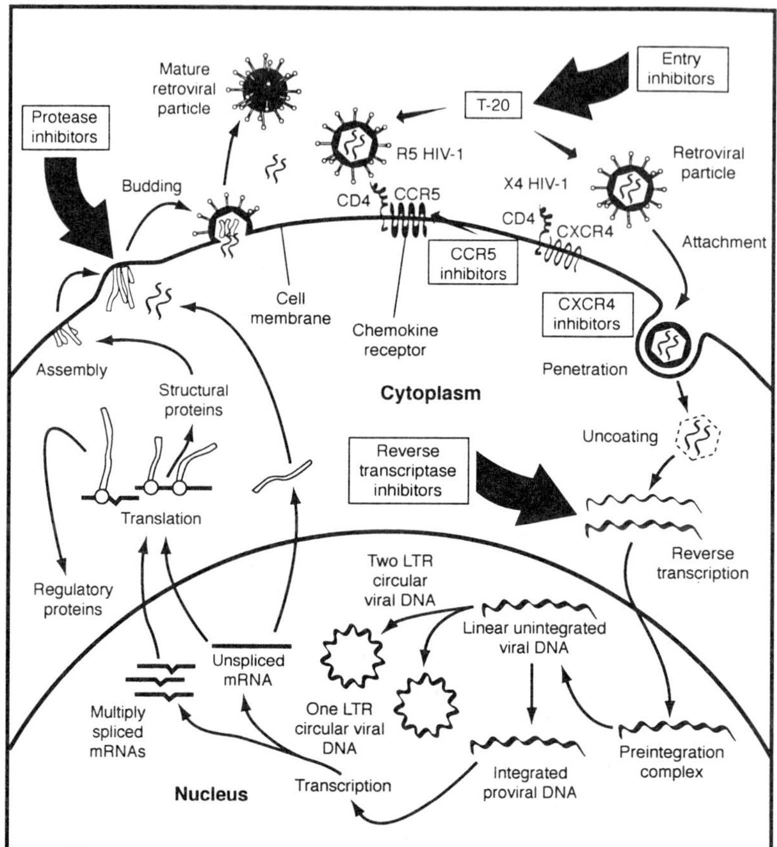

Figure 2 Chemokines, coreceptors and the HIV life cycle. HIV binds to susceptible cells via CD4 and a chemokine receptor. This fusion event is followed by viral entry, reverse transcription, integration, viral RNA synthesis and processing, viral protein synthesis, virion assembly, and budding. Current therapies, which are directed against viral reverse transcriptase and viral protease, are shown. HIV entry inhibitors would augment existing strategies by targeting viral envelope-CD4 or coreceptor interactions. [Adapted with permission from (2)].

A survey of the *CCR5* allele frequency found that about 1% of the Caucasian population is homozygous for a 32 base pair deletion in the coding region (29-31). The *Δ32* allele encodes a nonfunctional, truncated receptor protein that is rapidly degraded intracellularly and is not expressed on the cell surface. CCR5 was implicated as a critical factor in transmission or initial establishment of HIV infection when it was found that *CCR5-Δ32* homozygosity proved to be strongly, but not totally, protective against HIV-1 infection (32-34). Also, PBMCs from

CCR5-Δ32 homozygotes are refractory to *in vitro* infection by R5 (but not X4) viruses, are more sensitive to the HIV-1 blocking effects of recombinant chemokines, and make about 5-10-fold higher amounts of β-chemokines (29,35). In addition, CCR5 knock-out mice do not exhibit any overt pathology (36). As described in chapter 10, CCR5-*Δ32* homozygotes are generally similar to wild-type persons lending further support to the therapeutic targeting of the CCR5 receptor in individuals expressing two wild-type alleles.

More comprehensive studies of *CCR5-Δ32* allele frequency in HIV-1 progression showed that a single copy of the *CCR5-Δ32* allele was present in about 15% of the population and was not associated with protection from acquiring HIV-1 infection (31,37,38). However, the heterozygous phenotype modestly reduced the rate of disease progression in HIV-infected individuals. The attenuated course of disease is associated with reduced viral burdens and slower declines in the number of CD4+ T cells. PBMCs from *CCR5-Δ32* heterozygotes show markedly reduced surface expression of CCR5 and infectability by R5 viruses *in vitro* (39,40). These observations raise hope that deliberate manipulation of the CCR5 expression levels can significantly improve the prognosis of HIV-1-infected individuals. However, the *CCR5-Δ32* defect may not be the only factor influencing CCR5 expression; individuals with two wild-type *CCR5* alleles have a considerable range of CCR5 expression on their CD4+ T cells, and the number of receptors expressed influences the infectivity of these cells by R5 strains (39-41). Hence, the level of CCR5 expression on target cells, and the ability of different viral strains to use this receptor, may have a major impact on the replicative capacity of M-tropic virus in HIV-1 infected individuals.

The absolute requirement of coreceptors for HIV-1 infection, the antiviral properties of chemokines, and polymorphisms in chemokine receptor (42,43) and chemokine genes (44) that afford resistance to virus infection or delay disease progression underscore the relevance of these targets for antiviral drug development.

CHALLENGES TO THE DEVELOPMENT OF INHIBITORS TARGETING CHEMOKINE RECEPTORS

The development of therapeutic strategies targeted to the HIV-chemokine receptor interaction is in many ways subject to the same issues encountered in the development of therapies against HIV-encoded enzymes. These include the development of compounds that are orally bioavailable, affordable, and well tolerated by the patient. And in the era of HAART, as new therapies are developed, use will be in the context of existing antiviral agents, so the compatibility of new therapies with existing treatments must also be closely monitored.

The selection of the patient population in which to test the various inhibitors will be a critical determinant in the successful development of chemokine receptor-based therapies. CCR5 blockers, used in combination with other therapies, would be expected to have their greatest impact soon after transmission or during early chronic infection, as viruses isolated early after infection are most often homogeneous and M-tropic. In contrast, CXCR4 blockers would be expected to have their greatest effects in later stages of disease. Clearly, tailoring therapy to the tropism of the virus present in the individual patient, a strategy that is receiving greater attention as drug-resistant viruses emerge with current anti-retroviral agents, would provide greatest benefit.

Because chemokine receptors are host proteins, there are additional issues that must be addressed in the development of strategies that inhibit the function of these molecules. Toxicities that result from interference with the normal function of these molecules in lymphocyte development, trafficking, and inflammation must be closely monitored. It is possible that *CCR5-Δ32* homozygous individuals may have compensating immunological changes in other components of the chemokine/receptor system, so the consequences of experimentally manipulating CCR5 expression levels in individuals who functionally express protein remain unknown. Development of CXCR4 blockers is potentially even more problematic since deletion of the CXCR4 gene (45), or of the gene encoding its cognate chemokine ligand, SDF-1 (46), leads to severe hematopoietic and cardiac defects in the developing mouse embryo. The development of chemokine receptor blockers that interfere with HIV envelope, but not cognate ligand interactions with chemokine receptors, could potentially avoid this complication.

The virologic consequences of the selective pressures exerted by agents targeting chemokine receptors must also be closely monitored. Even when given in the context of other anti-viral agents, the low level of viral replication likely to be experienced by most patients may be sufficient to allow selection of viral variants that use alternative co-receptors or entry mechanisms. Drug failures are now being seen in a substantial minority of patients receiving current HAART regimens. There is no reason chemokine receptor blockers will escape these same limitations. This is a particular concern for CCR5 blockers, which have the potential to select for more pathogenic X4 viral strains. Of course, this selective pressure could also be used to advantage if CXCR4 blockers could be used to drive HIV tropism away from X4 usage. The issue of concern with R5 or X4 blockers is that the virus may mutate to use co-receptors other than CCR5 or CXCR4, with unknown consequences of disease pathogenesis. A possible example of natural selection for alternative co-receptor usage has recently emerged. It has been observed that approximately 85% of red-capped mangabeys harbor a 24 base-pair deletion in the CCR5 gene that precludes infection by CCR5-using SIV strains. Nevertheless, a red-capped mangabey with the 24 base-pair deletion has been identified that was naturally infected with an SIV isolate that uses CCR2b as its entry co-receptor (47). This observation suggests that CCR2b tropism may have been an adaptation by the virus to the selective pressure imposed by the CCR5 genetic defect. Although, this observation highlights the concern that therapies that target chemokine receptors may select for HIV variants with alternative tropisms, there is no evidence that this occurs with HIV under selective pressure of chemokine receptor antagonists.

Should any of these concerns prevent the development and testing of chemokine receptor inhibitors? Although these concerns must be addressed when therapeutically targeting chemokine receptors, G-protein-coupled receptors have provided successful targets for the development of therapeutic compounds for other uses, albeit not against infectious pathogens. For example, the drug cimetidine, which targets histamine receptors, has been used very commonly to treat gastritis and peptic ulcer disease (48). This is one of many examples of effective oral pharmaceuticals that should provide an impetus for the development of therapeutic agents that inhibit HIV entry.

NATURAL LIGAND AND PEPTIDE-BASED STRATEGIES

Chemokines are obvious therapeutic candidates because they compete with the HIV-1 envelope glycoprotein for binding to the chemokine receptors and down-regulate their cognate receptors, thereby interfering with entry/fusion. Certain chemokines may also affect levels of virus indirectly. For instance, RANTES interaction with CCR3 increases FasL expression on CD8+ effector cells, resulting in increased cytolytic activity against infected cells (49).

Therapeutic interventions based on administration or over-expression of these bioactive compounds must be approached cautiously because of the key role these molecules play in natural biological processes such as lymphocyte migration and inflammation (50). The activities of several of these chemokines, including SDF-1 and RANTES, are regulated by CD26, a dipeptidyl peptidase that is both secreted and expressed on the surface of many HIV-susceptible cell types (51). Its activity may serve to limit (52) or increase (51,53, 54) the anti-HIV-1 activity of certain chemokines. Although the effect of CD26 on RANTES-mediated HIV inhibition is controversial and has not been confirmed by all groups (55), the activity of CD26 could have an impact on the levels of active chemokines attainable *in vivo*, if these factors are used therapeutically. In addition, many of these chemokines have been shown to increase HIV replication under certain circumstances (56,57), making the outcome of *in vivo* administration of these compounds unpredictable.

These observations may help explain the conflicting results that have been obtained in studies examining the effect of β-chemokines on the virus *in vivo*. Several studies have suggested a protective role for β-chemokines in HIV-infection (35,58,59) as well as shown an inverse relationship between β-chemokine production and HIV plasma RNA load (60). However, other studies have shown an association of elevated levels of β-chemokines with HIV disease progression and low CD4 cell counts (61,62). Studies analyzing β-chemokine levels in the tissues of infected patients or an SIV experimental model have yielded more consistent data. Tissue distribution of β-chemokines during primary infection of macaques inoculated with SIV showed increased secretion of β-chemokines by bronchoalveolar lavage cells by the time of peak viremia, and increased RANTES gene expression in intestinal tissue (63,64). In addition, a recent cross-sectional study demonstrated a clear correlation between high cervical HIV-1 RNA levels and increased genital fluid concentration of β-chemokines. However, the association between β-chemokine concentration and virus load in plasma was not statistically significant (65). Because all of these studies are correlative, interpretation of chemokine effects on viral load is unclear. *In vitro* studies suggest that bioactive β-chemokines can have opposing effects on viral replication depending on how they are measured and the source and phenotype of the virus.

Because of the issues discussed above, current efforts are directed towards the identification and development of modified β-chemokines that block HIV infection without the inflammatory side effects or the HIV-1-stimulatory effects of the parent molecules. Mutational analysis by several groups has highlighted the importance of residues in the N-terminus of CC-chemokines in binding and activating chemokine receptors (66-68). N-terminal residues are also critical to the formation of dimers, the most common conformation observed in most three-dimensional analyses of wild-type proteins of the CC-chemokine family (69-74). It is therefore understandable that the biologically inactive CC-chemokines identified to date have focused on alterations in this critical region of the molecule.

Five β-chemokine derivatives that bind CCR5 with diminished cellular signaling capabilities have been reported. These are RANTES (9-68) and RANTES (3-68), in which the first 8 or the first 2 N-terminal amino acids of RANTES have been deleted, respectively (75); Met-RANTES, in which a methionine is appended to the N-terminus of RANTES (76); aminooxypentane (AOP)-RANTES (77); and nonanoyl (NNY)-RANTES (78). Additional RANTES derivatives with improved affinity and ability to inhibit HIV replication are also under development (R. Offord, personal communication). Initially, these chemokine derivatives were thought to inhibit HIV by a process of competitive inhibition for viral binding. However, it now appears more likely that the effects on HIV replication are mediated predominantly by inhibitor-mediated coreceptor down-regulation. In support of this hypothesis, AOP-RANTES induces down-regulation of CCR5 (55), whereas MCP-3, which binds to CCR5 with nearly the same affinity as RANTES, fails to induce receptor down-regulation and has negligible effects on HIV replication *in vitro* (79). AOP-RANTES and NNY-RANTES have been shown to inhibit HIV replication *in vivo* in SCID mice reconstituted with human peripheral blood cells (hu PBL-SCID mice). Further, NNY-RANTES was able to prevent HIV infection in a subset of hu-PBL mice challenged with an R5 HIV isolate (78). However, in NNY-RANTES-treated mice that became infected on challenge with an R5 virus, HIV emerged that was resistant to the therapeutic agent and exhibited an altered tropism for CXCR4.

Strategies that capitalize on biologically inactive versions of the CXCR4 ligand SDF-1 are not as advanced as those based on RANTES derivatives. In part, this is because modifications that inactivate RANTES do not have a similar effect on SDF-1. For instance, the addition of a methionine residue at the N-terminus, a strategy that significantly diminishes the biologic activity of RANTES, enhances the intracellular signaling activity of SDF-1 (80). However, two N-terminal truncations of SDF-1, or versions in which substitutions have been made at the N-terminus, have been examined and found to lack CXCR4 signaling capacity while retaining significant binding affinity for the receptor (69). In addition, several peptides have been identified that block the interaction of HIV with CXCR4 yet are not homologous to SDF-1. T22 is an 18-amino acid peptide derived from the hemocyte debris of the horseshoe crab. It specifically blocks membrane fusion and infection by X4 viruses as well as chemotaxis in response to SDF-1 (81). ALX40-4C, a 9 D-amino acid peptide, also blocks HIV envelope and SDF-1 interactions with CXCR4 (82). More recently, a 14-amino acid peptide related to T22, termed T134, has been described (83). This peptide has improved HIV-1 inhibitory activity *in vitro*, as well as the ability to inhibit HIV-1 X4 variants that are resistant to AMD3100, a small molecule CXCR4 antagonist (see below). All of these peptides have a high net positive charge, suggesting that they may interact with CXCR4 through electrostatic interactions, as has been proposed for the positively charged SDF-1 core (84). Structure/function studies suggest that ALX40-4C and the SDF-1 core interact with CXCR4 at different sites (85), offering an opportunity for synergistic inhibition. It remains to be determined whether these peptides inhibit HIV by competitive blocking or, as appears to be the case with SDF-1, by receptor down-modulation.

Although the initial laboratory data on the ability of these compounds to inhibit HIV is promising, the chief obstacles to their clinical utility, as stated above, will include the immunologic consequences of blocking a single coreceptor, as well as the ability of the virus to evade a single target. In a different vein, because HIV is spread predominantly through sexual transmission and CCR5 appears to be critical to transmission and initial establishment of HIV infection, there is a clear impetus to examine CCR5 blockers as topical microbicides (preparations for intravaginal or intrarectal use). Investigators are beginning to evaluate several of these compounds for their potential use as transmission blockers (R. Offord, M. Lederman, personal communication). Many of the pharmacologic issues associated with intravenous administration of a peptide inhibitor would be obviated with their use in topical formulations. Moreover, other entry inhibitors that are independent of chemokine receptor interactions, such as T20 (see below) might also be considered for use as topical microbicides. These inhibitors could provide protection against R5 isolates, as well as X4 isolates, which in rare instances have been found to be responsible for establishment of initial infection (86).

SMALL MOLECULE INHIBITORS

The first described nonpeptide antagonist directed against CCR5 is a compound named TAK-779, a small molecule of molecular weight 531 daltons. TAK-779 inhibits the replication of R5, but not X4, HIV clinical isolates at concentrations of <10nM. TAK-779 specifically inhibits the binding of ^{125}I-RANTES to CCR5, but not to other chemokine receptors. Furthermore, the inhibitory effect of TAK-779 is selective for CCR5 and not for RANTES because it has no effect on ^{125}I-RANTES binding to CCR1 and RANTES induced Ca^{2+} mobilization in CHO/CCR1 cells (87). Recent unpublished studies have determined that TAK-779 blocks gp120-CCR5 association and membrane fusion by binding near the extracellular surface of CCR5 within a cavity formed between transmembrane helices 1, 2, 3 and 7 (87a). Whether TAK-779 turns out to be a viable drug will depend on its pharmacological properties, but its binding site within the transmembrane domain represents a viable target for a range of small molecule inhibitors of CCR5 function. Thus, CCR5 targeted small molecules may be of value in other clinical conditions such as inflammatory, or autoimmune diseases, or asthma (88,89). Since chemokine receptors are structurally conserved, similar pockets in the transmembrane domains of other chemokine receptors could well serve as targets for antagonists of this pharmacologically important receptor family.

A compound named NSC 651016 has been reported to antagonize CXCR4 and CCR5 mediated syncytia formation and fusion of HIV. Detailed studies have shown that the mechanism of inhibition of NSC 651016 is due to specific interaction with chemokine receptors, leading to receptor internalization and an attenuated chemotactic response (90).

The most effective nonpeptide inhibitor of CXCR4 described to date is a small molecule, AMD3100. This compound is a member of the heterocyclic family of compounds called bicyclams. The anti-viral properties of AMD3100 have been known since 1992 when it was shown to inhibit HIV-1 and HIV-2 infection prior to initiation of reverse transcriptase, but its mechanism of action was unknown. Recent studies have shown that AMD3100 blocks HIV entry and membrane fusion and prevents the anti-CXCR4 mAb 12G5 from binding to its target receptor (91). It also inhibits binding of SDF-1α to CXCR4 and subsequent signal transduction, but does not itself cause signaling. Thus, AMD3100 prevents CXCR4 functioning as both an HIV coreceptor, and a CXC-chemokine receptor (92). The binding site for this molecule has been localized to the extracellular domain (ECL), particularly anionic resides within the second extracellular loop. In one published report, addition of AMD3100 to peripheral blood mononuclear cells infected with X4 or R5X4 viruses exerted sufficient selective pressure such that the emerging virus exhibited an R5 genotype and phenotype (93). When *in vivo* experiments were performed in SCID-hu mice, AMD3100 was effective in preventing the replication of X4 isolates, but had no inhibitory effect on the replication of R5 isolates. Interestingly, AMD3100 proved effective in partially suppressing the replication of dual-tropic R5X4 isolates in the mice, the recovered viruses were unable to use CXCR4 and had lost their pathogenic SI phenotype. AMD3100 is currently being evaluated in a Phase I pharmacokinetic study of 12 healthy uninfected human volunteers.

Overall, compounds like AMD3100 provide proof of principle that effective small molecule antagonists of HIV entry can be developed. However, AMD3100 is strongly cationic and, because CXCR4 is negatively charged, the interactions between inhibitor and receptor are probably substantially electrostatic rather than truly biochemical in nature. Nevertheless, these molecules can serve as the starting point for further medicinal chemistry refinements and the development of second-generation therapeutic or prophylactic agents to inhibit HIV entry.

A principle challenge to the ultimate success of small molecule antagonists is the ability of HIV to quickly mutate and evade a single drug targeted at a single chemokine receptor. Already, an AMD3100 escape mutant of HIV-1 $_{LAI}$ has been made *in vitro* (92,94,95). Studies are in progress to determine whether the resistant virus can still interact with CXCR4 (but in an AMD3100-insentive manner) or whether it has evolved to use a different coreceptor. The escape mutant is no longer sensitive to inhibition by SDF-1α, perhaps indicating the latter as a more likely possibility. Theoretically, some viruses may be able to use CXCR4 without interference by AMD3100, as suggested by the virus strain and cell type dependence of the *in vitro* antiviral activity of the 12G5 monoclonal antibody to CXCR4. The reasons for the finding are not fully understood, but may relate to the way that different HIV envelopes interact with CXCR4 (96,97).

MONOCLONAL ANTIBODIES

Monoclonal antibodies (mAbs) provide powerful tools to probe the structural and functional relationships of viral entry. These antibodies also may be useful therapeutically by binding to CCR5 and CXCR4 and blocking receptor interaction with HIV envelope. There are several mAbs directed against CXCR4 (98); the best characterized of these is 12G5 (99). This mAb exerts its anti-viral effect by binding and blocking the second extracellular domain of CXCR4, a domain that is essential for both chemokine and virus binding. The efficiency of 12G5 inhibition of viral entry has been reported to be both cell and isolate dependent (96,97), though the precise mechanism of the inhibition is unknown (100).

Recently, investigators have also reported success in generating mAbs to CCR5 (101-103) some of which inhibited both cell-cell fusion and HIV entry (101). A particularly interesting anti-CCR5 mAb is 2D7 (102). This antibody recognizes the second extracellular domain of CCR5 and blocks the binding of RANTES, MIP-1α, and MIP-1β, as well as infection by M-tropic and dual-tropic HIV strains, suggesting that binding elements in this domain are common to both gp120 and chemokines. In contrast, antibodies binding to the NH2 terminal region of CCR5 block infection, but have no effect on chemokine activity.

As described above, a potential problem with the use of mAb receptor antagonists, as with other chemokine receptor inhibitors, is that the virus may mutate to use an alternate co-receptor. In a series of experiments to evaluate the consequences of receptor evasion, hu-PBL-SCID mice were infected with the R5 virus, JR-CSF and treated with 2D7 mAb. The effect of the mAb treatment on viral replication was assessed by the measurement of plasma HIV RNA levels (104). Administration of 2D7 mAb even at high doses (1mg) only transiently controlled *in vivo* viral replication. Moreover, virus isolated from 2 of the 5 antibody-treated mice could replicate in *CCR5-Δ32* homozygous donors cells, demonstrating that the virus had mutated to use another co-receptor. Further, sequencing studies of a single viral clone from the antibody treated animal revealed the presence of mutations in the V4 and C4 regions close to the receptor binding site. This report suggests that co-receptor switching may occur rapidly under selective pressure of CCR5-blocking agents, and that it may be necessary to simultaneously block multiple co-receptors to prevent HIV entry. One caveat of the SCID-hu model that was used to perform the proof-of-concept studies is that human immune system engraftment in these mice is limited to peripheral lymphocytes and not lymphoid tissue. As a result, immune-based mechanisms that normally suppress emergence of X4 viruses in humans may not operate in these mice. In humans, the frequency with which X4 viruses emerge in individuals who express reduced levels of CCR5 protein because they are heterozygous for the *CCR5-Δ32* allele is no greater than in individuals with homozygous wild type alleles (105). Therefore, deliberate efforts to reduce surface expression levels of CCR5 are not certain to drive the rapid emergence of X4 viruses, especially in the presence of the selection pressure that normally suppresses these viruses. More relevant information may come from non-human primate studies and ultimately from carefully controlled human clinical trials.

Potential problems with the use of mAbs as therapeutic tools include the expense of generating sufficient quantities of the reagents for clinical application, accessibility of the targeted cellular population to this relatively large molecule, the necessity for parenteral administration, and the potential immunogencity associated with murine-derived reagents. The last problem may be overcome with the availability of humanized mAbs. In addition, the possible effects of these agents on the targeted cell population beyond simple receptor blockade, such as receptor down-regulation or clearance of receptor-expressing cells, must be taken into account. Resolution of these issues will determine the use of these reagents as potential therapies or as transmission blockers. Importantly, these natural products offer the benefit of inducing fewer of the toxic side effects that are sometimes associated with small molecule therapeutics.

GENE THERAPY TO PREVENT CHEMOKINE RECEPTOR EXPRESSION

The intent of HIV gene therapy is to provide the patient with cells that have been rendered resistant to the virus by some type of genetic alteration. The strategy is based on the premise that disease progression can be improved if sufficient numbers of resistant cells are given to the patient to sustain normal immune functions. The strategy further presupposes that HIV-induced damage to uninfected cells can be minimized with attainable levels of gene-altered cells. Since mature CD4+ T cells and macrophages, the two most common targets for HIV infection, are relatively short-lived, most current gene therapy strategies focus on the hematopoietic stem cell as the cellular target for gene therapy. The approach has many technological issues that require resolution before it can be considered a viable treatment option. These include: the low efficiency of transduction with most currently available gene therapy vectors (mostly virus-based); the difficulty of obtaining sufficient numbers of stem cells; and the requirement for individually tailored treatment regimens that require the ex vivo manipulation of large numbers of cells. A further complication is the inability of large numbers of stem cells to engraft in the patient without concomitant use of myelo-reducing or ablating regimens that are hypothesized to increase the efficiency of stem cell engraftment. This requirement makes the technique ethically appropriate for HIV-infected individuals only in cases, such as AIDS lymphoma, where such regimens would be used in the normal care of the patient (106). Other issues that must be addressed include the potential immunogenicity of selectable marker genes that are included in most gene therapy vectors, which could impose limits on the life span of gene modified cells *in vivo*, and the current inability to target cells *in vivo* with gene therapy vectors. An additional problem in targeting CXCR4 is that this protein is a critical component of normal lymphoid development (see above). However, it is possible that CXCR4 function is dispensable after embryogenesis and that CXCR4-directed gene therapy strategies may be tolerated in mature cells and a mature host.

A number of gene therapy approaches are moving forward that specifically target chemokine receptor expression. If the issues mentioned above can be resolved, these strategies are likely to play a role in the armamentarium of treatment options for HIV-infected patients.

Intrakines

In this approach, chemokines are appended to endoplasmic reticulum (ER) retention signals that result in the intracellular expression of the chemokine. The best constructs have been able to substantially diminish expression of their targeted receptors presumably by retaining the receptor in the ER where it is rapidly degraded. The initial finding that intracellularly expressed chemokines, so-called 'intrakines', can specifically retain their cognate receptors, preventing cell surface receptor expression and rendering cell lines resistant to HIV infection (107,108) has now been confirmed using RANTES intrakine-transduced peripheral blood lymphocytes (109). In the latter studies, RANTES or a RANTES derivative that was unable to induce intracellular signaling following interaction with its cognate receptor, were used to specifically down-regulate CCR5. In addition to rendering cells resistant to M-tropic HIV infection, a finding of importance to the clinical development of this concept is that the transduced primary cells maintained basic biological functions, including antigen-specific proliferation and cytokine production. The promiscuity of RANTES for interaction with several chemokine receptors, such as CCR1, CCR3 and CCR10, is a confounding variable in the clinical development of this particular intrakine that can potentially be addressed with chemokines such as MIP-1β that target CCR5 more specifically. In addition, it is important to ensure that the retained chemokine is not secreted by the gene-modified cell, a common problem with several chemokine constructs expressing ER retention signals (G. Nabel, personal communication) that could result in inflammatory side effects *in vivo*. This problem might be addressed using different retention signals. Alternatively, intrakines could be developed in which the chemokine has been rendered defective in intracellular signaling capacity. In the latter approach, inflammatory side effects would not be expected even if leakage occurred, due to the defect in signaling capacity of the chemokine. RANTES variants have already been developed with these characteristics (109). MIP-1 β and SDF-α variants would be appropriate additions to this array.

Ribozymes

Ribozymes are enzymatic RNA molecules that can be designed to specifically recognize and cleave other RNAs. By disrupting the normal coding sequence of the RNA molecule, ribozymes can prevent or diminish the translation of proteins encoded by the targeted sequence. The first studies to target HIV were directed at inhibition of HIV gag expression (110) and to sequences in the 5' LTR of the HIV genome (111). Several groups have developed ribozymes targeted to CCR5 (112,113 and J Rossi, personal communication). Where reported (112), ribozyme effects on CCR5 expression have not been dramatic (a 60% reduction in a cell line co-transfected with CCR5 and a 20-fold molar excess of plasmid encoding the ribozyme) and have not yet been analyzed for effects on HIV infectivity. Attempts to improve ribozyme expression or intracellular localization, or to pair ribozyme and other HIV-inhibitory strategies, may be required to advance this concept.

Other Approaches

Several other gene therapy approaches that have been used to target other genes or proteins important for HIV replication might also be adapted to chemokine receptor inhibition. Intrabodies are intracellular antibodies that bind to and prevent expression and function of their target molecules. This strategy has been used to document the feasibility of targeting HIV-encoded proteins to prevent HIV replication. Similar approaches have been used to target the IL-2 receptor (114) and might also be used with chemokine receptor-targeted antibodies to prevent expression of HIV co-receptors. Antisense methods might also be considered, in which the therapeutic gene would bind to and prevent translation of chemokine receptor mRNA.

EX VIVO MANIPULATION OF CCR5 PROTEIN EXPRESSION

Novel strategies are being implemented to sequester or prevent the expression of chemokine receptors to make cells resistant to infection with M-tropic strains of HIV. An intriguing laboratory finding is that activation of CD4+ T cells with immobilized antibodies to the cell surface molecules CD3 and CD28 results in a population of CD4+ memory cells that have down-modulated transcription of CCR5. These cells produce factors that inhibit both M-tropic and T-tropic HIV replication. These CD4+ cells resist infection with R5 viruses, but remain sensitive to infection with CXCR4-using viruses (115,116). Resistance of the stimulated cells to HIV infection is temporary, with re-acquisition of HIV infectability occurring within one week after the stimuli are removed.

These findings illustrate that CCR5 levels can be experimentally manipulated and support studies in HIV-infected individuals to examine the safety and efficacy of administering CD4+ T cells in which CCR5 expression is diminished. A clinical trial was conducted in which HIV+ subjects were infused with 3 doses of their own CD4+ cells, which had been previously treated with anti-CD3 and anti-CD28 mAbs. Two out of three participants in this trial experienced sustained increases in CD4+ cells for greater than 4 months post-infusion (116). Although the protocol is unlikely to have wide clinical application because of the expense and cumbersome nature of the treatment strategy, the preliminary data suggest that manipulation of the CD28 signal transduction pathway as a means of decreasing expression of CCR5 may have therapeutic potential.

FUSION INHIBITORS TARGETING VIRAL PROTEINS

In addition to blocking agents targeted at the chemokine receptors, investigational antiretroviral compounds that block both virus-to-cell and cell-to-cell membrane fusion by binding directly to viral envelope offer promise as potentially useful therapeutics. The HIV envelope protein is initially made as a precursor polyprotein that is proteolytically cleaved into gp120 and gp41. Each envelope glycoprotein spike on the viral surface is thought to consist of a trimer of three gp120 exterior envelope glycoproteins and three gp41 transmembrane envelope glycoproteins. The gp120 moiety comprises the outer, exposed surface of the trimer and is responsible for binding of the virus to its target cell receptors, whereas the gp41 is thought to be responsible for fusing the viral and target cell membranes.

A working model for the entry process involves multiple steps beginning with the binding of gp120 to CD4 and a chemokine receptor, resulting in a conformational change in the envelope structure and culminating in fusion of host and viral membranes. Interactions of the viral protein and the host receptor are thought to trigger a conformational change in the gp41 portion that is buried in the interior of the complex resulting in its exposure and the formation of a transient species termed a "prehairpin" intermediate. The prehairpin intermediate resolves to a trimer-of-hairpins structure that likely represents the fusion active state of gp41 (117,118). The structure of the trimer has been studied by X-ray diffraction (119,120). The core structure is a six-helix bundle, in which three C-terminal helices pack around three central N-terminal helices.

Recent publications have utilized the high-resolution structures of gp41 in a structure-based approach to design inhibitors that block HIV infection by preventing gp41 activation. One of the first agents found to disrupt HIV's fusogenic machinery was a fragment of gp41 itself, a peptide known as T-20. It does this by binding to the transient prehairpin intermediate at the N-terminal hydrophobic inner core just proximal to the membrane-spanning domain and inhibiting conformational changes that drive membrane fusion (121). T-20 was discovered several years ago as a conserved 36 amino acid peptide in gp41 for use as a vaccine candidate. Although it failed as a viable vaccine candidate, it demonstrated potent anti-viral activity (122,123). The fact that T-20 can act in a dominant negative fashion by binding to a required intermediate along the pathway to viral fusiondemonstrates its singular mechanism of action. The fact that it is effective in subjects with high baseline viral loads and a history of extensive antiretroviral treatment demonstrates its therapeutic potential.

T-20 has successfully completed a Phase I study of safety, dosage, and antiviral activity (124). A Phase II study to assess pharmacokinetic and immunological consequences of 16 weeks of T-20 administration to HIV-infected adults also showed positive results. In this study, 33 of 55 heavily pre-treated patients who were given 50 mg of T-20 twice daily by subcutaneous injection in combination with oral antiretroviral agents responded with one log reduction of HIV in the blood. Twenty of the 55 patients had undetectable levels of virus. Thus, to date this trial has shown that T-20 can provide a virologic benefit through week 16 to the majority of patients. Furthermore, the drug is well tolerated and does not induce detectable anti-T-20 antibodies (125). The latter point is particularly important since T-20 is a foreign peptide that could potentially stimulate an immune response, which in turn could compromise T-20's bioavailability or activity.

While the initial laboratory and clinical data on the ability of T-20 to block a transient membrane fusion intermediate are encouraging, there are potential problems. T-20 is relatively large (36 amino acids), expensive to manufacture, unable to penetrate the blood brain barrier, short lived (half-life of about 2 hours), and likely to exhibit limited oral bioavailability. In its current form the drug must be administered intravenously or subcutaneously. However, delivery methods using a portable infusion pump, similar to that used by diabetics, are in development. Another potential problem is the ability of HIV to mutate and for virus variants to emerge that avoid the selective pressure exerted by the drug. Preliminary *in vitro* tests indicate that resistant variants can emerge, even though resistance is slow to develop because this agent targets a conserved viral peptide (126). Resistant virus is being used to develop new peptide analogs. Two such agents show early clinical promise: T-1249 and peptide 2. Because T-20 inhibits virus replication at a unique site it is unlikely to exhibit cross-resistance with existing treatments, nor is it likely to pose problems because of a previous history of antiretroviral treatment.

A second attractive site for designing smaller T-20-like peptides is to target the deep, transient, hydrophobic cavity in the inner core of the gp41 ectodomain formed by the coiled N-helices. Based on the crystal structure of the gp41 core, the prehairpin intermediate is expected to contain three prominent, symmetry-related pockets on the surface of the central trimeric structure. In recent work, a simplified version of this cavity has been engineered, designated IQN17, by fusing a soluble, trimeric coiled coil (GCN4-pIQI) to 17 residues of the relevant gp41 region. This in effect produces a stable gp41 intermediate (127). Recent work shows that this pocket can accommodate small, circular D-peptides that inhibit viral fusion. The IQN17 reagent was used as bait to select D-peptide ligands from a random pool and the D-peptides selected bound within the pocket on the authentic gp41 structure, and successfully inhibited membrane fusion. D-amino acids are unnatural and resistant to proteolytic cleavage, which increases their stability *in vivo*. The present set of D-peptide inhibitors are not very potent, with IC50 values in the 10-100 μM range. However, this is only the first step in the drug development pathway and future derivatives of these D-peptides are likely to exhibit enhanced potency.

These pockets are expected to be attractive drug targets for several reasons. First, the dimensions of the pockets are of a suitable size for targeting with a small molecule of approximately 500 daltons and historic data suggests that successful oral pharmaceuticals do not exceed 1000 daltons in size. Second, mutagenesis studies have shown that the N-peptide residues forming the pocket are critical for HIV infectivity (123,128). In accord with these results, studies of inhibitory peptides that target the N-peptide region show that inhibitory activity depends on the peptide's ability to bind to the pocket (129). Third, the HIV pocket is highly conserved among different HIV strains, so a drug targeted against this pocket should be effective against various strains, decreasing the likelihood of resistant strains.

These studies validate the feasibility of targeting the gp41 pocket to inhibit the HIV envelope glycoprotein, and set the stage for the development of a new class of orally bioavailable anti-HIV drugs that inhibit viral entry into cells. The pocket-blocking peptides exhibit lower antiviral potency than the longer T-20 like peptides, an expected consequence of contacting a smaller surface on the gp41 target. A further reduction in size of these peptides will be necessary to create a clinically practical therapeutic. To satisfy the dual requirements of potency and reduced size, the next generation of these drugs will probably need to exploit the potential of nonpeptide molecules to fill the pocket more efficiently than the natural peptide analogs. These drugs would complement the current antiretroviral regimen, since they would interfere with protein-protein interactions as opposed to enzyme activity.

The development of soluble forms of the N peptide trimer opens the door to the use of a wide variety of empirical methods to identify potential nonpeptide inhibitors of the interaction between the N and C peptides within the trimer. Screening of combinatorial chemical libraries of nonnatural molecules coupled to segments of C-like peptides has recently been employed to identify new moieties that interact with the N pocket (130). In the future, it is likely that soluble trimers alone or in combination with specific pocket binding molecules will facilitate the discovery of more potent pocket-filling molecules.

CONCLUSIONS AND FUTURE DIRECTIONS

It is estimated that more than 30 million people worldwide are now currently infected with HIV. Heterosexual transmission rates are on the rise and with increasing rates of treatment failure and the emergence of resistant virus, the development of therapeutic strategies based on HIV-cell surface interactions offers new directions with the possibility of improvements in standard of care. Only further studies *in vitro* and *in vivo* can determine whether the potential obstacles to the development of these strategies, discussed in this chapter, are surmountable. Table 1 summarizes the strategies that have been described in this chapter that target aspects of the viral entry process.

In the era of HAART, it is expected that any entry inhibitor, whether coreceptor targeted or otherwise, will be combined with existing reverse transcriptase and protease inhibitors, to target multiple steps in HIV replication and maximally suppress HIV replication. Because the speed with which mutations are generated is directly dependent on HIV replication rate, the simultaneous administration of multiple drugs should slow the emergence of phenotypic variants or other escape mutants, making it difficult for the virus to genetically elude therapy.

In addition to its impact on the development of coreceptor inhibitors as antivirals, the discovery of coreceptors has served to focus HIV vaccine and topical microbicide efforts as well. The interaction of gp120 with chemokine receptors is an obvious step to target in preventive strategies since it involves the interaction of gp120 with invariant host molecules that participate in the very first step in viral replication. The discovery that HIV transmission occurs primarily by R5 viruses has focused envelope-based protective approaches on CCR5-using isolates. In addition, the observation that CCR5 co-receptor usage is a common feature of many isolates across multiple HIV clades offers promise that a common structural

TABLE 1 Status of anti-HIV therapeutic strategies for blocking HIV entry and fusion.

Strategy	Therapy	Target	Status
Chemokines, modified chemokines, and peptides	met-RANTES	CCR5	Preclinical
	AOP-RANTES	CCR5	Preclinical
	NNY-RANTES	CCR5	Preclinical
	SDF-1 variants	CXCR4	Preclinical
	T22, T134	CXCR4	Preclinical
	ALX40-4C	CXCR4	Preclinical
Small molecule antagonists	AMD3100	CXCR4	Phase I human trials
	TAK-779	CCR5	Preclinical
	NSC 65016	CXCR4, CCR5	Preclinical
Monoclonal antibodies	Various	CCR5, CXCR4	Preclinical
Gene therapy	Ribozymes	CCR5, CXCR4	Preclinical
	Intrakines	CCR5, CXCR4	Preclinical
	Single chain (sFv)	CCR5, CXCR4	Concept
	mAbs	CCR5, CXCR4	Concept
	Antisense		Concept
Immune restoration	Down-regulation of CCR5 on CD4+ T cells	CCR5	Phase I human trials
Fusion inhibitors	T20	gp41	Phase II human trials
	T1249	gp41	Preclinical
	Peptide 2	gp41	Preclinical

feature can be identified to serve as an immunogen and induce protective immunity against diverse HIV isolates. Indeed, encouraging results have been obtained recently using immunogens that appear to freeze the viral envelope in a conformation that may exist only after interaction of the virus with cell surface CD4 (131), or CD4 and the chemokine receptor CCR5 (132). In the latter study, a cell-based vaccine elicited antibody responses in mice that were capable of neutralizing 23 of 24 primary isolates, including M-tropic and T-tropic representatives from five prevalent and geographically distinct HIV clades. If these results can be extended to humans, they suggest that immunization with envelopes from one or a small number of HIV isolates, when presented in an appropriate conformation, may induce protective responses against a diverse array of primary HIV-1 strains.

ACKNOWLEDGMENTS

We thank Drs. Carl Dieffenbach, Susan Plaeger, Nava Sarver and Karl Salzwedel for providing comments on the manuscript.

REFERENCES

1. Cairns JS, D'Souza MP. Chemokines and HIV-1 second receptors: the therapeutic connection. Nat Med. 1998;4:563-8.
2. Michael NL, Moore JP. HIV-1 entry inhibitors: evading the issue. Nat Med. 1999;5:740-2.
3. Maddon PJ, Dalgleish AG, McDougal JS, Clapham PR, Weiss RA, Axel R. The T4 gene encodes the AIDS virus receptor and is expressed in the immune system and the brain. Cell. 1986;47:333-48.
4. McDougal JS, Kennedy MS, Sligh JM, Cort SP, Mawle A, Nicholson JK. Binding of HTLV-III/LAV to T4+ T cells by a complex of the 110K viral protein and the T4 molecule. Science. 1986;231:382-5.
5. Feng Y, Broder CC, Kennedy PE, Berger EA. HIV-1 entry cofactor: functional cDNA cloning of a seven-transmembrane, G protein-coupled receptor. Science. 1996;272:872-7.
6. Dragic T, Litwin V, Allaway GP, et al. HIV-1 entry into CD4+ cells is mediated by the chemokine receptor CC-CKR-5. Nature. 1996;381:667-73.
7. Deng H, Liu R, Ellmeier W, et al. Identification of a major co-receptor for primary isolates of HIV-1. Nature. 1996;381:661-6.
8. Alkhatib G, Combadiere C, Broder CC, et al. CC CKR5: a RANTES, MIP-1alpha, MIP-1beta receptor as a fusion cofactor for macrophage-tropic HIV-1. Science. 1996;272:1955-8.
9. Doranz BJ, Rucker J, Yi Y, et al. A dual-tropic primary HIV-1 isolate that uses fusin and the beta-chemokine receptors CKR-5, CKR-3, and CKR-2b as fusion cofactors. Cell. 1996;85:1149-58.
10. Choe H, Farzan M, Sun Y, et al. The beta-chemokine receptors CCR3 and CCR5 facilitate infection by primary HIV-1 isolates. Cell. 1996;85:1135-48.

11. Cocchi F, DeVico AL, Garzino-Demo A, Arya SK, Gallo RC, Lusso P. Identification of RANTES, MIP-1 alpha, and MIP-1 beta as the major HIV-suppressive factors produced by CD8+ T cells. Science. 1995;270:1811-5.
12. Bleul CC, Farzan M, Choe H, et al. The lymphocyte chemoattractant SDF-1 is a ligand for LESTR/fusin and blocks HIV-1 entry. Nature. 1996;382:829-33.
13. Oberlin E, Amara A, Bachelerie F, et al. The CXC chemokine SDF-1 is the ligand for LESTR/fusin and prevents infection by T cell line-adapted HIV-1. Nature. 1996;382:833-5.
14. Roos MT, Lange JM, de Goede RE, et al. Viral phenotype and immune response in primary human immunodeficiency virus type 1 infection. J Infect Dis. 1992;165:427-32.
15. Schuitemaker H, Koot M, Kootstra NA, et al. Biological phenotype of human immunodeficiency virus type 1 clones at different stages of infection: progression of disease is associated with a shift from monocytotropic to T-cell-tropic virus population. J Virol. 1992;66:1354-60.
16. Connor RI, Ho DD. Human immunodeficiency virus type 1 variants with increased replicative capacity develop during the asymptomatic stage before disease progression. J Virol. 1994;68:4400-8.
17. Tersmette M, Gruters RA, de Wolf F, et al. Evidence for a role of virulent human immunodeficiency virus (HIV) variants in the pathogenesis of acquired immunodeficiency syndrome: studies on sequential HIV isolates. J Virol. 1989;63:2118-25.
18. Tersmette M, Lange JM, de Goede RE, et al. Association between biological properties of human immunodeficiency virus variants and risk for AIDS and AIDS mortality. Lancet. 1989;1:983-5.
19. Tersmette M, de Goede RE, Al BJ, et al. Differential syncytium-inducing capacity of human immunodeficiency virus isolates: frequent detection of syncytium-inducing isolates in patients with acquired immunodeficiency syndrome (AIDS) and AIDS-related complex. J Virol. 1988;62:2026-32.
20. Berger EA, Doms RW, Fenyo EM, et al. A new classification for HIV-1. Nature. 1998;391:240.
21. Wyatt R, Kwong PD, Desjardins E, et al. The antigenic structure of the HIV gp120 envelope glycoprotein. Nature. 1998;393:705-11.
22. Combadiere C, Salzwedel K, Smith ED, Tiffany HL, Berger EA, Murphy PM. Identification of CX3CR1. A chemotactic receptor for the human CX3C chemokine fractalkine and a fusion coreceptor for HIV-1. J Biol Chem. 1998;273:23799-804.
23. Horuk R, Hesselgesser J, Zhou Y, et al. The CC chemokine I-309 inhibits CCR8-dependent infection by diverse HIV-1 strains. J Biol Chem. 1998;273:386-91.
24. Deng HK, Unutmaz D, Kewalramani VN, Littman DR. Expression cloning of new receptors used by simian and human immunodeficiency viruses. Nature. 1997;388:296-300.
25. Alkhatib G, Liao F, Berger EA, Farber JM, Peden KW. A new SIV co-receptor, STRL33. Nature. 1997;388:238.
26. Richman DD, Bozzette SA. The impact of the syncytium-inducing phenotype of human immunodeficiency virus on disease progression. J Infect Dis. 1994;169:968-74.
27. Berger EA. HIV entry and tropism: the chemokine receptor connection. AIDS. 1997;11 Suppl A:S3-16.
28. Simmons G, Wilkinson D, Reeves JD, et al. Primary, syncytium-inducing human immunodeficiency virus type 1 isolates are dual-tropic and most can use either Lestr or CCR5 as coreceptors for virus entry. J Virol. 1996;70:8355-60.

29. Liu R, Paxton WA, Choe S, et al. Homozygous defect in HIV-1 coreceptor accounts for resistance of some multiply-exposed individuals to HIV-1 infection. Cell. 1996;86:367-77.
30. Samson M, Libert F, Doranz BJ, et al. Resistance to HIV-1 infection in caucasian individuals bearing mutant alleles of the CCR-5 chemokine receptor gene. Nature. 1996;382:722-5.
31. Dean M, Carrington M, Winkler C, et al. Genetic restriction of HIV-1 infection and progression to AIDS by a deletion allele of the CKR5 structural gene. Hemophilia Growth and Development Study, Multicenter AIDS Cohort Study, Multicenter Hemophilia Cohort Study, San Francisco City Cohort, ALIVE Study. Science. 1996;273:1856-62.
32. Biti R, Ffrench R, Young J, Bennetts B, Stewart G, Liang T. HIV-1 Infection in an Individual Homozygous for the CCR5 Deletion Allelle. Nat Med. 1997;3:252-3.
33. O'Brien TR, Winkler C, Dean M, et al. HIV-1 infection in a man homozygous for CCR5 delta 32. Lancet. 1997;349:1219.
34. Balotta C, Bagnarelli P, Violin M, et al. Homozygous delta 32 deletion of the CCR-5 chemokine receptor gene in an HIV-1-infected patient. AIDS. 1997;11:F67-71.
35. Paxton WA, Martin SR, Tse D, et al. Relative resistance to HIV-1 infection of CD4 lymphocytes from persons who remain uninfected despite multiple high-risk sexual exposure. Nat Med. 1996;2:412-7.
36. Zhou Y, Kurihara T, Ryseck RP, et al. Impaired macrophage function and enhanced T cell-dependent immune response in mice lacking CCR5, the mouse homologue of the major HIV-1 coreceptor. J Immunol. 1998;160:4018-25.
37. Huang Y, Paxton WA, Wolinsky SM, et al. The role of a mutant CCR5 allele in HIV-1 transmission and disease progression. Nat Med. 1996;2:1240-3.
38. Zimmerman PA, Buckler-White A, Alkhatib G, et al. Inherited resistance to HIV-1 conferred by an inactivating mutation in CC chemokine receptor 5: studies in populations with contrasting clinical phenotypes, defined racial background and quantified risk. Mol Med. 1997;3:22-35.
39. Moore JP. Coreceptors: implications for HIV pathogenesis and therapy. Science. 1997;276:51-2.
40. Wu L, Paxton WA, Kassam N, et al. CCR5 levels and expression pattern correlate with infectability by macrophage-tropic HIV-1, in vitro. J Exp Med. 1997;185:1681-91.
41. Paxton WA, Kang S, Liu R, et al. HIV-1 infectability of CD4+ lymphocytes with relation to beta-chemokines and the CCR5 coreceptor. Immunol Lett. 1999;66:71-5.
42. Mummidi S, Ahuja SS, McDaniel B, Ahuja SK. The human CC chemokine receptor 5 (CCR5) gene: multiple transcripts with 5'-end heterogeneity, dual promoter usage, and evidence for polymorphisms within the regulatory regions and non-coding exons. J Biol Chem. 1997; 272(49):30662-71.
43. Smith MW, Dean M, Carrington M, et al. Contrasting genetic influence of CCR2 and CCR5 variants on HIV-1 infection and disease progression. Hemophilia Growth and Development Study (HGDS), Multicenter AIDS Cohort Study (MACS), Multicenter Hemophilia Cohort Study (MHCS), San Francisco City Cohort (SFCC), ALIVE Study. Science. 1997;277:959-65.
44. Winkler C, Modi W, Smith MW, et al. Genetic Restriction of AIDS Pathogenesis by an SDF-1 Chemokine Gene Variant. Science. 1998;279:389-93.

45. Zou YR, Kottmann AH, Kuroda M, Taniuchi I, Littman DR. Function of the chemokine receptor CXCR4 in haematopoiesis and in cerebellar development. Nature. 1998;393:595-9.
46. Nagasawa T, Nakajima T, Tachibana K, et al. Molecular cloning and characterization of a murine pre-B-cell growth-stimulating factor/stromal cell-derived factor 1 receptor, a murine homolog of the human immunodeficiency virus 1 entry coreceptor fusin. Proc Natl Acad Sci U S A. 1996;93:14726-9.
47. Chen Z, Kwon D, Jin Z, et al. Natural infection of a homozygous delta24 CCR5 red-capped mangabey with an R2b-tropic simian immunodeficiency virus. J Exp Med. 1998;188:2057-65.
48. Hill SJ, Ganellin CR, Timmerman H, et al. International Union of Pharmacology. XIII. Classification of histamine receptors. Pharmacol Rev. 1997;49:253-78.
49. Hadida F, Vieillard V, Mollet L, Clark-Lewis I, Baggiolini M, Debre P. Cutting edge: RANTES regulates Fas ligand expression and killing by HIV- specific CD8 cytotoxic T cells. J Immunol. 1999;163:1105-9.
50. Melchers F, Rolink AG, Schaniel C. The role of chemokines in regulating cell migration during humoral immune responses. Cell. 1999;99:351-4.
51. Proost P, De Meester I, Schols D, et al. Amino-terminal truncation of chemokines by CD26/dipeptidyl-peptidase IV. Conversion of RANTES into a potent inhibitor of monocyte chemotaxis and HIV-1-infection. J Biol Chem. 1998;273:7222-7.
52. Shioda T, Kato H, Ohnishi Y, et al. Anti-HIV-1 and chemotactic activities of human stromal cell-derived factor 1alpha (SDF-1alpha) and SDF-1beta are abolished by CD26/dipeptidyl peptidase IV-mediated cleavage. Proc Natl Acad Sci U S A. 1998;95:6331-6.
53. Schols D, Proost P, Struyf S, et al. CD26-processed RANTES(3-68), but not intact RANTES, has potent anti-HIV-1 activity [published erratum appears in Antiviral Res 1999 Jan;40(3):189-90]. Antiviral Res. 1998;39:175-87.
54. Oravecz T, Pall M, Roderiquez G, et al. Regulation of the receptor specificity and function of the chemokine RANTES (regulated on activation, normal T cell expressed and secreted) by dipeptidyl peptidase IV (CD26)-mediated cleavage. J Exp Med. 1997;186:1865-72.
55. Mack M, Luckow B, Nelson PJ, et al. Aminooxypentane-RANTES induces CCR5 internalization but inhibits recycling: a novel inhibitory mechanism of HIV infectivity. J Exp Med. 1998;187:1215-24.
56. Schmidtmayerova H, Sherry B, Bukrinsky M. Chemokines and HIV replication. Nature. 1996;382:767.
57. Kinter A, Catanzaro A, Monaco J, et al. CC-chemokines enhance the replication of T-tropic strains of HIV-1 in CD4(+) T cells: role of signal transduction. Proc Natl Acad Sci U S A. 1998;95:11880-5.
58. Paxton WA, Dragic T, Koup RA, Moore JP. The beta-chemokines, HIV type 1 second receptors, and exposed uninfected persons. AIDS Res Hum Retroviruses. 1996;12:1203-7.
59. Saha K, Bentsman G, Chess L, Volsky DJ. Endogenous production of beta-chemokines by CD4+, but not CD8+, T-cell clones correlates with the clinical state of human immunodeficiency virus type 1 (HIV-1)-infected individuals and may be responsible for blocking infection with non-syncytium-inducing HIV-1 in vitro. J Virol. 1998;72:876-81.

60. Ferbas J, Giorgi JV, Amini S, et al. Antigen-specific production of RANTES, MIP-1a and MIP-1B in vitro is a correlate of reduced HIV burden in vivo. J Infect Dis.; 2000;182:1247-50.
61. Tartakovsky B, Turner D, Vardinon N, Burke M, Yust I. Increased intracellular accumulation of macrophage inflammatory protein 1beta and its decreased secretion correlate with advanced HIV disease. J Acquir Immune Defic Syndr Hum Retrovirol. 1999;20:420-2.
62. Polo S, Veglia F, Malnati MS, et al. Longitudinal analysis of serum chemokine levels in the course of HIV-1 infection. AIDS. 1999;13:447-54.
63. Ndolo T, Rheinhardt J, Zaragoza M, Smit-McBride Z, Dandekar S. Alterations in RANTES gene expression and T-cell prevalence in intestinal mucosa during pathogenic or nonpathogenic simian immunodeficiency virus infection. Virology. 1999;259:110-8.
64. Caufour P, le Grand R, Cheret A, et al. Secretion of beta-chemokines by bronchoalveolar lavage cells during primary infection of macaques inoculated with attenuated nef-deleted or pathogenic simian immunodeficiency virus strain mac251. J Gen Virol. 1999;80:767-76.
65. Iversen AK, Fugger L, Eugen-Olsen J, et al. Cervical human immunodeficiency virus type 1 shedding is associated with genital beta-chemokine secretion. J Infect Dis. 1998;178:1334-42.
66. Gong JH, Clark-Lewis I. Antagonists of monocyte chemoattractant protein 1 identified by modification of functionally critical NH2-terminal residues. J Exp Med. 1995;181:631-40.
67. Gong JH, Uguccioni M, Dewald B, Baggiolini M, Clark-Lewis I. RANTES and MCP-3 antagonists bind multiple chemokine receptors. J Biol Chem. 1996;271:10521-7.
68. Pakianathan DR, Kuta EG, Artis DR, Skelton NJ, Hebert CA. Distinct but overlapping epitopes for the interaction of a CC-chemokine with CCR1, CCR3 and CCR5. Biochemistry. 1997;36:9642-8.
69. Crump MP, Gong JH, Loetscher P, et al. Solution structure and basis for functional activity of stromal cell- derived factor-1; dissociation of CXCR4 activation from binding and inhibition of HIV-1. EMBO J. 1997;16:6996-7007.
70. Lubkowski J, Bujacz G, Boque L, Domaille PJ, Handel TM, Wlodawer A. The structure of MCP-1 in two crystal forms provides a rare example of variable quaternary interactions. Nat Struct Biol. 1997;4:64-9.
71. Fairbrother WJ, Reilly D, Colby TJ, Hesselgesser J, Horuk R. The solution structure of melanoma growth stimulating activity. J Mol Biol. 1994;242:252-70.
72. Handel TM, Domaille PJ. Heteronuclear (1H, 13C, 15N) NMR assignments and solution structure of the monocyte chemoattractant protein-1 (MCP-1) dimer. Biochemistry. 1996;35:6569-84.
73. Chung CW, Cooke RM, Proudfoot AE, Wells TN. The three-dimensional solution structure of RANTES. Biochemistry. 1995;34:9307-14.
74. LiWang AC, Cao JJ, Zheng H, Lu Z, Peiper SC, LiWang PJ. Dynamics study on the anti-human immunodeficiency virus chemokine viral macrophage-inflammatory protein-II (VMIP-II) reveals a fully monomeric protein. Biochemistry. 1999;38:442-53.
75. Polo S, Nardese V, De Santis C, et al. Two analogues of the C-C chemokine RANTES with CCR5-antagonistic activity and enhanced HIV-inhibitory potency. J Human Virol. 1999;2:Abstract #105.

76. Proudfoot AE, Power CA, Hoogewerf AJ, et al. Extension of recombinant human RANTES by the retention of the initiating methionine produces a potent antagonist. J Biol Chem. 1996;271:2599-603.
77. Simmons G, Clapham PR, Picard L, et al. Potent inhibition of HIV-1 infectivity in macrophages and lymphocytes by a novel CCR5 antagonist. Science. 1997;276:276-9.
78. Mosier DE, Picchio GR, Gulizia RJ, et al. Highly potent RANTES analogues either prevent CCR5-using human immunodeficiency virus type 1 infection in vivo or rapidly select for CXCR4-using variants. J Virol. 1999;73:3544-50.
79. Blanpain C, Migeotte I, Lee B, et al. CCR5 binds multiple CC-chemokines: MCP-3 acts as a natural antagonist. Blood. 1999;94:1899-905.
80. Yang OO, Swanberg SL, Lu Z, et al. Enhanced inhibition of human immunodeficiency virus type 1 by Met- stromal-derived factor 1beta correlates with down-modulation of CXCR4. J Virol. 1999;73:4582-9.
81. Murakami H, Nakajima T, Koyanagi Y, et al. A small molecule CXCR4 inhibitor that blocks T cell line-tropic HIV-1 infection. J Exp Med. 1997;186:1389-93.
82. Doranz BJ, Grovit-Ferbas K, Sharron M, et al. A small-molecule inhibitor directed against the chemokine receptor CXCR4 prevents its use as an HIV-1 coreceptor. J Exp Med. 1997;186:1395-400.
83. Arakaki R, Tamamura H, Premanathan M, et al. T134, a small-molecule CXCR4 inhibitor, has no cross-drug resistance with AMD3100, a CXCR4 antagonist with a different structure. J Virol. 1999;73:1719-23.
84. Dealwis C, Fernandez EJ, Thompson DA, Simon RJ, Siani MA, Lolis E. Crystal structure of chemically synthesized [N33A] stromal cell-derived factor 1alpha, a potent ligand for the HIV-1 "fusin" coreceptor. Proc Natl Acad Sci U S A. 1998;95:6941-6.
85. Luo Z, Zhou N, Luo J, Hall JW, Huang Z. The role of positively charged residues in CXCR4 recognition probed with synthetic peptides. Biochem Biophys Res Commun. 1999;263:691-5.
86. Michael NL, Nelson JA, Kewalramani VN, et al. Exclusive and persistent use of the entry coreceptor CXCR4 by human immunodeficiency virus type 1 from a subject homozygous for CCR5 delta32. J Virol. 1998;72:6040-7.
87. Baba M, Nishimura O, Kanzaki N, et al. A small-molecule, nonpeptide CCR5 antagonist with highly potent and selective anti-HIV-1 activity. Proc Natl Acad Sci U S A. 1999;96:5698-703.
87a. Dragic T, Trkola A, Thompson DA, Cormier EG, Kajumo FA, Maxwell E, Lin SW, Ying W, Smith SO, Sakmar TP, Moore JP. A binding pocket for a small molecule inhibitor of HIV-1 entry within the transmembrane helices of CCR5. Proc Natl Acad Sci U S A. 2000;97:5639-44.
88. Premack BA, Schall TJ. Chemokine receptors: gateways to inflammation and infection. Nat Med. 1996;2:1174-8.
89. Hall IP, Wheatley A, Christie G, McDougall C, Hubbard R, Helms PJ. Association of CCR5 delta32 with reduced risk of asthma. Lancet. 1999;354:1264-5.
90. Howard OM, Korte T, Tarasova NI, et al. Small molecule inhibitor of HIV-1 cell fusion blocks chemokine receptor- mediated function. J Leukoc Biol. 1998;64:6-13.
91. Donzella GA, Schols D, Lin SW, et al. AMD3100, a small molecule inhibitor of HIV-1 entry via the CXCR4 co-receptor. Nat Med. 1998;4:72-7.
92. Schols D, Este JA, Henson G, De Clercq E. Bicyclams, a class of potent anti-HIV agents, are targeted at the HIV coreceptor fusin/CXCR-4. Antiviral Res. 1997;35:147-56.

93. Este JA, Cabrera C, Blanco J, et al. Shift of clinical human immunodeficiency virus type 1 isolates from X4 to R5 and prevention of emergence of the syncytium-inducing phenotype by blockade of CXCR4. J Virol. 1999;73:5577-85.
94. De Vreese K, Reymen D, Griffin P, et al. The bicyclams, a new class of potent human immunodeficiency virus inhibitors, block viral entry after binding. Antiviral Res. 1996;29:209-19.
95. De Vreese K, Kofler-Mongold V, Leutgeb C, et al. The molecular target of bicyclams, potent inhibitors of human immunodeficiency virus replication. J Virol. 1996;70:689-96.
96. McKnight A, Wilkinson D, Simmons G, et al. Inhibition of human immunodeficiency virus fusion by a monoclonal antibody to a coreceptor (CXCR4) is both cell type and virus strain dependent. J Virol. 1997;71:1692-6.
97. Strizki JM, Turner JD, Collman RG, Hoxie J, Gonzalez-Scarano F. A monoclonal antibody (12G5) directed against CXCR-4 inhibits infection with the dual-tropic human immunodeficiency virus type 1 isolate HIV-1(89.6) but not the T-tropic isolate HIV-1(HxB). J Virol. 1997;71:5678-83.
98. Hori T, Sakaida H, Sato A, et al. Detection and delineation of CXCR-4 (fusin) as an entry and fusion cofactor for T-tropic HIV-1 by three different monoclonal antibodies [published erratum appears in J Immunol 1999 Jul 15;163(2):1092]. J Immunol. 1998;160:180-8.
99. Endres MJ, Clapham PR, Marsh M, et al. CD4-independent infection by HIV-2 is mediated by fusin/CXCR4. Cell. 1996;87:745-56.
100. Brelot A, Heveker N, Pleskoff O, Sol N, Alizon M. Role of the first and third extracellular domains of CXCR-4 in human immunodeficiency virus coreceptor activity. J Virol. 1997;71:4744-51.
101. Olson WC, Rabut GE, Nagashima KA, et al. Differential inhibition of human immunodeficiency virus type 1 fusion, gp120 binding, and CC-chemokine activity by monoclonal antibodies to CCR5. J Virol. 1999;73:4145-55.
102. Wu L, LaRosa G, Kassam N, et al. Interaction of chemokine receptor CCR5 with its ligands: multiple domains for HIV-1 gp120 binding and a single domain for chemokine binding. J Exp Med. 1997;186:1373-81.
103. Hill CM, Kwon D, Jones M, et al. The amino terminus of human CCR5 is required for its function as a receptor for diverse human and simian immunodeficiency virus envelope glycoproteins. Virology. 1998;248:357-71.
104. Poignard P, Peng T, Sabbe R, Newman W, Mosier DE, Burton DR. Blocking HIV-1 co-receptor CCR5 in the hu-PBL-SCID mouse leads to a co-receptor switch. 6th Conference on Retroviruses and Opportunistic Infections Conference Presentation. 1999;Chicago, IL.
105. Michael NL, Chang G, Louie LG, et al. The Role of Viral Phenotype and CCR-5 gene Defects in HIV-1 Transmission and Disease Progression. Nat Med. 1997;3:338-40.
106. Zaia JA, Cairns JS, Sarver N. Genetic modification and transplantation of hematopoietic cells for treatment of HIV infection. In: Forman SJ, Blume KG, Thomas ED, eds. Hematopoietic cell transplantation. Boston: Blackwell Scientific Publications, 1998.
107. Chen JD, Bai X, Yang AG, Cong Y, Chen SY. Inactivation of HIV-1 chemokine co-receptor CXCR-4 by a novel intrakine strategy. Nat Med. 1997;3:1110-6.
108. Yang AG, Bai X, Huang XF, Yao C, Chen SY. Phenotypic knockout of chemokine CCR5 coreceptor by intrakines for HIV-1 therapy. Proc Natl Acad Sci U S A. 1997; 94(21):11567-72.

109. Yang AG, Zhang X, Torti F, Chen SY. Anti-HIV type 1 activity of wild-type and functional defective RANTES intrakine in primary human lymphocytes. Hum Gene Ther. 1998;9:2005-18.
110. Sarver N, Cantin EM, Chang PS, et al. Ribozymes as potential anti-HIV-1 therapeutic agents. Science. 1990;247:1222-5.
111. Yu M, Ojwang J, Yamada O, et al. A hairpin ribozyme inhibits expression of diverse strains of human immunodeficiency virus type 1 [published erratum appears in Proc Natl Acad Sci U S A 1993 Sep 1;90(17):8303]. Proc Natl Acad Sci U S A. 1993;90:6340-4.
112. Gonzalez MA, Serrano F, Llorente M, Abad JL, Garcia-Ortiz MJ, Bernad A. A hammerhead ribozyme targeted to the human chemokine receptor CCR5. Biochem Biophys Res Commun. 1998;251:592-6.
113. Goila R, Banerjea AC. Sequence specific cleavage of the HIV-1 coreceptor CCR5 gene by a hammer-head ribozyme and a DNA-enzyme: inhibition of the coreceptor function by DNA-enzyme. FEBS Lett. 1998;436:233-8.
114. Richardson JH, Hofmann W, Sodroski JG, Marasco WA. Intrabody-mediated knockout of the high-affinity IL-2 receptor in primary human T cells using a bicistronic lentivirus vector. Gene Ther. 1998;5:635-44.
115. Levine BL, Mosca JD, Riley JL, et al. Antiviral effect and ex vivo CD4+ T cell proliferation in HIV-positive patients as a result of CD28 costimulation. Science. 1996;272:1939-43.
116. Carroll RG, Riley JL, Levine BL, et al. Differential regulation of HIV-1 fusion cofactor expression by CD28 costimulation of CD4+ T cells. Science. 1997;276:273-6.
117. Blacklow SC, Lu M, Kim PS. A trimeric subdomain of the simian immunodeficiency virus envelope glycoprotein. Biochemistry. 1995;34:14955-62.
118. Lu M, Blacklow SC, Kim PS. A trimeric structural domain of the HIV-1 transmembrane glycoprotein. Nat Struct Biol. 1995;2:1075-82.
119. Chan DC, Fass D, Berger JM, Kim PS. Core structure of gp41 from the HIV envelope glycoprotein. Cell. 1997;89:263-73.
120. Weissenhorn W, Dessen A, Harrison SC, Skehel JJ, Wiley DC. Atomic structure of the ectodomain from HIV-1 gp41. Nature. 1997;387:426-30.
121. Chan DC, Kim PS. HIV entry and its inhibition. Cell. 1998;93:681-4.
122. Wild C, Oas T, McDanal C, Bolognesi D, Matthews T. A synthetic peptide inhibitor of human immunodeficiency virus replication: correlation between solution structure and viral inhibition. Proc Natl Acad Sci U S A. 1992;89:10537-41.
123. Wild CT, Shugars DC, Greenwell TK, McDanal CB, Matthews TJ. Peptides corresponding to a predictive alpha-helical domain of human immunodeficiency virus type 1 gp41 are potent inhibitors of virus infection. Proc Natl Acad Sci U S A. 1994;91:9770-4.
124. Kilby JM, Hopkins S, Venetta TM, et al. Potent suppression of HIV-1 replication in humans by T-20, a peptide inhibitor of gp41-mediated virus entry. Nat Med. 1998;4:1302-7.
125. Lalezari J, Eron J, Carlson M, et al. Sixteen week analysis of heavily pre-treated patients receiving T-20 as a component of multi-drug slavage therapy. 39th Interscience Conference on Antimicrobial Agents and Chemotherapy. 1999;Abstract #LB-18.
126. Rimsky LT, Shugars DC, Matthews TJ. Determinants of human immunodeficiency virus type 1 resistance to gp41- derived inhibitory peptides. J Virol. 1998;72:986-93.

127. Eckert DM, Malashkevich VN, Hong LH, Carr PA, Kim PS. Inhibiting HIV-1 entry: discovery of D-peptide inhibitors that target the gp41 coiled-coil pocket. Cell. 1999;99:103-15.
128. Weng Y, Weiss CD. Mutational analysis of residues in the coiled-coil domain of human immunodeficiency virus type 1 transmembrane protein gp41. J Virol. 1998;72:9676-82.
129. Chan DC, Chutkowski CT, Kim PS. Evidence that a prominent cavity in the coiled coil of HIV type 1 gp41 is an attractive drug target. Proc Natl Acad Sci U S A. 1998;95:15613-7.
130. Ferrer M, Kapoor TM, Strassmaier T, et al. Selection of gp41-mediated HIV-1 cell entry inhibitors from biased combinatorial libraries of non-natural binding elements. Nat Struct Biol. 1999;6:953-60.
131. Devico A, Silver A, Thronton AM, Sarngadharan MG, Pal R. Covalently crosslinked complexes of human immunodeficiency virus type 1 (HIV-1) gp120 and CD4 receptor elicit a neutralizing immune response that includes antibodies selective for primary virus isolates. Virology. 1996;218:258-63.
132. LaCasse RA, Follis KE, Trahey M, Scarborough JD, Littman DR, Nunberg JH. Fusion-competent vaccines: broad neutralization of primary isolates of HIV. Science. 1999;283:357-62.
133. Fauci AS. Host factors and the pathogenesis of HIV-induced disease. Nature. 1996;384:529-34.

Index

About the Editor

Thomas R. O'Brien is a Senior Investigator in the Viral Epidemiology Branch of the National Cancer Institute, Rockville, Maryland. The author, coauthor, or editor of numerous scientific articles, book chapters, and books, he is a member of the American Association for the Advancement of Science. The recipient of many awards from the U.S. Public Health Service, the National Cancer Institute, and the Centers for Disease Control and Prevention, Dr. O'Brien received the B.A. degree from the University of Michigan, Ann Arbor, the M.D. degree from the University of Michigan School of Medicine, Ann Arbor, and the M.P.H. degree from the Harvard School of Public Health, Boston, Massachusetts.

ISBN 0-8247-0636-6

90000

9 780824 706364

INTENSITY-MODULATED RADIATION THERAPY

Series in Medical Physics

Series Editors:

Other books in the series

The Physics of Medical Imaging
S Webb (ed)

The Physics of Three-Dimensional Radiation Therapy: Conformal Radiotherapy, Radiosurgery and Treatment Planning
S Webb

The Physics of Conformal Radiotherapy: Advances in Technology
S Webb

Medical Physics and Biomedical Engineering
B H Brown, R H Smallwood, D C Barber, P V Lawford and D R Hose

Biomedical Magnetic Resonance Technology
C-N Chen and D I Hoult

Rehabilitation Engineering Applied to Mobility and Manipulation
R A Cooper

Physics for Diagnostic Radiology, second edition
P P Dendy and B H Heaton

Linear Accelerators for Radiation Therapy, second edition
D Greene and P C Williams

Health Effects of Exposure to Low-Level Ionizing Radiation
W R Hendee and F M Edwards (eds)

Monte Carlo Calculations in Nuclear Medicine
M Ljungberg, S-E Strand and M A King (eds)

Introductory Medical Statistics, third edition
R F Mould

The Design of Pulse Oxymeters
J G Webster (ed)

Ultrasound in Medicine
F A Duck, A C Baker and H C Starritt (eds)

Of related interest

From the Watching of Shadows: The Origins of Radiological Tomography
S Webb